Water Intake, Body Water Regulation and Health

Water Intake, Body Water Regulation and Health

Special Issue Editors
William M. Adams
Evan C. Johnson

MDPI • Basel • Beijing • Wuhan • Barcelona • Belgrade

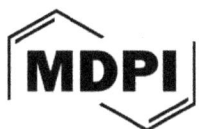

Special Issue Editors
William M. Adams
University of North Carolina at Greensboro
USA

Evan C. Johnson
University of Wyoming
USA

Editorial Office
MDPI
St. Alban-Anlage 66
4052 Basel, Switzerland

This is a reprint of articles from the Special Issue published online in the open access journal *Nutrients* (ISSN 2072-6643) from 2018 to 2020 (available at: https://www.mdpi.com/journal/nutrients/special_issues/water_intake).

For citation purposes, cite each article independently as indicated on the article page online and as indicated below:

LastName, A.A.; LastName, B.B.; LastName, C.C. Article Title. *Journal Name* **Year**, *Article Number*, Page Range.

ISBN 978-3-03928-656-0 (Pbk)
ISBN 978-3-03928-657-7 (PDF)

© 2020 by the authors. Articles in this book are Open Access and distributed under the Creative Commons Attribution (CC BY) license, which allows users to download, copy and build upon published articles, as long as the author and publisher are properly credited, which ensures maximum dissemination and a wider impact of our publications.

The book as a whole is distributed by MDPI under the terms and conditions of the Creative Commons license CC BY-NC-ND.

Contents

About the Special Issue Editors vii

Evan C. Johnson and William M. Adams
Water Intake, Body Water Regulation and Health
Reprinted from: *Nutrients* **2020**, *12*, 702, doi:10.3390/nu12030702 1

Colleen X. Muñoz and Michael Wininger
Unexplained Variance in Hydration Study
Reprinted from: *Nutrients* **2019**, *11*, 1828, doi:10.3390/nu11081828 3

Alexander Basov, Liliia Fedulova, Mikhail Baryshev and Stepan Dzhimak
Deuterium-Depleted Water Influence on the Isotope $^2H/^1H$ Regulation in Body and Individual Adaptation
Reprinted from: *Nutrients* **2019**, *11*, 1903, doi:10.3390/nu11081903 14

Rogelio González-Arellanes, Rene Urquidez-Romero, Alejandra Rodríguez-Tadeo, Julián Esparza-Romero, Rosa-Olivia Méndez-Estrada, Erik Ramírez-López, Alma-Elizabeth Robles-Sardin, Bertha-Isabel Pacheco-Moreno and Heliodoro Alemán-Mateo
High Hydration Factor in Older Hispanic-American Adults: Possible Implications for Accurate Body Composition Estimates
Reprinted from: *Nutrients* **2019**, *11*, 2897, doi:10.3390/nu11122897 33

Joseph C. Watso and William B. Farquhar
Hydration Status and Cardiovascular Function
Reprinted from: *Nutrients* **2019**, *11*, 1866, doi:10.3390/nu11081866 43

Kurt J. Sollanek, Robert W. Kenefick and Samuel N. Cheuvront
Osmolality of Commercially Available Oral Rehydration Solutions: Impact of Brand, Storage Time, and Temperature
Reprinted from: *Nutrients* **2019**, *11*, 1485, doi:10.3390/nu11071485 64

Zachary J. Schlader, David Hostler, Mark D. Parker, Riana R. Pryor, James W. Lohr, Blair D. Johnson and Christopher L. Chapman
The Potential for Renal Injury Elicited by Physical Work in the Heat
Reprinted from: *Nutrients* **2019**, *11*, 2087, doi:10.3390/nu11092087 74

Caroline J. Smith
Pediatric Thermoregulation: Considerations in the Face of Global Climate Change
Reprinted from: *Nutrients* **2019**, *11*, 2010, doi:10.3390/nu11092010 99

Tamara Hew-Butler, Valerie Smith-Hale, Alyssa Pollard-McGrandy and Matthew VanSumeren
Of Mice and Men—The Physiology, Psychology, and Pathology of Overhydration
Reprinted from: *Nutrients* **2019**, *11*, 1539, doi:10.3390/nu11071539 123

Lawrence E. Armstrong and Evan C. Johnson
Water Intake, Water Balance, and the Elusive Daily Water Requirement
Reprinted from: *Nutrients* **2018**, *10*, 1928, doi:10.3390/nu10121928 137

William M. Adams, Lesley W. Vandermark, Luke N. Belval and Douglas J. Casa
The Utility of Thirst as a Measure of Hydration Status Following Exercise-Induced Dehydration
Reprinted from: *Nutrients* **2019**, *11*, 2689, doi:10.3390/nu11112689 162

About the Special Issue Editors

William M. Adams is currently an Assistant Professor in the Department of Kinesiology at the University of North Carolina at Greensboro where he also serves as the Program Director for the M.S. in Athletic Training Program and Director of the Hydration, Environment and Thermal. (H.E.A.T.) Stress Lab. Dr. Adams' research interests are focused on optimizing human health and performance. Specifically, his interests lie in determining the role of habitual fluid intake on health and wellness, investigating the various facets of exertional heat stroke, and maximizing athletic performance. He has been either a lead or co-author of over 60 publications in both peer-reviewed scientific journals and edited textbooks on topics related to exertional heat stroke, maximizing athletic performance in the heat, hydration on human health and performance, and preventing sudden death in sport and physical activity.

Evan C. Johnson is an Assistant Professor within the Division of Kinesiology and Health at the University of Wyoming and a member of the Human Integrated Performance Laboratory. The overarching theme of Evan's research is low-cost Interventions for health. Primarily, his research has two main foci: (1) the measurement and influence of water intake on health outcomes and (2) the renal response to physical activity coupled with alterations in thermoregulation. Outside of hydration research, Evan is dedicated to enhancing the presentation skills of our future scientific leaders through the application of new and evidenced-based pedagogical techniques, as well as increasing the diversity of ideas within our field by serving as an advocate for the promotion of underrepresented groups.

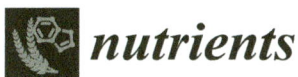

Editorial

Water Intake, Body Water Regulation and Health

Evan C. Johnson [1],* and William M. Adams [2]

1. Human Integrated Physiology Laboratory, Division of Kinesiology and Health, University of Wyoming, Laramie, WY 82071, USA
2. Hydration, Environment and Thermal Stress Lab, Department of Kinesiology, University of North Carolina at Greensboro, Greensboro, NC 27412, USA; wmadams@uncg.edu
* Correspondence: evan.johnson@uwyo.edu

Received: 29 February 2020; Accepted: 3 March 2020; Published: 6 March 2020

The biological feedback provided by human water intake upon our physiology is grossly under-investigated. The delicate regulation of intake and imperceptible changes to physiological processes makes it easy for the casual observer to overlook the acute and chronic impacts of water consumption on human health and performance. Given this gap, we aim to bring a special edition of Nutrients to highlight some of the growing areas of interest that fall under the broad umbrella of "water intake, body water regulation and health".

As with any research topic, investigators must begin with, and be able to constantly update, their understanding of the appropriate measurement of their target phenomenon. Three of the manuscripts within this Special Issue will help the researchers of tomorrow to do just that. Drs. Muñoz and Wininger provide us with "food for thought" when considering the utilization of the National Health and Nutrition Examination Survey (NHANES) for hydration-related investigations [1]. Additionally, Dr. Basov and colleagues review the influence of deuterium-depleted water on isotope regulation, an important topic for those looking to apply D_2O application for the measurement of water intake and/or turnover [2]. Relatedly, Dr. González-Arellanes and co-authors present evidence of how chronic high-volume water consumption can affect body composition measurement via D_2O dilution while also introducing the influence that age, sex, and ethnicity may play in being able to accurately assess total body water [3].

Although still under-investigated, the influence of water intake on dimensions of health has been increasing within recent literature. Rightly so, a further understanding of health behaviors related to something as fundamental as water intake can have a substantial impact on public health. First, Drs. Watso and Farquhar provide a comprehensive review discussing current evidence and physiological mechanisms that tie water intake to cardiovascular function [4]. A separate study presented by Drs. Sollanek, Kenefick, and Cheuvront reviews the osmolality standards of several commercially available rehydration solutions [5], which has relevance to treatment standards within countries in need of rehydration plans for combatting diseases such as malaria. Tangential to water intake, is the influence that body water has upon the human body's ability to thermoregulate. Papers by Dr. Schlader and colleagues [6] and Dr. Smith [7] address this aspect of water homeostasis through a mechanistic review of how physical labor in the heat presents risk for renal injury, and a novel focus regarding pediatric thermoregulation in the face of increasing ambient temperature due to climate change, respectively. Lastly, among our health focused papers, is a wonderful review by Dr. Hew-Butler which examines the other side of the water intake coin; what happens to the body when too much water is consumed [8]? The career achievements of all of the above authors make these manuscripts not to be missed for those interested in the influence of water intake on health.

In conclusion, the co-editors of this Special Issue, together with our collaborators, introduce two papers on hydration biomarkers; a topic that is continuously evolving within scientific literature. The manuscript by Drs. Armstrong and Johnson provides background on the evidence behind the current water intake guidelines and introduces a novel biomarker, copeptin, along with providing the history of how this biomarker came to be established in the water intake literature [9]. Drs. Adams, Vandermark, Belval, and Casa present our final manuscript on how the perception of thirst can be properly used to evaluate hydration status within exercise investigations [10]. To read this paper alongside Dr. Hew-Butlers will provide fantastic context for early-career scientists to emeritus scientists.

We thank the readers for seeking out this Special Issue. We are honored to be able to collect the works from a diversified group of leaders within the field of human physiology. The data, thoughts, and ideas presented in this Special Issue are a sign of wonderful times ahead in our field!

References

1. Muñoz, C.X.; Wininger, M. Unexplained Variance in Hydration Study. *Nutrients* **2019**, *11*, 1828.
2. Basov, A.; Fedulova, L.; Baryshev, M.; Dzhimak, S. Deuterium-Depleted Water Influence on the Isotope $^2H/^1H$ Regulation in Body and Individual Adaptation. *Nutrients* **2019**, *11*, 1903. [CrossRef] [PubMed]
3. González-Arellanes, R.; Urquidez-Romero, R.; Rodríguez-Tadeo, A.; Esparza-Romero, J.; Méndez-Estrada, R.-O.; Ramírez-López, E.; Robles-Sardin, A.-E.; Pacheco-Moreno, B.-I.; Alemán-Mateo, H. High Hydration Factor in Older Hispanic-American Adults: Possible Implications for Accurate Body Composition Estimates. *Nutrients* **2019**, *11*, 2897. [CrossRef] [PubMed]
4. Watso, J.C.; Farquhar, W.B. Hydration Status and Cardiovascular Function. *Nutrients* **2019**, *11*, 1866. [CrossRef] [PubMed]
5. Sollanek, K.J.; Kenefick, R.W.; Cheuvront, S.N. Osmolality of Commercially Available Oral Rehydration Solutions: Impact of Brand, Storage Time, and Temperature. *Nutrients* **2019**, *11*, 1485. [CrossRef] [PubMed]
6. Schlader, Z.J.; Hostler, D.; Parker, M.D.; Pryor, R.R.; Lohr, J.W.; Johnson, B.D.; Chapman, C.L. The Potential for Renal Injury Elicited by Physical Work in the Heat. *Nutrients* **2019**, *11*, 2087. [CrossRef] [PubMed]
7. Smith, C.J. Pediatric Thermoregulation: Considerations in the Face of Global Climate Change. *Nutrients* **2019**, *11*, 2010. [CrossRef] [PubMed]
8. Hew-Butler, T.; Smith-Hale, V.; Pollard-McGrandy, A.; VanSumeren, M. Of Mice and Men—The Physiology, Psychology, and Pathology of Overhydration. *Nutrients* **2019**, *11*, 1539. [CrossRef] [PubMed]
9. Armstrong, L.E.; Johnson, E.C. Water Intake, Water Balance, and the Elusive Daily Water Requirement. *Nutrients* **2018**, *10*, 1928. [CrossRef] [PubMed]
10. Adams, W.M.; Vandermark, L.W.; Belval, L.N.; Casa, D.J. The Utility of Thirst as a Measure of Hydration Status Following Exercise-Induced Dehydration. *Nutrients* **2019**, *11*, 2689. [CrossRef] [PubMed]

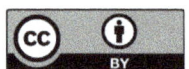

© 2020 by the authors. Licensee MDPI, Basel, Switzerland. This article is an open access article distributed under the terms and conditions of the Creative Commons Attribution (CC BY) license (http://creativecommons.org/licenses/by/4.0/).

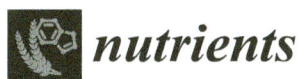 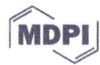

Article

Unexplained Variance in Hydration Study

Colleen X. Muñoz [1] and Michael Wininger [2,3,4,*]

[1] Department of Health Sciences and Nursing, University of Hartford, West Hartford, CT 06117, USA
[2] Department of Rehabilitation Sciences, University of Hartford, West Hartford, CT 06117, USA
[3] Department of Biostatistics, Yale University, New Haven, CT 06510, USA
[4] Cooperative Studies Program, Department of Veterans Affairs, West Haven, CT 06516, USA
* Correspondence: wininger@hartford.edu; Tel.: +1-860-768-5787

Received: 4 June 2019; Accepted: 30 July 2019; Published: 7 August 2019

Abstract: With the collection of water-intake data, the National Health and Nutrition Examination Survey (NHANES) is becoming an increasingly popular resource for large-scale inquiry into human hydration. However, are we leveraging this resource properly? We sought to identify the opportunities and limitations inherent in hydration-related inquiry within a commonly studied database of hydration and nutrition. We also sought to critically review models published from this dataset. We reproduced two models published from the NHANES dataset, assessing the goodness of fit through conventional means (proportion of variance, R^2). We also assessed model sensitivity to parameter configuration. Models published from the NHANES dataset typically yielded a very low goodness of fit $R^2 < 0.15$. A reconfiguration of variables did not substantially improve model fit, and the goodness of fit of models published from the NHANES dataset may be low. Database-driven inquiry into human hydration requires the complete reporting of model diagnostics in order to fully contextualize findings. There are several emergent opportunities to potentially increase the proportion of explained variance in the NHANES dataset, including novel biomarkers, capturing situational variables (meteorology, for example), and consensus practices for adjustment of co-variates.

Keywords: hydration; water intake; obesity; modeling; database; NHANES; chronic disease; big data

---

1. Introduction

Water intake and hydration status are evolving as increasingly important points of focus in far-reaching corners of medicine and public health. Investigators in search of phenotypic risk factors and as a possible strategy for mitigating disease burden and progression have targeted total water intake practices in myriad diseases including hyperglycemia [1,2], obesity [3–8], diabetes mellitus [5,6,9–12], metabolic syndrome [6,13], cardiovascular diseases [14–18], chronic kidney disease [5,19–23], cystic renal disease [24–26], and bladder cancer [27–29]. Given the extensive foundational research linking total water intake to other high-relevance morbidities, it is exciting that the National Center for Health Statistics collects water intake data. However, are we leveraging this resource optimally?

In this article, we explore model design in database-supported hydration inquiry. We contrast model diagnostics and explore optimization scenarios by reproducing two recently published regression models related to hydration. In particular, we look into regression models in hydration, published by others, by way of the model goodness of fit parameter, the R^2. The coefficient of determination ($0 \leq R^2 \leq 1$) is a standard measure for how well scatter data fit to their model regressor; it is the proportion of explained variation relative to total variation. A low R^2 value indicates a large proportion of unexplained variance; a high R^2 indicates that much of the variance observed in the data are explained by effects described in the model.

Our interest was to replicate two recently-published models in order to ascertain their goodness of fit. We also wanted to extend these published works by assessing the sensitivity of the model goodness to parameter selection. The models studied here are mutually similar but distinct, making use of different variables in both prediction and response, but both had a similar design in that regression models were designed to test specific hypotheses within a large, publicly available dataset. Our objective was to critically review the state of the art—and identify opportunities to enhance—database-driven inquiry into human hydration.

2. Methods and Results

2.1. Study Selection

We took as exemplars two recently published papers: Rosinger et al. [3] and Chang et al. [4]. Both groups leveraged the same dataset (National Health and Nutrition Examination Survey (NHANES) 2009–2012), tested for associations between hydration and body composition, were posed as population studies (i.e., weighted analyses), and utilized a parallel design, i.e., tandem linear and logistic regression. Naturally, these papers differ in terms of co-variate selection, dataset filtering, the selection of predictor versus response variable, and the age-adjustment of hydration status. Full methodologies are described in the original manuscripts, but in short summary: The Rosinger et al. study ($n = 9528$) utilized urine osmolality (URXOAV) as the response variable, with the following predictor variables: Age (RIDAGEYR) stratified 20–39, 40–59, and ≥60 years; gender (RIAGENDR); race–ethnicity (RIDRETH1) re-coded into three groups (Non-Hispanic White, Non-Hispanic Black, and Hispanic); fasting session index (PHDSESN); physical activity (MINMODVIG) as low versus high-activity at 150 min of moderate or vigorous activity per week; caffeine intake (DR1TCAFF), stratified as low versus high-intake at 400 mg; alcohol consumed (DR1TALCO), total calories consumed (DR1TKCAL); diabetes status (DIQ010); and moisture-intake (DR1TMOIS) stratified at males <3700 g, females <2700 g, or lactating females <3800 g. The Chang et al. study ($n = 9601$) utilized BMI (BMXBMI) as a response variable, with urine osmolality, gender, race–ethnicity, the ratio of family income to poverty level (INDFMPIR), and age as continuous variables. Data were obtained de novo from the NHANES repository at CDC.gov. These studies were selected because they provided the right balance between comparability and mutual novelty, both had already been cited multiple times in their short history in print, and both papers were written in a way that facilitated replication.

2.2. Model Diagnostics

A detail not reported in either study was a model goodness of fit. We extracted the model fit as R^2 values, defined as 1 minus the ratio of residual deviance to null deviance. Our motivation for reporting R^2 is that this is an exquisitely important parameter used to contextualize analytical models. Both papers (Chang et al. and Rosinger et al.) presented significance values (*p*-values) for individual parameters, and these values are informative as to the existence of a relationship between two variables. However, neither paper reported a goodness of fit (R^2), so there was no way to draw an inference as to which group presented a more compelling model, or whether either model was tenable at all. A further review of models in this area of study revealed that it is the rare exception that a model goodness is published alongside the model results. Thus, there is an opportunity to provide valuable supporting information regarding our analytical approaches in the analysis of hydration datasets.

In total, eight models were considered: Two from Chang et al. and six from Rosinger et al. R^2 was low, ranging from 0.03 to 0.11. The models shown here reflect an extension of the original published analyses, starting with a reproduction of the models as originally published, using identical datasets and identical assumptions. We considered our replication successful when we were able to reproduce all linear regression coefficients described in Chang et al. to within 1% of their printed value, and we were able to reproduce all linear regression coefficients in the normal-weight dataset described in Rosinger et al., also to within 1%. Once we were able to confidently replicate these published findings by others, thus confirming their models as described, we felt comfortable extending their models. As an illustration, consider the univariate regressions shown in Figure 1. Both models yield a statistically significant relationship between predictor and response variables (both *p*-values were incalculably small, below the precision of the computer), but neither had an R^2 above 2.5%.

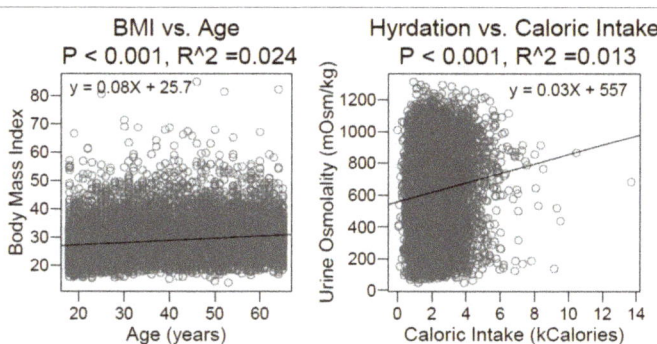

Figure 1. Univariate regressions from the National Health and Nutrition Examination Survey (NHANES) 2009–2010 and 2011–2012 datasets, based on Chang et al. (**Left**) and Rosinger et al. (**Right**). Both regressions have highly significant *p*-values but negligible R^2.

We note that the relationships demonstrated in these plots depart somewhat from those reported in the prior studies due to their use of multi-variate models and weighted regressions. We have shown unweighted univariate models for the sake of clarity in visualization. Nevertheless, these figures are useful as visual aids in demonstrating the low goodness of fit in these studies. Could the weakness of these models be explained by variable configuration? We tested this in three different variables.

2.3. Urine Osmolality and BMI

Rosinger et al. posed hydration (via urine osmolality) as a response variable adjusted for age via the linear transformation 831 mOsm/kg − 3.4 × (age − 20 years), per published guidance [30,31], and BMI as a trichotomous predictor: Normal, overweight, and obese (BMI <25, 25–30, and ≥30). Chang et al. posed hydration as a predictor variable without adjusting for age, and they treated body composition as a dichotomous quantity: Normal versus obese stratified at BMI ≥ 30.

In order to test model sensitivity to variable configuration, we assessed the goodness of fit on the published regression models with four different settings: Hydration status with and without age adjustment and BMI as a continuous versus categorical variable. For these four models, the threshold for adequate hydration was systematically altered over a range of urine osmolality values from 200 to 1100 mOsm/kg. Thus, eight models were tested in total: Four variants from Chang et al. and four from Rosinger et al.; the BMI as a continuous versus factor variable and hydration as an adjusted versus unadjusted variable.

We found that there were substantial differences in model fit depending on the defined threshold for adequate hydration status and that this relationship was opposite between the papers (R^2 maximized at extreme thresholds in models derived from Rosinger et al. versus optimization in mid-range values in models derived from Chang et al.). We also noted that age adjustment seemed to have had a profound impact on the Rosinger models but not on Chang's models—vice-versa for BMI as a continuous versus categorical measure (Figure 2). While not rigorously assessed, we suspect that this is most likely due to their respective positioning as outcome measures, as opposed to differences in datasets or inclusion of other co-variates.

A few remarks bear discussion regarding our methodology and interpretation. Firstly, Rosinger implemented separate models for each category. Here, we merged all data together and included BMI as a co-variate. While this changes the nature of the model, perturbing a single model facilitates interpretation versus three separate models, it allows for a direct contrast against Chang's results.

We specifically decided not to alter the stratification of BMI (Chang: Two-level; Rosinger: Three-level), as we felt it was valuable to retain this semblance of the published model. Additionally, we note that we intentionally tested urine osmolality ranges that were physiologically unrealistic: Stratifying at 200 mOsm/kg and 1100 mOsm/kg is unknown in the literature. While we were interested in a narrower range of strata (threshold 500–800 mOsm/kg), we felt it appropriate to test for model behavior beyond those benchmarks in order to fully describe the relationship between the model and its parameter configuration.

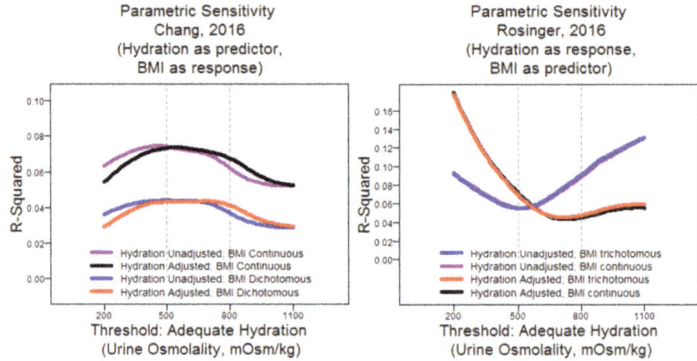

Figure 2. Model goodness (R^2) versus hydration threshold (via urine osmolality) in sensitivity analysis of two database studies on hydration in relation to body composition.

While it is certainly more common to consider hydration to be adequate at more moderate ranges of urine osmolality, we note that there are some respondents with values as or more extreme than this range (approximately 6% of respondents were below 200 mOsm/kg, and approximately 2% of respondents were above 1100 mOsm/kg), so while such extreme boundaries are unlikely to be useful in stratifying the general population, they are physiologically meaningful and might conceivably be of interest to those making inquiries about extreme hydration status levels. Our interest in such extreme thresholds was to explore the edge effects of the relationship between dichotomized hydration status and model goodness in order to verify that model performance is spectral and to provide perspective as to the impact of threshold selection outside of the historical range.

Lastly, we observed that the model fits were generally very weak: $R^2 \leq 0.10$ in all models in the interval between 500 and 800 mOsm/kg of urine osmolality. Separately, we assessed whether model fit would improve with urine osmolality as a continuous variable, and we found that the results were similar: $0.10 \leq R^2 \leq 0.12$ in all simulations of Rosinger's models and $0.05 \leq R^2 \leq 0.08$ in Chang's models (Figure 3).

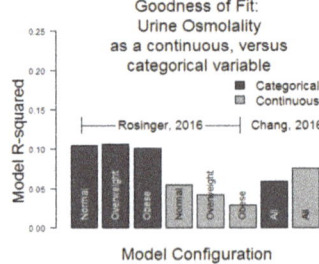

Figure 3. Model goodness (R^2) comparison, incorporating hydration as a continuous variable versus categorical variable $R^2 < 0.12$ in all models.

2.4. Water Intake

Rosinger's work categorizes respondents according to their water intake, with a two-level stratification, also accounting for sex (and within females: Lactation status). We tested other stratification approaches in order to test the sensitivity of the model to this parameter (Table 1).

Table 1. Goodness of fit of Rosinger et al. with various water intake stratifications used in previous publications. Cells contain R^2 values obtained from regression models built from the published model. Top row is the replicated model from Rosinger et al.; all other rows use same dataset and same model as Rosinger et al., but with the altered stratification of a single variable (water intake). Some stratifications showed an improved goodness of fit (R^2 greater than Rosinger et al.); some stratifications showed a degraded goodness of fit (R^2 less than Rosinger et al.). All models showed a generally weak model fit ($R^2 < 0.15$).

	Norm.	OWt	Obese	All	Strata (Water Intake (mL/day))
Rosinger, 2016 [3]	0.111	0.110	0.107	0.095	<2700 (F), <3700 (M), <3800 (Lactating F)
Armstrong, 2012 [32]	0.132	0.109	0.114	0.101	{0, 1507, 1745, 2109, 2507, 2945, 3407, ∞}
Armstrong, 2010 [33]	0.132	0.110	0.113	0.100	{0, 1382, 2008, 2048, 2453, 2614, 3261, ∞}
Johnson, 2015 [34]	0.127	0.108	0.107	0.099	{0, 1620, 3210, ∞}
Muñoz, 2015 [35]	0.126	0.106	0.111	0.099	{0, 1500, 2250, 3130, ∞}
Sontrop, 2013 [19]	0.114	0.109	0.112	0.097	{0, 2000, 4300}
Pross, 2014 [36]	0.101	0.095	0.093	0.084	{0, 1200, 2000, ∞}
Perrier, 2013 [37,38]	0.107	0.099	0.103	0.080	{0, 1200; 2000, 4000} [1]
Roussel, 2011 [1]	0.080	0.086	0.094	0.077	{0, 500, 1000, ∞}

Norm = Normal Weight; OWt = Overweight. Strata defined or inspired by recent studies in hydration inquiry.
[1] Middle hydration group (1200–2000 mL/d) and extremely hydrated (>4000 mL/d) censored.

Results were mixed: Some stratification designs yielded improved fits in the linear regressions based on Rosinger's model, while some designs yielded a weaker fit. We note that even the best model among the 32 created yielded $R^2 < 0.14$.

3. Discussion

3.1. Modeling

The papers analyzed here are not atypical in not having reported their R^2: We are unaware of any prior database studies in hydration where model fit is reported. However, they highlight the problematic emphasis of a significance test over a heuristic and more reflective of model goodness of fit [39]. The *p*-value does not provide information about whether the data are especially adherent to the regressor. The *p*-value indicates the relationship's existence, and R^2 indicates the relationship's precision.

Moreover, each point of inquiry will require its own assumptions and its own selection of response variables or outcome measures, co-variates, and data conditioning steps. It is not possible for this manuscript to serve as guidance for model design, and it is beyond the scope of this paper to critically review the designs adopted by others. Rather, we recognize the inherent variation in analytical approaches that have been published to date and that there is further variety to come. We do strongly encourage thoroughness in explaining variable selection, assumption declarations, and in reporting model goodness.

Regression models in the study of hydration face a substantial design challenge: Complex co-variate interdependencies. Total body water balance is a function of water gains (via beverages, foods and metabolic water) and losses (via sweat, urine, feces and respiratory losses). Those who expect these factors to be highly co-dependent will argue that a model containing multiple factors among this set to be poorly-posed for its inclusion of collinearities [40–42]. At the other extreme, those who view these factors to be acceptably independent will argue that database studies are unviable for their lack of collection of the many meaningful determinants of body water balance and that those few that are present will be inadequately supported and "over-interpreted" [43–46].

3.2. Asynchrony

The NHANES survey incorporates a variety of reporting windows. Dietary recall estimates consumption during the 24-h period prior to the examination center visit (midnight to midnight); physical activity reports incorporate the past seven days, past 30 days, and "in a typical week," which may synchronize poorly with the timing of dietary information; and urine samples are collected on the day of the examination center visit, where participants are randomly assigned to appointments in the morning, afternoon, or evening, which vary somewhat versus protocols for optimal hydration assessment [38] and canonical renal function testing [47]. Investigators may or may not find this sequence (survey, delay, then measure) serviceable; others may not recognize that these are not contemporaneous measurements and may mis-interpret the models altogether.

3.3. Biomarkers

Tools used to indicate hydration process and status have been disputed, and no gold standard currently exists for an appropriate assessment across all scenarios [31,48,49]. While elevated urine osmolality has much perceived utility as a hydration biomarker [34,37,50,51], some question its validity with single (spot) samples [52,53]. Urine osmolality has noteworthy interindividual variation [38,53] and is an ephemeral data point which measures hydration status in an instantaneous way. However, diet, physical activity, and phenotype are more enduring. Thus, there is great need for novel biomarkers to capture this hysteresis. One emergent marker, an arginine vasopressin (AVP) surrogate, copeptin, has shown preliminary promise as a water-balance indicator with robustness to various levels of hydration status and attenuation following an increased water intake intervention [54]. Copeptin has high molecular stability compared to AVP that aids in more accurate and less complicated measurement [55], and AVP and copeptin can distinguish acute and chronic water consumption variations [37,56], rendering this circulating protein a potentially attractive option to better characterize participants' water intake practices. While it is likely that there is no single substance or indicator with optimal responsiveness to daily hydration status [32], there is reason to continue searching for biomarkers with increasing fidelity to hydration status, as there is currently an unknown proportion of unexplained variance attributable to the biomarkers available currently.

3.4. Weather

NHANES currently does not collect information related to weather conditions at the time of data collection [57–60]. Seasonality corrections are common [32,61–64], although they are not universally justified [65,66], perhaps because of the complexity in adjusting for such a diffuse variable [67]. It would be feasible to document local weather conditions at or near to the time of survey response; this could be designed to capture weather in locales where the respondent habited in the preceding 24 h or to capture specific exposures, e.g., "Did you spend most of your time in a climate-controlled building or outdoors?" We observe that accounting for weather is not necessarily the sole province of future NHANES iterations: It is strictly possible to obtain zip-level geographic identifiers and date-of-survey information from restricted data (research data center) which could be cross-referenced against a historical weather database, although this requires some assumptions about a lack of travel.

3.5. Analytic Approach

Clearly, relationships between variables are labile to the way each variable is posed, and there are unlimited ways to create an analytical model. Should water intake be adjusted according to body composition, daily max ambient temperature, Mean temperature, or a composite measure accounting for time spent outdoors, total amount of direct sunlight, temperature and wind speed? Wearable sensors capable of recording climatic parameters are becoming increasingly prevalent [68–71], and perhaps large population investigations will soon have access to more accurate estimations of internal body temperature [72,73], sweat rate [74], and physical activity due to an increasingly robust infrastructure to support analysis of pedometers [75]. Furthermore, we recommend reporting the model goodness of fit as is conventional in modeling [76–78]. There are, as of yet, no published R^2 values for hydration models in public datasets; without knowing where our benchmarks lie, it is impossible to know whether our models are keeping pace with the field in terms of explained variance. Where these actions are practicable, investigators should make efforts to incorporate them; where these actions are inappropriate, researchers should justify their approach.

4. Conclusions

With continued investigation into hydration practices and health outcomes, optimal model design, statistical reporting, and database extensions are warranted. By manipulating two recently-published hydration models, we were able to show (1) a substantial variation in the model fit depending on parameter configurations and (2) a consistently weak model fit, i.e., $R^2 < 0.14$. We propose the inclusion of variables contributing to body water balance, which might increase the proportion of explained variance in a hydration study and mitigate artificial associations. In addition, consensus variable selection and stratification will increase comparability between studies. We make the following additional suggestions regarding targets for the advancement of the science and communication of results within the study of hydration: (1) The aggressive pursuit of promising biomarkers such as copeptin; (2) the creative utilization of assistive resources like meteorological databases; (3) the integration of advanced biostatistical techniques such as principal components analysis, survival analysis, time-series and longitudinal analysis; and (4) the detailed reporting of model goodness in any paper where modeling is employed. In particular, we recommend R^2 and not merely a model's *p*-value, as statistical significance is not nearly as informative as proportion of variance explained. Through the establishment of best practices and identification of new opportunities in hydration study, we anticipate that the maximum value can be obtained from database-driven inquiry, both past and future.

Author Contributions: Designed Research, C.X.M. and M.W.; conducted Research, C.X.M. and M.W.; data analysis and statistical analysis, M.W.; writing, C.X.M. and M.W.; responsibility for final content, C.X.M. and M.W.

Funding: Work was supported by internal grant from the College of Education, Nursing and Health Professions; University of Hartford.

Conflicts of Interest: The authors have no personal, professional, or financial relationships that might influence this work.

Ethics Statement: The procedures followed were in accordance with the ethical standards of the institution or regional committee on human experimentation and that approval was obtained from the relevant committee on human subjects and/or animal welfare.

Abbreviations

AVP	Arginine vasopressin
BMI	Body-mass index
d	Day
kg	Kilogram
mL	Milliliter
mOsm	Milliosmoles
NHANES	National Health and Nutrition Examination Survey
OWt	Overweight

References

1. Roussel, R.; Fezeu, L.; Bouby, N.; Balkau, B.; Lantieri, O.; Alhenc-Gelas, F.; Marre, M.; Bankir, L. Low water intake and risk for new-onset hyperglycemia. *Diabetes Care* **2011**, *34*, 2551–2554. [CrossRef] [PubMed]

2. Taveau, C.; Chollet, C.; Waeckel, L.; Desposito, D.; Bichet, D.G.; Arthus, M.F.; Magnan, C.; Philippe, E.; Paradis, V.; Foufelle, F.; et al. Vasopressin and hydration play a major role in the development of glucose intolerance and hepatic steatosis in obese rats. *Diabetologia* **2015**, *58*, 1081–1090. [CrossRef]
3. Rosinger, A.Y.; Lawman, H.G.; Akinbami, L.J.; Ogden, C.L. The role of obesity in the relation between total water intake and urine osmolality in US adults, 2009–2012. *Am. J. Clin. Nutr.* **2016**, *104*, 1554–1561. [CrossRef] [PubMed]
4. Chang, T.; Ravi, N.; Plegue, M.A.; Sonneville, K.R.; Davis, M.M. Inadequate Hydration, BMI, and Obesity Among US Adults: NHANES 2009–2012. *Ann. Fam. Med.* **2016**, *14*, 320–324. [CrossRef]
5. Tasevska, I.; Enhorning, S.; Christensson, A.; Persson, M.; Nilsson, P.M.; Melander, O. Increased Levels of Copeptin, a Surrogate Marker of Arginine Vasopressin, Are Associated with an Increased Risk of Chronic Kidney Disease in a General Population. *Am. J. Nephrol.* **2016**, *44*, 22–28. [CrossRef] [PubMed]
6. Enhorning, S.; Bankir, L.; Bouby, N.; Struck, J.; Hedblad, B.; Persson, M.; Morgenthaler, N.G.; Nilsson, P.M.; Melander, O. Copeptin, a marker of vasopressin, in abdominal obesity, diabetes and microalbuminuria: The prospective Malmo Diet and Cancer Study cardiovascular cohort. *Int. J. Obes. (2005)* **2013**, *37*, 598–603. [CrossRef]
7. Dennis, E.A.; Dengo, A.L.; Comber, D.L.; Flack, K.D.; Savla, J.; Davy, K.P.; Davy, B.M. Water consumption increases weight loss during a hypocaloric diet intervention in middle-aged and older adults. *Obesity* **2010**, *18*, 300–307. [CrossRef]
8. Stookey, J.D.; Constant, F.; Popkin, B.M.; Gardner, C.D. Drinking water is associated with weight loss in overweight dieting women independent of diet and activity. *Obesity* **2008**, *16*, 2481–2488. [CrossRef]
9. Enhorning, S.; Wang, T.J.; Nilsson, P.M.; Almgren, P.; Hedblad, B.; Berglund, G.; Struck, J.; Morgenthaler, N.G.; Bergmann, A.; Lindholm, E.; et al. Plasma copeptin and the risk of diabetes mellitus. *Circulation* **2010**, *121*, 2102–2108. [CrossRef]
10. Abbasi, A.; Corpeleijn, E.; Meijer, E.; Postmus, D.; Gansevoort, R.T.; Gans, R.O.; Struck, J.; Hillege, H.L.; Stolk, R.P.; Navis, G.; et al. Sex differences in the association between plasma copeptin and incident type 2 diabetes: The Prevention of Renal and Vascular Endstage Disease (PREVEND) study. *Diabetologia* **2012**, *55*, 1963–1970. [CrossRef]
11. Wannamethee, S.G.; Welsh, P.; Papacosta, O.; Lennon, L.; Whincup, P.H.; Sattar, N. Copeptin, Insulin Resistance, and Risk of Incident Diabetes in Older Men. *J. Clin. Endocrinol. Metab.* **2015**, *100*, 3332–3339. [CrossRef] [PubMed]
12. Johnson, E.C.; Bardis, C.N.; Jansen, L.T.; Adams, J.D.; Kirkland, T.W.; Kavouras, S.A. Reduced water intake deteriorates glucose regulation in patients with type 2 diabetes. *Nutr. Res.* **2017**, *43*, 25–32. [CrossRef]
13. Enhorning, S.; Struck, J.; Wirfalt, E.; Hedblad, B.; Morgenthaler, N.G.; Melander, O. Plasma copeptin, a unifying factor behind the metabolic syndrome. *J. Clin. Endocrinol. Metab.* **2011**, *96*, E1065–E1072. [CrossRef] [PubMed]
14. Tasevska, I.; Enhorning, S.; Persson, M.; Nilsson, P.M.; Melander, O. Copeptin predicts coronary artery disease cardiovascular and total mortality. *Heart* **2016**, *102*, 127–132. [CrossRef] [PubMed]
15. Melander, O. Vasopressin, from Regulator to Disease Predictor for Diabetes and Cardiometabolic Risk. *Ann. Nutr. AMP Metab.* **2016**, *68* (Suppl. 2), 24–28. [CrossRef]
16. Enhorning, S.; Hedblad, B.; Nilsson, P.M.; Engstrom, G.; Melander, O. Copeptin is an independent predictor of diabetic heart disease and death. *Am. Heart J.* **2015**, *169*, 549–556. [CrossRef] [PubMed]
17. Riphagen, I.J.; Boertien, W.E.; Alkhalaf, A.; Kleefstra, N.; Gansevoort, R.T.; Groenier, K.H.; van Hateren, K.J.; Struck, J.; Navis, G.; Bilo, H.J.; et al. Copeptin, a surrogate marker for arginine vasopressin, is associated with cardiovascular and all-cause mortality in patients with type 2 diabetes (ZODIAC-31). *Diabetes Care* **2013**, *36*, 3201–3207. [CrossRef] [PubMed]
18. Chan, J.; Knutsen, S.F.; Blix, G.G.; Lee, J.W.; Fraser, G.E. Water, other fluids, and fatal coronary heart disease: The Adventist Health Study. *Am. J. Epidemiol.* **2002**, *155*, 827–833. [CrossRef]
19. Sontrop, J.M.; Dixon, S.N.; Garg, A.X.; Buendia-Jimenez, I.; Dohein, O.; Huang, S.H.; Clark, W.F. Association between water intake, chronic kidney disease, and cardiovascular disease: A cross-sectional analysis of NHANES data. *Am. J. Nephrol.* **2013**, *37*, 434–442. [CrossRef]
20. Clark, W.F.; Sontrop, J.M.; Huang, S.H.; Moist, L.; Bouby, N.; Bankir, L. Hydration and Chronic Kidney Disease Progression: A Critical Review of the Evidence. *Am. J. Nephrol.* **2016**, *43*, 281–292. [CrossRef]

21. Clark, W.F.; Sontrop, J.M.; Huang, S.H.; Gallo, K.; Moist, L.; House, A.A.; Cuerden, M.S.; Weir, M.A.; Bagga, A.; Brimble, S.; et al. Effect of Coaching to Increase Water Intake on Kidney Function Decline in Adults With Chronic Kidney Disease: The CKD WIT Randomized Clinical Trial. *JAMA* **2018**, *319*, 1870–1879. [CrossRef]
22. Enhorning, S.; Christensson, A.; Melander, O. Plasma copeptin as a predictor of kidney disease. *Nephrol. Dial. Transplant.* **2019**, *34*, 74–82. [CrossRef] [PubMed]
23. Strippoli, G.F.; Craig, J.C.; Rochtchina, E.; Flood, V.M.; Wang, J.J.; Mitchell, P. Fluid and nutrient intake and risk of chronic kidney disease. *Nephrology* **2011**, *16*, 326–334. [CrossRef] [PubMed]
24. Sagar, P.S.; Zhang, J.; Luciuk, M.; Mannix, C.; Wong, A.T.Y.; Rangan, G.K. Increased water intake reduces long-term renal and cardiovascular disease progression in experimental polycystic kidney disease. *PLoS ONE* **2019**, *14*, e0209186. [CrossRef] [PubMed]
25. Wang, X.; Wu, Y.; Ward, C.J.; Harris, P.C.; Torres, V.E. Vasopressin directly regulates cyst growth in polycystic kidney disease. *J. Am. Soc. Nephrol. JASN* **2008**, *19*, 102–108. [CrossRef] [PubMed]
26. Torres, V.E.; Bankir, L.; Grantham, J.J. A case for water in the treatment of polycystic kidney disease. *Clin. J. Am. Soc. Nephrol. CJASN* **2009**, *4*, 1140–1150. [CrossRef] [PubMed]
27. Jiang, X.; Castelao, J.E.; Groshen, S.; Cortessis, V.K.; Shibata, D.K.; Conti, D.V.; Gago-Dominguez, M. Water intake and bladder cancer risk in Los Angeles County. *Int. J. Cancer* **2008**, *123*, 1649–1656. [CrossRef]
28. Braver, D.J.; Modan, M.; Chetrit, A.; Lusky, A.; Braf, Z. Drinking, micturition habits, and urine concentration as potential risk factors in urinary bladder cancer. *J. Natl. Cancer Inst.* **1987**, *78*, 437–440. [PubMed]
29. Villanueva, C.M.; Cantor, K.P.; King, W.D.; Jaakkola, J.J.; Cordier, S.; Lynch, C.F.; Porru, S.; Kogevinas, M. Total and specific fluid consumption as determinants of bladder cancer risk. *Int. J. Cancer* **2006**, *118*, 2040–2047. [CrossRef] [PubMed]
30. Cheuvront, S.N.; Ely, B.R.; Kenefick, R.W.; Sawka, M.N. Biological variation and diagnostic accuracy of dehydration assessment markers. *Am. J. Clin. Nutr.* **2010**, *92*, 565–573. [CrossRef]
31. Cheuvront, S.N.; Kenefick, R.W.; Charkoudian, N.; Sawka, M.N. Physiologic basis for understanding quantitative dehydration assessment. *Am. J. Clin. Nutr.* **2013**, *97*, 455–462. [CrossRef] [PubMed]
32. Armstrong, L.E.; Johnson, E.C.; Munoz, C.X.; Swokla, B.; Le Bellego, L.; Jimenez, L.; Casa, D.J.; Maresh, C.M. Hydration biomarkers and dietary fluid consumption of women. *J. Acad. Nutr. Diet.* **2012**, *112*, 1056–1061. [CrossRef] [PubMed]
33. Armstrong, L.E.; Pumerantz, A.C.; Fiala, K.A.; Roti, M.W.; Kavouras, S.A.; Casa, D.J.; Maresh, C.M. Human hydration indices: Acute and longitudinal reference values. *Int. J. Sport Nutr. Exerc. Metab.* **2010**, *20*, 145–153. [CrossRef] [PubMed]
34. Johnson, E.C.; Munoz, C.X.; Le Bellego, L.; Klein, A.; Casa, D.J.; Maresh, C.M.; Armstrong, L.E. Markers of the hydration process during fluid volume modification in women with habitual high or low daily fluid intakes. *Eur. J. Appl. Physiol.* **2015**, *115*, 1067–1074. [CrossRef] [PubMed]
35. Munoz, C.X.; Johnson, E.C.; McKenzie, A.L.; Guelinckx, I.; Graverholt, G.; Casa, D.J.; Maresh, C.M.; Armstrong, L.E. Habitual total water intake and dimensions of mood in healthy young women. *Appetite* **2015**, *92*, 81–86. [CrossRef] [PubMed]
36. Pross, N.; Demazieres, A.; Girard, N.; Barnouin, R.; Metzger, D.; Klein, A.; Perrier, E.; Guelinckx, I. Effects of changes in water intake on mood of high and low drinkers. *PLoS ONE* **2014**, *9*, e94754. [CrossRef] [PubMed]
37. Perrier, E.; Vergne, S.; Klein, A.; Poupin, M.; Rondeau, P.; Le Bellego, L.; Armstrong, L.E.; Lang, F.; Stookey, J.; Tack, I. Hydration biomarkers in free-living adults with different levels of habitual fluid consumption. *Br. J. Nutr.* **2013**, *109*, 1678–1687. [CrossRef] [PubMed]
38. Perrier, E.; Demazieres, A.; Girard, N.; Pross, N.; Osbild, D.; Metzger, D.; Guelinckx, I.; Klein, A. Circadian variation and responsiveness of hydration biomarkers to changes in daily water intake. *Eur. J. Appl. Physiol.* **2013**, *113*, 2143–2151. [CrossRef]
39. Wagenmakers, E.J. A practical solution to the pervasive problems of p values. *Psychon. Bull. AMP Rev.* **2007**, *14*, 779–804. [CrossRef]
40. Farrar, D.E.; Glauber, R.R. Multicollinearity in Regression Analysis: The Problem Revisited. *Rev. Econ. Stat.* **1967**, *49*, 92–107. [CrossRef]
41. Belsley, D.A. *Conditioning Diagnostics: Collinearity and Weak Data in Regression*; Wiley: New York, NY, USA, 1991.
42. Bollen, K.A. *Structural Equations with Latent Variables*; Wiley: New York, NY, USA, 1989.

43. Hart, R.A.; MacKay, D.I. Wage Inflation, Regional Policy and the Regional Earnings Structure. *Economica* **1977**, *44*, 267–281. [CrossRef]
44. Browne, M.W.; Cudeck, R. Alternative ways of assessing model fit. *Sociol. Methods Res.* **1992**, *21*, 230–258. [CrossRef]
45. Moore, G.P.; Perkel, D.H.; Segundo, J.P. Statistical analysis and functional interpretation of neuronal spike data. *Annu. Rev. Physiol.* **1966**, *28*, 493–522. [CrossRef] [PubMed]
46. Jaeger, B.C.; Edwards, L.J.; Das, K.; Sen, P. An R^2 statistic for fixed effects in the generalized linear mixed model. *J. Appl. Stat.* **2017**, *44*, 1086–1105. [CrossRef]
47. Jacobson, M.H.; Levy, S.E.; Kaufman, R.M.; Gallinek, W.E.; Donnelly, O.W. Urine osmolality. A definitive test of renal function. *Arch. Intern. Med.* **1962**, *110*, 83–89. [CrossRef]
48. Armstrong, L.E. Assessing hydration status: The elusive gold standard. *J. Am. Coll. Nutr.* **2007**, *26*, 575s–584s. [CrossRef]
49. Munoz, C.X.; Johnson, E.C.; Demartini, J.K.; Huggins, R.A.; McKenzie, A.L.; Casa, D.J.; Maresh, C.M.; Armstrong, L.E. Assessment of hydration biomarkers including salivary osmolality during passive and active dehydration. *Eur. J. Clin. Nutr.* **2013**, *67*, 1257–1263. [CrossRef]
50. Perrier, E.; Rondeau, P.; Poupin, M.; Le Bellego, L.; Armstrong, L.E.; Lang, F.; Stookey, J.; Tack, I.; Vergne, S.; Klein, A. Relation between urinary hydration biomarkers and total fluid intake in healthy adults. *Eur. J. Clin. Nutr.* **2013**, *67*, 939–943. [CrossRef]
51. Perrier, E.T.; Buendia-Jimenez, I.; Vecchio, M.; Armstrong, L.E.; Tack, I.; Klein, A. Twenty-four-hour urine osmolality as a physiological index of adequate water intake. *Dis. Mark.* **2015**, *2015*, 231063. [CrossRef]
52. Cheuvront, S.N.; Kenefick, R.W.; Zambraski, E.J. Spot Urine Concentrations Should Not be Used for Hydration Assessment: A Methodology Review. *Int. J. Sport Nutr. Exerc. Metab.* **2015**, *25*, 293–297. [CrossRef]
53. Cheuvront, S.N.; Munoz, C.X.; Kenefick, R.W. The void in using urine concentration to assess population fluid intake adequacy or hydration status. *Am. J. Clin. Nutr.* **2016**, *104*, 553–556. [CrossRef] [PubMed]
54. Lemetais, G.; Melander, O.; Vecchio, M.; Bottin, J.H.; Enhorning, S.; Perrier, E.T. Effect of increased water intake on plasma copeptin in healthy adults. *Eur. J. Nutr.* **2018**, *57*, 1883–1890. [CrossRef] [PubMed]
55. Morgenthaler, N.G.; Struck, J.; Alonso, C.; Bergmann, A. Assay for the measurement of copeptin, a stable peptide derived from the precursor of vasopressin. *Clin. Chem.* **2006**, *52*, 112–119. [CrossRef] [PubMed]
56. Szinnai, G.; Morgenthaler, N.G.; Berneis, K.; Struck, J.; Muller, B.; Keller, U.; Christ-Crain, M. Changes in plasma copeptin, the c-terminal portion of arginine vasopressin during water deprivation and excess in healthy subjects. *J. Clin. Endocrinol. Metab.* **2007**, *92*, 3973–3978. [CrossRef] [PubMed]
57. Sun, Z.; Tao, Y.; Li, S.; Ferguson, K.K.; Meeker, J.D.; Park, S.K.; Batterman, S.A.; Mukherjee, B. Statistical strategies for constructing health risk models with multiple pollutants and their interactions: Possible choices and comparisons. *Environ. Health Glob. Access. Sci. Sour.* **2013**, *12*, 85. [CrossRef] [PubMed]
58. Schleicher, R.L.; McCoy, L.F.; Powers, C.D.; Sternberg, M.R.; Pfeiffer, C.M. Serum concentrations of an aflatoxin-albumin adduct in the National Health and Nutrition Examination Survey (NHANES) 1999–2000. *Clin. Chim. Acta Int. J. Clin. Chem.* **2013**, *423*, 46–50. [CrossRef] [PubMed]
59. United States Environmental Protection Agency (USEPA). *Handbook for Use of Data from the National Health and Nutrition Examination Surveys (NHANES): A Goldmine of Data for Environmental Health Analyses*; United States Environmental Protection Agency (USEPA): Washington, DC, USA, 2003.
60. CDC/National Center for Health Statistics. National Health and Nutrition Examination Survey. In *Questionnaires, Datasets, and Related Documentation*; CDC/National Center for Health Statistics: Hyattsville, MD, USA.
61. Malisova, O.; Bountziouka, V.; Panagiotakos, D.; Zampelas, A.; Kapsokefalou, M. Evaluation of seasonality on total water intake, water loss and water balance in the general population in Greece. *J. Hum. Nutr. Diet.* **2013**, *26* (Suppl. 1), 90–96. [CrossRef]
62. McKenzie, A.L.; Perrier, E.T.; Guelinckx, I.; Kavouras, S.A.; Aerni, G.; Lee, E.C.; Volek, J.S.; Maresh, C.M.; Armstrong, L.E. Relationships between hydration biomarkers and total fluid intake in pregnant and lactating women. *Eur. J. Nutr.* **2017**, *56*, 2161–2170. [CrossRef]
63. Bougatsas, D.; Arnaoutis, G.; Panagiotakos, D.B.; Seal, A.D.; Johnson, E.C.; Bottin, J.H.; Tsipouridi, S.; Kavouras, S.A. Fluid consumption pattern and hydration among 8-14 years-old children. *Eur. J. Clin. Nutr.* **2017**, *72*, 420–427. [CrossRef]

64. Peacock, O.J.; Stokes, K.; Thompson, D. Initial hydration status, fluid balance, and psychological affect during recreational exercise in adults. *J. Sports Sci.* **2011**, *29*, 897–904. [CrossRef]
65. Bland, J.M.; Altman, D.G. Statistical methods for assessing agreement between two methods of clinical measurement. *Lancet* **1986**, *1*, 307–310. [CrossRef]
66. Heller, K.E.; Sohn, W.; Burt, B.A.; Eklund, S.A. Water consumption in the United States in 1994–96 and implications for water fluoridation policy. *J. Public Health Dent.* **1999**, *59*, 3–11. [CrossRef] [PubMed]
67. Wallis, K.F. Seasonal Adjustment and Relations between Variables. *J. Am. Stat. Assoc.* **1974**, *69*, 18–31. [CrossRef]
68. Fahrni, T.K.M.; Sommer, P.; Wattenhofer, R.; Welten, S. Sundroid: Solar radiation awareness with smartphones. In Proceedings of the 13th International Conference on Ubiquitous Computing, Beijing, China, 17–21 September 2011; pp. 365–374.
69. Kinkeldei, T.Z.C.; Cherenack, K.H.; Troster, G. A textile integrated system for monitoring humidity and tempterature. In Proceedings of the IEEE 16th International Solid-State Sensors, Actuators and Microsystems Conference, Beijing, China, 5–9 June 2011; pp. 1156–1159.
70. Yun, J.K.J. Deployment Support for Sensor Networks in Indoor Climate Monitoring. *Int. J. Distrib. Sens. Netw.* **2013**, *9*, 875802. [CrossRef]
71. Yamamoto, Y.; Harada, S.; Yamamoto, D.; Honda, W.; Arie, T.; Akita, S.; Takei, K. Printed multifunctional flexible device with an integrated motion sensor for health care monitoring. *Sci. Adv.* **2016**, *2*, e1601473. [CrossRef] [PubMed]
72. Feng, J.C.Z.; He, C.; Li, Y.; Ye, X. Development of an improved wearable device for core body temperature monitoring based on the dual heat flux principle. *Physiol. Meas.* **2017**, *38*, 652–668. [CrossRef]
73. Atallah, L.C.C.; Wang, C.; Bongers, E.; Blom, T.; Paulussen, I.; Noordergraaf, G. An ergonomic wearable core body temperature sensor. In Proceedings of the IEEE 15th International Conference on Wearable and Implantable Body Sensor Networks, Las Vegas, NV, USA, 4–7 March 2018.
74. Nyein, H.Y.Y.; Tai, L.C.; Ngo, Q.P.; Chao, M.; Zhang, G.B.; Gao, W.; Bariya, M.; Bullock, J.; Kim, H.; Fahad, H.M.; et al. A Wearable Microfluidic Sensing Patch for Dynamic Sweat Secretion Analysis. *ACS Sens.* **2018**, *3*, 944–952. [CrossRef]
75. Wininger, M.; Bjornson, K. Filtering for productive activity changes outcomes in step-based monitoring among children. *Physiol. Meas.* **2016**, *37*, 2231–2244. [CrossRef]
76. Hoyt, W.T.; Imel, Z.E.; Chan, F. Multiple regression and correlation techniques: Recent controversies and best practices. *Rehabil. Psychol.* **2008**, *53*, 321–339. [CrossRef]
77. Osborne, J.W. *Best Practices in Logistical Regression*, 1st ed.; SAGE Publications, Inc.: Thousand Oaks, CA, USA, 2015.
78. Osborne, J. *Best Practices in Quantitative Methods*; SAGE Publications Ltd.: Thousand Oaks, CA, USA, 2008.

 © 2019 by the authors. Licensee MDPI, Basel, Switzerland. This article is an open access article distributed under the terms and conditions of the Creative Commons Attribution (CC BY) license (http://creativecommons.org/licenses/by/4.0/).

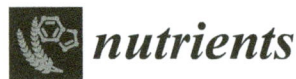

Review

Deuterium-Depleted Water Influence on the Isotope $^{2}H/^{1}H$ Regulation in Body and Individual Adaptation

Alexander Basov [1,2], Liliia Fedulova [3], Mikhail Baryshev [2] and Stepan Dzhimak [2,3,4,*]

1. Kuban State Medical University, 350063 Krasnodar, Russia
2. Kuban State University, 350040 Krasnodar, Russia
3. The V.M. Gorbatov Federal Research Center for Food Systems of Russian Academy of Sciences, 109316 Moscow, Russia
4. Federal Research Center the Southern Scientific Center of the Russian Academy of Sciences, 344006 Rostov-on-Don, Russia
* Correspondence: jimack@mail.ru; Tel.: +7-905-408-36-12

Received: 31 May 2019; Accepted: 13 August 2019; Published: 15 August 2019

Abstract: This review article presents data about the influence of deuterium-depleted water (DDW) on biological systems. It is known that the isotope abundances of natural and bottled waters are variable worldwide. That is why different drinking rations lead to changes of stable isotopes content in body water fluxes in human and animal organisms. Also, intracellular water isotope ratios in living systems depends on metabolic activity and food consumption. We found the $^{2}H/^{1}H$ gradient in human fluids ($\delta^{2}H_{saliva} \gg \delta^{2}H_{blood\ plasma} > \delta^{2}H_{breast\ milk}$), which decreases significantly during DDW intake. Moreover, DDW induces several important biological effects in organism (antioxidant, metabolic detoxification, anticancer, rejuvenation, behavior, etc.). Changing the isotope $^{2}H/^{1}H$ gradient from "$^{2}H_{blood\ plasma} > \delta^{2}H_{visceral\ organs}$" to "$\delta^{2}H_{blood\ plasma} \ll \delta^{2}H_{visceral\ organs}$" via DDW drinking increases individual adaptation by isotopic shock. The other possible mechanisms of long-term adaptation is DDW influence on the growth rate of cells, enzyme activity and cellular energetics (e.g., stimulation of the mitochondrion activity). In addition, DDW reduces the number of single-stranded DNA breaks and modifies the miRNA profile.

Keywords: deuterium; water; adaptation; DNA

---

1. Introduction

Non-radioactive isotopes of biogenic elements ($^{2}H/^{1}H$, $^{18}O/^{17}O/^{16}O$, $^{13}C/^{12}C$, $^{15}N/^{14}N$) have a significant influence on the rate of biochemical reactions, physiological processes, growth and development of unicellular and multicellular living organisms with different levels of energy metabolism and metabolic intensity rate [1–4].

Hydrogen and oxygen isotopes occupy a special place among all non-radioactive nutrients which are primarily included in addition to organic and inorganic compounds in the composition of water, as water is an essential solvent for all biological objects where the vast majority of biochemical reactions occur. In this regard, the importance of water for the implementation of physiological processes is extremely high, but it might vary and differ for each of its nine isotopologues: $^{1}H_{2}^{16}O$, $^{1}HD^{16}O$, $D_{2}^{16}O$, $^{1}H_{2}^{17}O$, $^{1}HD^{17}O$, $D_{2}^{17}O$, $^{1}H_{2}^{18}O$, $^{1}HD^{18}O$, $D_{2}^{18}O$. Some of them, which predominantly contain lighter isotopes, can have in certain concentrations a stimulating effect on functional activity of living systems [5], other isotopologues, including mainly heavy isotopes, are able to inhibit vital processes, especially at high concentrations of deuterium [6,7], and in some cases it was observed that variation of deuterium concentration (both increasing and decreasing its content in water) can enhance the functional activity of living systems [8]. In this regard it is very important to know about the peculiar features of use of certain isotopologues of water for regulation of metabolic processes in a body, and for monitoring of the anabolism and catabolism state of biological substances in various diseases [9].

The ratios of deuterium and protium in natural and bottled waters can vary by up to about two times, which is important to consider when people and animals migrate between continents and climatic zones. For example, the minimum deuterium content in natural water is observed in the ice of Antarctica: Standard Light Antarctic Precipitation (SLAP), which is $^2H_{SLAP}/^1H_{SLAP} = 89.0 \cdot 10^{-6}$ or 89 ppm, or −428.5‰ [10,11]; a somewhat higher content of deuterium (by 40%) is registered in Greenland ice and corresponds to the standard Greenland Ice Sheet Precipitation (GISP): $^2H_{GISP}/^1H_{GISP} = 124.6 \cdot 10^{-6}$ (124.6 ppm or −189.5‰ [12]); whereas the main standard for the content of deuterium in natural water, the Vienna Standard Mean Ocean Water (VSMOW), is: $^2H_{VSMOW}/^1H_{VSMOW} = 155.76 \cdot 10^{-6}$ (155.76 ppm or 0.0‰ [13]), which exceeds the values of $^2H_{SLAP}$ by 75%. It is necessary to note that the highest content of the natural deuterium (in Dababa +16‰) was found when studying the groundwater of the Sahel-Sahara region during the drought period [14–16].

Fluctuations of ^{18}O content are significantly lower than fluctuations of hydrogen isotopes content, and are equal to: $^{18}O_{SLAP}/^{16}O_{SLAP} = 1894 \cdot 10^{-6}$ (1894 ppm or −55.36‰ [16]); $^{18}O_{GISP}/^{16}O_{GISP} = 1955.4 \cdot 10^{-6}$ (1955.4 ppm or −24.76‰ [12]), which is only by 3% higher than standard $^{18}O_{SLAP}$; $^{18}O_{VSMOW}/^{16}O_{VSMOW} = 2005 \cdot 10^{-6}$ (2005 ppm or 0.0‰), at this value exceeds the value $^{18}O_{SLAP}$ by 5.9%, thus being significantly lower (by 12.7 times) than the differences in the ratio of similar standards ^2H and ^1H.

In the natural water sources some peculiar features were observed for a range of closed and freshwater water sources which feature significant differences from VSMOW as well as seasonal variations in isotopic composition of water. For example, in the surface waters of Kyambangunguru lake which is the part of Mbaka lakes, at the end of the dry season deuterium content was 16‰, oxygen-18 content was 3.4‰, while at the end of the rainy season the content of δ^2H was −7‰, content of $\delta^{18}O$ was equal to −0.8‰ [17]. Stable isotopic composition of water from the Antarctic subglacial Lake Vostok was: −59.0‰ (by 6% less $^{18}O_{VSMOW}$) for oxygen-18 and −455‰ (by 45% less $^2H_{VSMOW}$) for deuterium [18]. Isotopic composition of Lake Baikal, Siberia, varies only a little during a year, and is equal to: $\delta^{18}O = -15.8‰$, $\delta^2H = -123‰$, which is 1.6% and 12.3% less, than $^{18}O_{VSMOW}$ and $^2H_{VSMOW}$ respectively [19]. The variations of the isotopic composition in natural water sources are explained by displacement of isotopic equilibrium in range of cases as a result of phase transitions in the water cycle, which leads to fractionation in nature, primarily of $^2H/^1H$ and $^{18}O/^{17}O/^{16}O$ [20,21]. All this leads to a two-stage decrease in content of heavy isotopologues in water vapor: first due to a decrease in their concentration in the water evaporating from the surface of the seas and oceans, and then during partial condensation when precipitation forms (most expressed at their first fall, which also depends on terrain features, geographical and climatic conditions, precipitation frequency, etc. [22]). In this regard snow and rain falling far from the place of their evaporation are characterized by a high content of light water molecules ($^1H_2{}^{16}O$). Furthermore, the flora consumes this water, however as a result of transpiration it gradually enriches this water with ^2H and ^{18}O, leading to introduction of these isotopes into organic compounds [23,24]. This, for instance, explains the significant difference in isotopic composition of juices freshly squeezed from fruits and vegetables grown in various geographic regions [25–27]. In its turn water in healthy animal tissues is enriched with isotopes from two main sources: ingested/drinking water and water formed during oxidation of reducing equivalents during the metabolism of food substrates, including the reduced form of nicotinamide adenine dinucleotide (NAD) in the mitochondrial respiratory chain [28–31]. Moreover, the share of intracellular water synthesized de novo can reach more than 50% [32,33], that occurs with the active interaction of mitochondria, endoplasmic reticulum and peroxisome [34]. In the last organelle production of metabolic water (for example: its catalase converts H_2O_2-excess into H_2O иmolecular oxygen) increases under some pathological and specific conditions, such as high-fat diet (especially including very-long-chain and methyl-branched fatty acids), administration of hypolipidemic drugs (like clofibrate), ingestion of xenobiotics, development of inflammation, and others. Peroxisomal oxidase H_2O_2-production achieves about 1/3 of all cellular hydrogen peroxide [35], and oxygen consumption in peroxisomes can be about 1/5 of all O_2 in cells of metabolic active tissues. Additional pathways of isotopic fractionation in the animal world are perspiration and respiration processes [29], for example due to the release of carbon dioxide, which is highly enriched by ^{18}O [36]. The release of carbon dioxide is caused by the fact than in a body there is an exchange of oxygen atom between CO_2 and H_2O with participation of carbonic anhydrase, while fractionation of ^{18}O depends on time of interaction and pressure of carbon dioxide [37,38]. It is necessary to note that the carbonyl and carboxyl groups of organic substrates are the most active in oxygen atoms exchanging with intracellular water, whereas hydroxyl groups do not participate in oxygen-18 fractionation processes under physiological conditions [39]. At the same time the exchange of protons and deuterons is much more active in live organisms, since functional groups –OH, –NH_3^+, =NH, –SH easily dissociate, affecting the isotopic composition of the liquid medium [40], and although the carbon-related hydrogen which is most commonly found in live objects is stable (with a small exception of hydrogen atoms in composition of CH_2-groups adjacent to carbonyl groups), it is also able to indirectly affect the isotopic composition of water during the oxidation of organic substrates [1,41].

It should be pointed out that fluctuations in isotopic composition of water in a human body can have a wider range, both in connection with the consumption of not only water from surface water sources [42], but from water obtained from any other origin (artesian, glacial, mineral springs), and due to the characteristics of the food ration, for example the predominant consumption of lipid-based nutrients [43]. During study of isotopic composition of samples of bottled and packaged waters of the world, several scientific groups defined the following range of fluctuations: δ^2H from −147‰ to 15‰ and $\delta^{18}O$ from −19.1‰ to 3.0‰ [44–46]. Although as it was shown earlier the bottled mineral waters usually have insignificant differences in deuterium content and even smaller fluctuations in concentration of oxygen-18, modern technologies allow us to obtain deuterium-depleted water (DDW) (with deuterium content till δ^2H = −968‰) and oxygen-18 depleted water (reduction till 26.1% in comparison with $^{18}O_{VSMOW}$) [47–51].

The use of this water can have a significant impact on the isotopic composition and functional activity of both a healthy organism and in various diseases [43,52].

2. Biological Effects of Deuterium-Depleted Water (DDW)

To date a great number of works have been published, where both the activating and inhibitory effects of DDW on various levels of the organization of living matter (molecular, organoid, cellular, tissue and organismic) are described. Below the various results of studies of DDW effect on biological objects will be discussed.

2.1. Activating Influence of DDW at Molecular and Organoid Levels

In one research there was demonstrated an ability of DDW to activate transcription factors (DAF-16 and SOD-3 (extracellular superoxide dismutase [Cu-Zn]), previously inhibited by the introduction of Mn in a *Caenorhabditis elegans*), which were responsible for expression of antioxidant enzymes (superoxide dismutase) and lifespan of *C. elegans*. It is necessary to note that introduction of DDW with δ^2H = −422‰ regulated DAF-16 pathway, restored the activity of SOD (at the background of manganese intoxication) and lifespan of worms till the control reference values without changing of DAF-2 levels [53].

In other research on rats it was shown that the use of DDW containing deuterium δ^2H = −807‰ for 60 days led to the stimulation of the antioxidant protection system in erythrocytes, the stimulation of which was accompanied by an increase in the restored GSH (glutathione) and activity of SOD, while a decrease in catalase activity was found in absence of significant changes in the activity of glutathione peroxidase, glutathione reductase. At the same time less prolonged consumption of DDW by animals (within 30 days) led to prooxidant effects, which were accompanied by stimulation of glutathione reductase and catalase activity, while no changes in SOD activity were observed at the background of increase in malondialdehyde content in blood [54].

The study of the 12-week-old normotensive *Wistar-Kyoto* rats and spontaneously hypertensive rats revealed the ability of DDW with deuterium content $\delta^2H = -646‰$ to increase insulin levels and to lower down the levels of lipids (triglycerides and cholesterol) in the blood of normotensive Wistar-Kyoto rats. At the same time DDW increased the NO· synthase (nitric oxide synthase) activity in the left ventricle of both normotensive Wistar-Kyoto and spontaneously hypertensive rats, although it reduced inducible isoform of nitric oxide synthase (iNOS) protein expression and activity of synthase NO· in the aorta only in spontaneously hypertensive rats. These effects of the exchange of NO· persisted even against the introduction into the drinking ration of a 15% solution of fructose for 6 weeks. That can be explained by the influence of DDW on the terminal complex of mitochondrial electron transport chain, which reduces molecular oxygen into deuterium-depleted water. That, in turn, can change the rate of fatty acid oxidation and gluconeogenesis in a body, including by modifying the level of signaling molecules (reactive oxygen species, NO· and others) [55]. The similar model considered in one of the research works [56] indicates probability of the fact that under conditions of a liquid medium depleted in deuterium, the mechanism of its biological action may be related to the operation of the tricarboxylic acids cycle, because the enzymes localized inside the mitochondria are involved in the fractionation of deuterium. The violation of mitochondrial function due to cell exposure to hypoxia, acidosis, or other pathogenic factors, may reduce the content of a deuterium-free form of reduced nicotinamide adenine dinucleotide phosphate (NADPH), and consequently reduce transfer of ^1H (H-transfer carried out in transhydrogenase reaction by NAD(P)$^+$ transhydrogenase (EC 1.6.1.1): NADPH + NAD$^+$ <=> NADP$^+$ + NADH) in NADPH, thus reducing the reserves of the universal reducing equivalent [57], irreplaceable for many anabolic processes, and creating the prerequisites for mutation rate increase along with occurrence of further dysplastic processes or a decrease in the mass of organs and the whole organism. A possible mechanism of these phenomena may be the change in transportation of ^1H atoms formed in mitochondria during the beta-oxidation of fatty acids with a lower content of deuterium and atoms of ^2H, concentration of which is higher in water and glucose, entering the cytosol from the extracellular environment, leading in general to an increase in the intracellular ratio $^2H/^1H$ [58–60]. The higher values of this ratio can lead to changes in the speed and, rarely, to changes in the direction of biochemical reactions in a body, which can also be characterized by impaired replication processes and repair of DNA, which leads to disruption in synthesis of mRNA, and, consequently, of proteins, creating metabolic prerequisites for reducing of body mass and adaptation. Thus, in cells with mitochondria with impaired transfer of ^1H atom it is possible to regulate the production of high-energy compounds by reducing the concentration of deuterium in the drinking ration, which eventually corrects cell growth, cell division and functional impairment [61]. As a result, a drop in deuterium concentration in cytoplasmic water contributes, among other things, to the normalization of the phenotype of cells with impaired regulation of metabolism. All this leads, for example, to a decrease in the speed of cancer cells division (up to the speed of normal cells division) [62]. The above assumption can be confirmed by the results of a study of the effect of water with different deuterium content on chemical, biological and physical parameters of biological objects [63] (in the experiment the following waters were used: DDW ($\delta^2H = -968‰$); water with natural content of deuterium ($\delta^2H = -101‰$); D$_2$O (99.99%)). Biological objects demonstrated the characteristics of reactivity at various levels of the organization of biota. It was found that for biological molecules of different classes in the medium with different concentrations of deuterium there were distinctive features of the response to the isotopic composition of the medium: for nucleic acids it was shown that the mutation rate constant for L-galactose was slowed down in D$_2$O, whereas the rate of lysozyme activity of destabilase-lysozyme increased by 2 times in a liquid medium c$\delta^2H = -968‰$, while in D$_2$O no changes in activity of destabilase-lysozyme were found. In a two-phase heterogeneous system the kinetics of dissolution of the active ingredients approximately matched with the expected kinetic isotope effect ($k^1H/k^2H > 1$), which confirms the significant contribution of the isotopic composition of water to the process of organic substances dissolution in this water. However, it was noted that the most expressed ^{2}H/^{1}H-effect was observed in the cell system, where the speed of transition from the active to the immobilized state in *S. ambigua* cells increased 800 times in a medium with δ^2H = −968‰ in comparison with a medium in which δ^2H = −101‰ [63].

Particular attention must be drawn to the possible effect of isotopic composition of the medium on the molecular dynamics of the DNA molecule which under natural conditions has one deuterium atom for every 6400 hydrogen atoms and that ratio can lead to a change in the frequency of DNA molecule mutations during living systems evolution [64]. It has been shown that singular replacements of protium atom by deuterium in hydrogen bonds between pairs of nitrogenous bases of the DNA molecule lead to change in the frequency of occurrence of its open states, which in their turn are an obligatory condition for functional activity for the molecule, including facilitating specific intermolecular DNA protein interactions during transcription, folding and replication [65]. It was found that the probability of occurrence of open states between nitrogenous bases in double-stranded DNA depends on concentration of deuterium in the liquid medium surrounding the molecule, and on the magnitude of the energy of hydrogen bonds rupture. When the energy of hydrogen bonds rupture is equal to $0.335 \cdot 10^{-22}$ J the almost linear decrease in probability of appearance of open states between nitrogen bases in double-stranded DNA (for the first 10 base pairs of the gene encoding alpha 17 interferon) is observed within the range δ^2H from −743‰ to 0.0‰ in liquid medium surrounding a molecule. In this case the probability of hydrogen bonds rupture between nitrogenous bases in case of introduction of even one deuterium atom into the DNA molecule exceeds the probability of a similar rupture in the same molecule containing only protium atoms, which indicates a stability decrease in DNA molecular structure. If the energy of hydrogen bonds rupture is equal to $0.345 \cdot 10^{-22}$ J, within the range δ^2H from −743‰ till 0.0‰ in the liquid medium surrounding the DNA molecule there is almost a linear increase in the probability of open states occurrence between its nitrogenous bases. However, the probability of breaking hydrogen bonds between nitrogenous bases in the case of a deuterium atom introduction into DNA molecule does not exceed the likelihood of a similar rupture in the same molecule containing only protium atoms [66].

One more research work shows the influence of DDW with δ^2H = −679‰ on the efficiency of immunocompetent proteins extraction from the immune organs of *Sus scrofa*: spleen, thymus and lymph nodes [67]. At the same time, protein–peptide complexes were fractionated using the methods of step-by-step ultrafiltration and gel filtration method. It was shown that the extraction of proteins from the studied samples in solution with δ^2H = −679‰ provides a nearly twofold increase in the amount of extractable proteins and peptides, which can be caused by change in the ionic strength of this solution along with variation of ^{2}H amount in the medium. The main protein components of the extracts were 8 fractions, which contained from 11% to 20% of the total protein material, at that was visually detectable on two-dimensional electrophoresis [68]. The extracted proteins were the members of the family α- and β-chains of hemoglobin, and only in one case the presence of profilin 1 (actin-binding protein) was detected. Other fractions of hemoglobins were post-translationally modified. In a fraction of hemoglobin β-chains we observed the deimination of amino acid residues (Q) of glutamine or (N) asparagine, and their combination was varied in various fractions. Thus the obtained results indicate that the use of fragmented cells of pig immunocompetent organs isolated in the medium with modified ^{2}H/^{1}H composition as a base matrix allows creating innovative immunostimulating active complexes by improving the quality and safety of livestock products [69].

In addition, there are peculiar features of hydrogen and oxygen isotopes' fractionation for carbohydrates, for example for cellulose. A correlation was shown between the values of water δ^{18}O in leaves and stems [70], while the equilibrium of isotopic composition ^{18}O/^{16}O had specific temperature dependence, which changed little in temperatures of 20–30 °C (averaging 26‰) but increased to 31‰ at lower temperatures [71]. Either the existence of specific oxygen isotope composition in glucose derived from cellulose has been experimentally confirmed [72], when δ^{18}O in the sample of glucose synthesized with the help of gluconeogenesis, differs from the sample obtained by photosynthesis, at least for the C-6 position. At the same time, it should be pointed out that the relatively low value of $\delta^{18}O$ lactose, at least in part, is also a consequence of the aforementioned temperature sensitivity of isotopic fractionation [71] and is explained by the higher body temperature of an animal in comparison with the temperature of the plant leaves and stems.

2.2. Activating Influence of DDW at the Cell and Tissue Levels

The activating influence of DDW at the cell and tissue levels has been noted in a number of research works on the biological objects of animal and plant origin. For example, one of these research works showed the effect of $^2H/^1H$ for the life span of the unicellular biosensor *S. ambigua*, which had a parabolic pattern. In addition, the research observed the stimulating influence of DDW on the proliferative potential of cell culture (human dermal fibroblasts) in early passages [73]. Dynamics of the cell doubling index in the growth medium prepared on the base of DDW with $\delta^2H = -807‰$ showed a higher proliferation potential compared to water with normal isotopic composition: $\delta^2H = -37‰$ [5].

Another research shows the effect of liquid growth medium with $\delta^2H = -904‰$ for the speed of proliferation of human cultured adipose-derived stem cells which speed was characterized by cytotoxicity compared with the medium with the natural deuterium content ($\delta^2H = -37‰$). While that the presence of $\delta^2H = -518‰$ in medium led to a postponed (by one day) increase of migration and metabolic activity of adipose-derived stem cells [74,75]. Similar changes in cellular activity can also be explained by deuterium replacing with protium in HO–, HS– and H_3N^+–groups of macromolecules, especially in active and allosteric centers of enzymes, as well as by decrease of HDO (or $^1HO^2H$) concentration in hydration shell of proteins and nucleic acids, which can change their thermodynamic and, therefore, thermokinetic parameters, stimulating metabolic and mitogenic processes in cells [76].

During study of influence of water $c\delta^2H = -839‰$ for rate of survival of DLD-1 cell line, it was found that DDW was able to stimulate mitochondrial activity and enhance apoptosis of DLD-1cells line [77]. Moreover, the miRNA pattern, which was isolated from exosomes, had significant differences in cells that were incubated in the liquid medium with $\delta^2H = -839‰$, in comparison with the medium with δ^2H within the range from $-76‰$ till $0‰$.

Experimental possibility of influence for activity of mitochondria isolated from rat liver using DDW with δ^2H within the range from $-705‰$ till $-665‰$ and $\delta^{18}O$ within the range from $-135‰$ till $-11‰$ has been confirmed in some research [78,79]. In that research it was found that in case of reduction of ^2H and ^{18}O content in the incubation medium the higher generation (by 35%) of hydrogen peroxide by mitochondria isolated from rats liver that consumed the water with low deuterium concentration was observed. The revealed change in functional activity of mitochondria indicates the ability of the animals' organism to adapt to the deuterium-depleted drinking ration, that possibly is due to the formation of the transmembrane isotope gradient $^2H/^1H$, which induces preadaptation of living system. The mechanism of the biological effect of the altered ratio of hydrogen stable isotopes can be explained by the direct relationship with the work cycle tricarboxylic acids. This is explained by the fact that the enzymes of the tricarboxylic acid cycle, localized in internal volume of mitochondria, provide for redistribution of deuterium between the cytoplasmic and mitochondrial water pools [56]. At the same time the reduction of δ^2H in cytoplasmic water contributes, among other things, to normalization of cells phenotype with impaired metabolism regulation, for example, for cancer cell lines [80].

It is necessary to note the universal nature of deuterium low concentrations effect in cellular structures, as evidenced by change in metabolic and growth activity not only of animal cells, but also in cells of plant origin. For example, it was shown that incubation of corn seedlings (*Zeamays L.*) in DDW $\delta^2H = -839‰$ led to formation of airy cavities in the internal structure of a root [81]. In comparison with the control reference sample started in water $\delta^2H = -69‰$ it was found that deuterium-depleted water determines the best development of the absorbent bristles and increase in number of leading bundles and central vessels in the metaxylem. Also the change in ultrastructural and physiological characteristics of *Beta vulgaris* var. Conditiva seedlings was also shown under the term of hyperhydricity as a result of using the cultural medium with $\delta^2H = -839‰$ [82]. The structural changes (leaves and hypocotyls) characterized by modification of fluoroplastics, mixoplasma, tonoplast and nuclei, were related to hyperhydricity and were significantly less when *Beta vulgaris* var. Conditiva was grown in DDW.

2.3. Activating Influence of DDW for Organs and Organismic Level

More significant changes in comparison with molecular, organoid and cellular levels were observed during the study of DDW effects on internal organs and the organism as a whole. For example, the dependence of neuropsychiatric disorders (depressions) among the population on deuterium content in drinking water was researched. The correlation between the deuterium content in tap water and the level of depressions in US regions was researched. The increase of depressions frequency by 1.8% ($p = 0.0016$) along with increase of deuterium concentration in tap water for every $\delta^2H = 64‰$ was observed. The results were confirmed in experiments on laboratory animals, which on the background of simulated chronic stress, consumed water with $\delta^2H = -411‰$ (in control reference group animals consumed water with $\delta^2H = -99‰$). As a result, it was shown that the frequency of depressive-like signs was reduced in mice that consumed DDW [83], which is explained by its effect on the activity of serotonergic mechanisms of regulation of the nervous tissue functioning. The sensitivity of the central nervous system to fluctuations in the isotopic composition of water is confirmed by experiments on the Wistar rats, which consumed water with δ^2H within the range from $-827‰$ to $-807‰$. They demonstrated, in comparison with the rats who drank water with δ^2H within the range from $-69‰$ to $-37‰$, the reduction of fear and anxiety in unfamiliar environment [84]. In another research by the same authors the Wistar rats who consumed DDW showed an improvement in long-term memory and absence of short-term memory differences compared with animals that consumed water with a natural concentration of deuterium [85]. The decrease of HDO in the drinking ration also had a beneficial effect on prooxidant–antioxidant system of a brain during acute hypoxia in laboratory animals [86]. Studies have shown that in case of consuming DDW ($\delta^2H = -665‰$) for 8 weeks, there is a decrease of deuterium content in the blood plasma by 317‰ as well as in the brain of laboratory animals by 209‰, compared with the control group consuming natural water. Furthermore, DDW consumption in rat hypoxia modeling improves the functioning of antioxidant protection enzymes (catalase, superoxide dismutase, glutathione peroxidase and glutathione reductase) in the blood, increasing its antioxidant potential by 20%, while decreasing the intensity of free radical oxidation in plasma and the rate of peroxide modification of biomolecules in the red blood cells. Also in brain tissues of rats consuming DDW there was no disruption in catalase and superoxide dismutase functioning, and an increase (by 71%) in concentration of restored thiol-containing compounds, which reduce the risk of nerve cells damage under hypoxia. The presence of a neuroprotective effect is also confirmed by higher (by 32%) antioxidant activity of lyophilized brain tissue, as well as by a lower intensity of free radical oxidation (by 13%) and by the speed of oxidative modification of biomolecules (by 16%) in these tissues. The latter proves the feasibility of using the neuroprotective effects of DDW in case of cerebral circulation violations in experimental and clinical practice [87].

To influence nervous tissue, water with modified isotopic composition can affect the aging rate of the whole organism. For example, white outbred female rats of presenile age (20–22 months) consumed DDW ($\delta^2H = -704‰$) as drinking water for five weeks and it led to development of the expressed geroprotective effect, manifested in the appearance of recovery signs in the estrous cycle, as well as in the improvement of coat condition compared with the same parameters in animals exposed to drinking water with $\delta^2H = -37‰$. At the same time the rats that drank DDW showed development of persistent anti-stress adaptive responses of their bodies to calm and enhanced activation as well as increase in bactericidal activity of their skin. Thus in experiments on mammals the direct confirmation of DDW's geroprotective properties was obtained, and the relation between geroprotective and anti-stress effects was shown when DDW was used in the drinking ration. The study revealed a more expressed decrease of deuterium content in the rats' blood plasma (by 33.2%) in comparison with the change of deuterium content in visceral organs (liver—by 7.2%, kidney—by 9.7%, heart—by 7.3%). These changes led to formation of the experimental group of a new isotope $^2H/^1H$ gradient in the animals' organisms, in which δ^2H "visceral organs" > δ^2H"blood plasma", what is the opposite of physiological $^2H/^1H$ gradient, where δ^2H "visceral organs" < δ^2H"blood plasma" [88]. As the animals consumed food with unchanged isotopic composition under the experimental conditions, the observed changes are due only to the consumption of DDW. At the same time the decrease of deuterium content in blood plasma leads to decrease in its content in visceral organs also, obviously, due to replacement of deuterium with protium in hydroxyl (–OH) and thiol (–SH) groups, as well as in primary and secondary amino groups (–NH$_2$, =NH). The deuterium substitution by protium in active and allosteric centers of enzymes can alter the speed of catalytic reactions as a result of decrease in activation energy of transition states of the "enzyme-substrate" complex, which can serve as a basis for development of the organism's metabolic adaptation and lead to occurrence of anti-stress reactions at the system level. In case of substitution of deuterium by protium, not only energy of covalent chemical bonds changes, but there are also differences in the intermolecular interaction forces (for example, due to change in hydrogen bonds energy) between some singular molecules [89]. The noted systemic changes, indicating the restoration of neuroendocrine regulation impaired in animals of pre-senile age, are apparently caused by a decrease of deuterium in blood and visceral organs (liver, kidney, heart), and also by the ease of DDW use as a nutritional factor, which allows us to consider it as a promising solution for holistic geriatric care in a presenile period of ontogenesis. The presence of isotopic gradient $^2H/^1H$ was also confirmed in the study of biological fluids in humans. So women who gave birth showed significant differences in natural conditions in δ^2H of blood plasma (average δ^2H = −74‰), oral fluid (average δ^2H = 26‰) and breast milk (average δ^2H = −91‰), which led to formation of isotopic gradient $^2H/^1H$ (δ^2H oral fluid >> δ^2H blood plasma > δ^2H breast milk) [90]. These differences in the isotopic composition to a certain extent are caused by peculiarities of the biochemical composition of biological fluids; they are directly interrelated with the mass fraction of water ($R_{Spearman}$ = 0.81, $p < 0.0001$), and also negatively correlate with protein content ($R_{Spearman}$ = −0.55, $p < 0.0005$), carbohydrates ($R_{Spearman}$ = −0.80, $p < 0.0001$) and lipids ($R_{Spearman}$ = −0.82, $p < 0.0001$). This indicates the dependence of the deuterium concentration on the mass fraction of water and the content of carbohydrate and lipid substrates, which are characterized by approximately the same high rate $R_{Spearman}$. This data can be explained by the lowest intensity of isotope exchange $^2H/^1H$ in hydrophobic (non-polar) radicals of lipids, which even under terms of water consumption with different isotopic composition make a stable contribution to the final concentration of deuterium in the cell. In addition, these relations between the content of biomolecules and deuterium must be taken into account while developing non-invasive methods for monitoring the content of heavy non-radioactive isotopes in a body, including deuterium, since the biochemical composition of biological fluids can be variable depending on the person's lifestyle (diet, physical activity and other factors). It is not possible to explain completely the differences in content of $^2H/^1H$ isotopes only by characteristics of biochemical composition of these biological fluids and, apparently, there are additional mechanisms for regulation of isotopic metabolism in a body [91]. Among the possible mechanisms for isotopes fractionation, the presence of histohematic barriers shall be taken into account, including hematosalivar and hemato-lactation barriers, whose function is to ensure selective permeability for organic and inorganic molecules. Differences in intensity of metabolic processes in various tissues can make their contribution to difference in the isotopic composition in biological fluids [92], for example along with increased energy production there is an increased formation of water inside the cells from hydrogen isotopes which are part of biological oxidation substrates, i.e., different classes of organic compounds. At the same time, the metabolic water that formed intracellularly can significantly differ in deuterium content from extracellular water replenished in a body mainly as part of the diet [33]. It was also found that in case of consuming of DDW with δ^2H = −615‰ by women it is possible to achieve a significant reduction in deuterium concentration in blood plasma (average δ^2H = −175‰), oral fluid (average δ^2H = −134‰) and also in breast milk but in less volume (average δ^2H = −183‰), which leads to significant decrease of the described isotopic gradient $^2H/^1H$ (δ^2H oral fluid > δ^2H blood plasma ≥ δ^2H breast milk) [90].

Changes in the direction and level of expression of isotopic gradients in a body can affect various periods of ontogenesis, including its morphofunctional parameters and activity of biochemical processes, providing short-term and long-term adaptation [78]. These body reactions can increase survival and life functions longevity [89]. The geroprotective influence of DDW was also confirmed on organisms with different levels of organization, including *Caenorhabditis elegans* (*C. elegans*), which were placed into the liquid medium with $\delta^2H = -422‰$ and $\delta^2H = -229‰$. It was found that in case of Mn-induced reduction of worms lifespan against the background of DAF-16 and SOD-3 inhibition, the use of DDW restored their expression and increased the lifespan of *C. elegans* [53].

The ability of water with a low content of heavy stable isotopes of hydrogen and oxygen ^{18}O to neutralize the harmful environmental effects on a body has been shown in a number of research works devoted to study of not only chemical toxicants [93], but also to physical factors, for example, X-rays radiation [94]. The mice after exposure to γ-radiation ^{60}Co at dose 1.0 Gray showed reduction of aging rate and reduction of frequency of lens opacities formation cases. In addition, the mature males of the *Balb/c* line which consumed water с$\delta^{18}O= -206‰$ and $\delta^2H = -730‰$ and were exposed to radiation ^{60}Co at dose 0.50 Gray showed accelerated recovery of the thymus, spleen, and bone marrow in comparison with mice from the control reference group that consumed water with $\delta^{18}O = -18‰$ and $\delta^2H = -103‰$ [95]. After X-ray exposure, the mice which consumed water with $\delta^2H = -807‰$ and natural ^{18}O content showed a protective effect on spleen structure accompanied by immune stimulation with an increase of megakaryocytes quantity [96]. In general, the mechanism of the protective effect of water with low content of HDO and $^1H_2^{18}O$ is explained by its ability to stimulate the processes of proliferation, especially in radiosensitive tissues, which reduces damage to the body during sublethal irradiation [97]. While using of heavy water, radioprotective mechanisms is related to inhibition of catabolism and free radical oxidation of proteins, and also nucleic acids in radiosensitive organs and tissues.

It is planned to use the mechanisms of radioprotective action of water with depleted concentrations of heavy stable isotopes ^{18}O and ^2H described above during travel by humans in outer space [98,99].

2.4. Inhibitory Influence of DDW on Molecular and Organoid Level

Besides the activating effect of water with a modified isotopic composition, which is described in more researches, more often under physiological conditions and in the adaptation of the organism, the ability of DDW to inhibit certain metabolic reactions in the body is noted in a number of scientific works devoted to study of aspects of pathological metabolic states. Hence it is known that hydrogen ions are transported through the plasma membrane through the H^+-ATPase (adenosin triphosphatase), which cannot transfer deuterium atoms with the same ease as protium atoms [100]. Therefore, it is possible, that once the cell eliminates ions H^+ to increase the pH by activating the Na^+-H^+ transport [101–103], the $^2H/^1H$ ratio is increased in the intercellular substance. So it is possible that the $^2H/^1H$ ratio will also regulate the cell cycle [104] if it reaches a certain threshold, thus triggering molecular mechanisms that transfer the cell into the S phase.

One of the possible mechanisms of DDW influence on the cell cycle can be carried out through the suppression of individual genes expression. Thus it was found that the water $\delta^2H = -679‰$ inhibited the cells proliferation at the G0/G1 stage and the S phase cell population [105]. Moreover, female mice which consumed water $\delta^2H = -839‰$ showed significant suppression of 7,12-dimethylbenz[a]anthracene (DMBA)-induced expression of Bcl2, Kras, and Myc [52]. In the other research the rats that consumed DDW ($\delta^2H = -615‰$) found a significant decrease in blood plasma of both the total amount of glycoproteins and their degree of glycosylation, which may reflect two processes: decrease of tumor-associated proteins expression, as well as decrease of healthy tissues detritus against the background of anticancer drugs use: Vinblastine, Cyclophosphamide, 5-Fluorouracil and Farmarubicine, due to introduction of DDW into the drinking ration [106].

Probably, DDW can selectively stress tumor cells [104], including its ability to regulate the activity of key genes in cell cycle without, however, interfering with metabolic processes in healthy tissues. This assumption is also confirmed by the fact that CBA/Ca-sensitive inbred mice's consumption of drinking ration with $\delta^2H = -865‰$ resulted in (DMBA)-induced expression of c-myc, Ha-rasand p53 gene, which play a key role in the development of tumor cells. When evaluating the expression of RNA 48 h after exposure to a carcinogen, the expression of all the genes mentioned above was inhibited in various organs: spleen, lung, thymus, kidney, liver and lymph nodes [107].

2.5. The Inhibitory Influence of DDW at the Cellular and Tissue Levels

The inhibitory influence of DDW on cell proliferation has been established for cells with impaired metabolism, including in the neoplastic process. Thus it was shown that, in addition to expression of the gene regulating the cell cycle, DDW can change the activity of antioxidant defense enzymes, while inhibition of human breast cancer cell line (MCF7) was observed as the most expressed in the medium $\delta^2H = -807‰$. At the same time the activity of antioxidant protection enzymes (catalase, superoxide dismutase) and malondialdehyde content in MCF-7 cells changed. In general, the analysis of the cell cycle shows the ability of deuterium in low concentrations to cause a cell cycle stop during the G1/S transition [105]. Also changes in prooxidant-antioxidant system functional activity of nervous tissue cells against the background of their incubating in medium with $\delta^2H = -679‰$ led to decrease in mitochondrial potential of cerebellar neurons and their increased mortality rate during glucose deprivation and temperature stress (39 °C) [87].

Inhibition of cell growth with impaired metabolism was confirmed in research that studied 3-(4,5-dimethylthiazol-2-yl)-2,5-diphenyl tetrazolium bromide (MTT)-based cytotoxicity for cell lines: AGS (human gastric adenocarcinoma), MDA-MB231(human breast adenocarcinoma), U-87MG (glioblastoma multiform), PC-3 (human prostate adenocarcinoma) where DDW (within the δ^2H range from −743‰ to −486‰) increased the inhibitory effect of paclitaxel on the cell lines of the mammary gland, prostate, stomach cancer and glioblastoma, and the effect was more expressed in cases of mammary gland and prostate [108].

In addition, the incubation medium $\delta^2H = -807‰$ significantly decreased the growth rate of fibroblast cell line. In the same research the inhibition of different human breast adenocarcinoma (MDA-MB-231 and MCF-7) cells growth in female CBA/Ca mice. The above described changes in cell lines growth rate can be caused by the effect of $^2H/^1H$ ratio, reduction of which results inter alia to the following:

—increasing of time required by the cell to achieve the threshold ratio of deuterium/protium, which ratio triggers cell division;

—neutralization of oncogenic activity of ATPase gene, which can behave as an oncogene in mammalian cells along with increased concentrations of deuterium in the medium. Therefore, the reduced removal of protons from the cell slow down their proliferation by reducing the deuterium/protium ratio [109];

—decreasing in proliferation, as even a small decrease in deuterium concentration in the intercellular substance is able to inhibit cell growth, because it does not allow the intracellular concentration of deuterium to raise up to the threshold level [61].

Moreover, DDW ($\delta^2H = -679‰$) influenced not only the proliferation, but also the migration of tumor cell lines (nasopharyngeal carcinoma and MC3T3-E1). At the same time activation of normal preosteoblast cell MC3T3-E1 growth was observed when it was cultured in DDW. The analysis of the cell cycle showed the ability of DDW to cause the cell cycle to stop during the G1/S transition, reducing the cells number in S-phase and contributing to increase of cells number in the G1 phase in tumor cells (nasopharyngeal carcinoma), also DDW suppressed the expression of the proliferating cell nuclear antigen matrix metalloproteinase 9 [80]. Similar results with changes in cell cycle phases were obtained in research on the human lung carcinoma cell line A549 and human embryonic lung fibroblasts HLF-1 with incubation in DDW (δ^2H = −679‰). It was shown that reduction of ^{2}H/^{1}H ratio in medium led to DDW-induced cellular apoptosis [110].

2.6. Inhibitory Influence of DDW for Organs and Organism Level

The effects of water with modified isotopic composition on gene expression, the activity of enzymes of nonspecific defense, mitochondrial activity, cell proliferation and cell migration described above allow us understanding the individual systemic processes associated with DDW introduction into drinking diet. The inhibitory effect of deuterium concentration reducing in a body is mainly associated with decrease in tumor growth and metastasis rate, whereas healthy organs usually do not experience a negative effect when DDW is consumed by living organisms.

For example, in a clinical research that included 129 patients with small tumors (small cells and small cell lung cancers) who consumed DDW in addition to conventional chemotherapy and radiation therapy, an increase in median survival time was noted. That increase was 25.9 months in males and 74.1 months in female patients [52]. The other research demonstrated an increase in survival rate of patients with lung cancer and brain metastases who consumed the drinking ration with a final δ^2H of −839‰ for at least 3 months. Also the decrease of metastatic spread in these patients was observed [111]. Also 91 patients with prostate cancer were examined. These patients consumed DDW with a progressively lowering deuterium content in water from −326‰ to −839‰. During this process the patients' tumors volumes decreased as well as the level of prostate-specific antigen, which decreases in correlation with the consumption of DDW [112].

Moreover, while modeling tumors (H460 cells) by its injecting to *Balb/c* mice drinking DDW (δ^2H = −679‰), within 60 days inhibition of the tumor was observed (approximately 30%) in comparison with the group that had the same model of tumor and did not receive DDW [110].

At the same time, some studies presented convincing data which showed expressed difference between therapy effect of the same nutritive substance in the cell line (in vitro) and in animals with orthotopic tumor. An interesting explanation of this matter was recently published in the article, which contemplated metabolic water as influenced factor to growth rate of cancer cells [113], that based on some sequential suggestions about metabolic pathways in brain tumors:

(1) glioma cells (in vivo) are metabolically flexible to use beta-hydroxybutyrate in catabolism (in contradict of RG2 and 9L glioma models [114]) as do healthy cells of the contralateral brain areas;

(2) under a natural condition ketogenic diet, which containing 91% fat and 9% protein [115], can increase production intracellular water about two times compared with carbohydrates, that occurs due to cooperate mitochondrial and peroxisomal lipid-substratum oxidation to H_2O [116];

(3) in cells, between cytoplasmic and mitochondrial pools, the isotope (^{2}H/^{1}H) ratio change can take place, which leads to a decrease in deuterium content especially via oxidation long-chain unsaturated fatty acids in ^1H_2O in mitochondria with recycling matrix water by citric acid cycle's enzymes [56];

(4) deuterium reduction in matrix water can regulate not only functional activity of mitochondria, but also speed of other cellular processes caused by transfer DDW to the cytosol, and as result of the foregoing, cell ATP-production [78,79] and interfacial protein interactions are changed and, consequently, cellular rate of growth can be various due to deuterium loaded in molecular structures of living cell.

Nevertheless, the using of ketogenic diet in tumor therapy can be accompanied by a decrease in vivo in the intensity of fatty acid β-oxidation. It is possible, because speed of short-chain fatty acids (C_6-C_{10}) β-oxidation in mitochondria is higher than cooperative "peroxisomal-mitochondrial" long-chain and unsaturated fatty acid oxidation [117]. Therefore, during long-lasting lipid loading, it is can be probably to drop down ATP-production especially under intracellular O_2 fault (for example, produced by circulatory disorders of tumor), acetyl-CoA deficiency forming, accumulate ketogenic substrates (β-hidroxibutiryl-CoA and acetoacetyl-CoA), decrease pH and other processes, but deuterium depletion does not occur in the cytosol water. In contrast of mitochondrial ^1H_2O-production, the DDW consumption more significantly changes deuterium content in cytosol and less dependent on non-physiological cell conditions, so it can be used more effectively in adjuvant therapy.

3. Conclusions

This review demonstrated the important role of water isotopic composition to ensure the passing of many biochemical reactions, regulation of energy metabolism and functional activity of mitochondria, changes in the speed of the cell cycle, increase the body's adaptation and stimulate a number of vital processes in healthy tissues. At the same time some of the biological effects of DDW described above (antioxidant, antidepressant, anticancer, hypoglycemic, etc.) can be used in therapy of various diseases in humans. The stimulating effect on living systems of different levels of organization (molecular, organoid, cellular, tissue, organ and organism levels) is mainly produced by water with δ^2H within the range from −229‰ to −679‰ and $\delta^{18}O$ within the range from −135‰ to −206‰.

Nevertheless, it shall be noted that the consumption of water with a modified isotopic composition which has a significant deviation from the natural concentrations of ^2H and ^{18}O isotopes is also accompanied by stress effect on a body. This can be caused, for example, by a sharp change of isotope $^2H/^1H$ gradient from "$\delta^2H_{blood\ plasma} > \delta^2H_{visceral\ organs}$" to "$\delta^2H_{blood\ plasma} \ll \delta^2H_{visceral\ organs}$", therefore, the consumption of the drinking ration with δ^2H below −679‰ by living organisms may lead to isotopic shock [118], which has, inter alia, an inhibitory effect on biological processes and inhibits in some cases the growth, division and migration of cells, including cells of tumoral origin. The presence of an isotopic gradient in human biological fluids is confirmed by differences in the content of deuterium in the series: $\delta^2H_{saliva} \gg \delta^2H_{blood\ plasma} > \delta^2H_{breast\ milk}$ ($^2H/^1H$ gradient was equal to 117‰). At the same time while drinking deuterium-depleted water it is possible to achieve a significant reduction in the described isotope $^2H/^1H$ gradient by 58%: $\delta^2H_{saliva} > \delta^2H_{blood\ plasma} \geq \delta^2H_{breast\ milk}$ ($^2H/^1H$ gradient was equal to 49‰). In addition to the drinking diet, the proportion of proteins, lipids and carbohydrates in the consumed food, which proportion is associated with oxidation of organic compounds in mitochondria. At the same time, the greatest decrease of deuterium content in intracellular water is achieved with increase of lipid-containing nutrients proportion in the diet. So, cooperative influence of the drinking/ingested DDW and diet (containing lipogenic sources with certain deuterium/protium ratio [113], which is naturally lower than it takes place in the food carbohydrates and proteins [90,91]) can be used for treatment based on the compartmentalized deuterium disequilibrium and changing of intracellular isotope $^2H/^1H$ gradient, especially in previously drug-treated cells [119]. Besides, the results of the studies make it possible to point to the ability of DDW to increase the potential of the protective systems of the human body, mainly with its preventive consumption at the stage of preparing the living system for the expected stress. Therefore, in clinical practice, DDW usage in the acute period of the development of pathology requires caution in connection with the risk of a synergistic negative effect on the body's defense systems (both from the DDW side and from the pathological process [76,93]). Based on the foregoing, it is possible to recommend that people consume DDW during a period of remission of some chronic diseases, or when preparing the organism for extreme impacts (for example, high sports activities), and using it as a geroprotective nutritional factor of holistic geriatric care in presenile period [89]. The DDW also can be used as synergistic anti-inflammatory agent against sepsis with modulated oxidative stress/antioxidant parameters [120], as adjuvant to conventional anticancer treatment [52,105,111], moreover, DDW drinking is effective against hypoxia of the central nervous system and for the prevention of individuals with depression [83–87].

Also the influence of DDW for nucleic acids is noted, including its ability to increase the intensity of mitochondrial activity and autophagy as well as to alter and miRNA transcriptomic pattern in cells of some tumors [77,121]. Due to this, DDW can be used as adjuvant therapy for cancer treatment.

In its turn the influence of DDW on the molecular dynamics of DNA can be explained by several mechanisms. It is known, that decrease of deuterium concentration in functionally active regions of a DNA molecule may increase the rate of transcription and replication [98]. The latter effect can be caused by the influence of deuterium on the probability of occurrence of open states between complementary pairs of nitrogenous bases, which can significantly change the speed of reading genetic information. In the physiological range, the deuterium atom increases the probability for rupture the bond between the complementary nitrogenous bases by 0.22%–0.60%, which reflects its ability to slow down the reading speed of genetic information in transcription processes, narrowing down the range of regulatory mechanisms for persistent exposure during the cell cycle of the low-intensity adverse factor and leading to a decrease in the adaptive capacity of the cell [65].

At the same time in the case of occurrence of conditions weakening the strength of hydrogen bonds between bases in DNA molecule, the presence of a deuterium atom increases the rate of occurrence of open states, thus increasing the risk of mutations due to the greater availability of nitrogenous bases to the damaging effects of adverse external factors. The latter effect confirms the possibility of increasing the frequency of spontaneous mutations mediated by influence of deuterium atoms on the molecular dynamics of double-stranded DNA, which can play a significant role in the evolution of living organisms. All this is stipulated by the disparity of thermodynamic/kinetic effects associated with substitution of deuterium with protium in the DNA molecule, which indicates the ability of $^2H/^1H$ exchange to regulate the speed of vital processes of biologically active systems (for example, in reading of genetic information). Thus, the probability that living organisms have special mechanisms at different levels of organization that make long-term adaptation to pronounced fluctuations in $^2H/^1H$ ratio in the environment is not excluded [66]. Therefore even if only one protium atom is substituted by deuterium in the DNA molecule and at the same average DNA replication rate, some individual periodic decelerations can occur and accelerations equivalent in this case to the total intensity, although in general they are level with each other, but they are able to change the in-line reading pattern of genetic information which leads to a general accumulation of errors in the reproduction of genetic information, accompanied by a transition of quantitative changes (a number of replication failures) into qualitative defects (mutations) leading to persistent disorders of the genome in living beings, including inherited disorders.

Besides, when DDW is consumed, there is a decrease of HDO molecule content in the hydration shell of nucleic acids and proteins, which is also accompanied by changes in the biological activity of these macromolecules, for example, due to a higher frequency and amplitude of oscillations of atomic groups formed only from light isotopes. These rearrangements of biochemical processes in tissues with high metabolic activity are able to affect the morphofunctional parameters and long-term adaptation of the whole organism.

The considered biological effects that occur when the deuterium content in the organism decreases are important not only for slowing down aging and correcting biochemical disorders in humans in their natural environment, but also offer a perspective in the near future to use DDW during flights in outer space. In addition, it is known that water ice in the polar reservoirs of Mars is enriched in deuterium to at least 7000‰ [122], therefore, in the future it is necessary to study the possibility of correcting the negative effects of such water on living systems with DDW.

Author Contributions: Conceptualization, A.B. and S.D.; methodology, L.F.; software, A.B and L.F.; validation, A.B., L.F. and S.D.; formal analysis, M.B.; investigation, A.B. and S.D.; resources, L.F.; writing—original draft preparation, A.B., L.F. and S.D.; writing—review and editing, A.B., M.B. and S.D.; supervision, S.D.; project administration, M.B.; funding acquisition, L.F.

Funding: This work was supported by the Russian Science Foundation (RSF) project No. 15-16-00008.

Conflicts of Interest: The authors declare no conflict of interest.

References

1. Schmidt, H.L.; Robins, R.J.; Werner, R.A. Multi-factorial in vivo stable isotope fractionation: Causes, correlations, consequences and applications. *Isot. Environ. Health Stud.* **2015**, *51*, 155–199. [CrossRef] [PubMed]
2. Shchepinov, M.S. Reactive Oxygen Species, Isotope Effect, Essential Nutrients, and Enhanced Longevity. *Rejuvenation Res.* **2007**, *10*, 47–60. [CrossRef] [PubMed]

3. Li, X.; Snyder, M.P. Yeast longevity promoted by reversing aging-associated decline in heavy isotope content. *Npj Aging Mech. Dis.* **2016**, *2*, 16004. [CrossRef] [PubMed]
4. Xie, X.; Zubarev, R.A. Isotopic Resonance Hypothesis: Experimental Verification by Escherichia coli Growth Measurements. *Sci. Rep.* **2015**, *5*, 9215. [CrossRef] [PubMed]
5. Syroeshkin, A.; Antipova, N.; Zlatska, A.; Zlatskiy, I.; Skylska, M.; Grebennikova, T.; Goncharuk, V. The effect of the deuterium depleted water on the biological activity of the eukaryotic cells. *J. Trace Elements Med. Biol.* **2018**, *50*, 629–633. [CrossRef] [PubMed]
6. Abilev, S.K.; Smirnova, S.V.; Igonina, E.V.; Parmon, V.N.; Yankovsky, N.K. Deuterium Oxide Enhances Escherichia coli SOS Response Induced by Genotoxicants. *Dokl. Biol. Sci.* **2018**, *480*, 85–89. [CrossRef] [PubMed]
7. Krumbiegel, P. Large deuterium isotope effects and their use: A historical review. *Isot. Environ. Health Stud.* **2011**, *47*, 1–17. [CrossRef] [PubMed]
8. Lobyshev, V.I. Biphasic response of biological objects on variation of low deuterium concentration in water. *Int. J. High Dilution Res.* **2018**, *17*, 12–13.
9. O'Brien, D.M. Stable Isotope Ratios as Biomarkers of Diet for Health Research. *Annu. Rev. Nutr.* **2015**, *35*, 565–594. [CrossRef]
10. Wit, J.; Straaten, C.; Mook, W. Determination of the Absolute Hydrogen Isotopic Ratio of V-SMOW and SLAP. *Geostand. Geoanalytical Res.* **1980**, *4*, 33–36. [CrossRef]
11. Hidenori, G. Origin of Earth's oceans: An assessment of the total amount, history and supply of water. *Geochem. J.* **2016**, *50*, 27–42. [CrossRef]
12. Hut, G. *Consultants' Group Meeting on Stable Isotope Reference Samples for Geochemical and Hydrological Investigations*; IAEA: Vienna, Austria, 1985.
13. Hagemann, R.; Nief, G.; Roth, E. Absolute isotopic scale for deuterium analysis of natural waters. Absolute D/H ratio for SMOW. *Tellus* **1970**, *22*, 712–715. [CrossRef]
14. Risi, C.; Bony, S.; Vimeux, F.; Frankenberg, C.; Noone, D.; Worden, J. Understanding the Sahelian water budget through the isotopic composition of water vapor and precipitation. *J. Geophys. Res. Space Phys.* **2010**, *115*, 24110. [CrossRef]
15. Abderamane, H.; Ketchemen-Tandia, B.; Nlend, B.Y.; Arrakhais, A.B. Hydrogeochemical and isotopic characterization of the groundwater in the Dababa area (Chad). *Afr. J. Environ. Sci. Technol.* **2016**, *10*, 451–466. [CrossRef]
16. Gat, J.R.; Gonfiantini, R. *Stable Isotope Hydrology: Deuterium and Oxygen-18 in the Water Cycle*; International Atomic Energy Agency: Vienna, Austria, 1981; p. 339.
17. Delalande, M.; Bergonzini, L.; Massault, M. Mbaka lakes isotopic (18O and 2H) and water balances: Discussion on the used atmospheric moisture compositions. *Isot. Environ. Health Stud.* **2008**, *44*, 71–82. [CrossRef] [PubMed]
18. Ekaykin, A.A.; Lipenkov, V.Y.; Kozachek, A.V.; Vladimirova, D.O. Stable water isotopic composition of the Antarctic subglacial Lake Vostok: Implications for understanding the lake's hydrology. *Isot. Environ. Health Stud.* **2016**, *52*, 1–9. [CrossRef] [PubMed]
19. Seal, R.R.; Shanks, W.C. Oxygen and hydrogen isotope systematics of Lake Baikal, Siberia: Implications for paleoclimate studies. *Limnol. Oceanogr.* **1998**, *43*, 1251–1261. [CrossRef]
20. Good, S.P.; Noone, D.; Kurita, N.; Benetti, M.; Bowen, G.J. D/H isotope ratios in the global hydrologic cycle. *Geophys. Res. Lett.* **2015**, *42*, 5042–5050. [CrossRef]
21. Bowen, G.J. A Faster Water Cycle. *Science* **2011**, *332*, 430–431. [CrossRef]
22. Craig, H. Isotopic Variations in Meteoric Waters. *Science* **1961**, *133*, 1702–1703. [CrossRef]
23. White, J.W.C. *Stable Hydrogen Isotope Ratios in Plants: A Review of Current Theory and Some Potential Applications*; Springer Science and Business Media LLC: Berlin, Germany, 1989; Volume 68, pp. 142–162.
24. Barbour, M.M. Stable oxygen isotope composition of plant tissue: A review. *Funct. Plant Biol.* **2007**, *34*, 83–94. [CrossRef]
25. Magdas, D.A.; Feher, I.; Dehelean, A.; Cristea, G.; Magdas, T.M.; Puscas, R.; Marincaş, O. Isotopic and elemental markers for geographical origin and organically grown carrots discrimination. *Food Chem.* **2018**, *267*, 231–239. [CrossRef] [PubMed]

26. Bykov, I.M.; Dzhimak, S.S.; Basov, A.A.; Arcybasheva, O.M.; Shashkov, D.; Baryshev, M.G. [Comparative characteristics of the isotopic D/H composition and antioxidant activity of freshly squeezed juices from fruits and vegetables grown in different geographical regions]. *Vopr. Pitan.* **2015**, *84*, 89–96. [PubMed]
27. Magdas, D.A.; Puscas, R. Stable isotopes determination in some Romanian fruit juices. *Isot. Environ. Health Stud.* **2011**, *47*, 372–378. [CrossRef] [PubMed]
28. Kohn, M.J. Predicting animal δ18O: Accounting for diet and physiological adaptation. *Geochim. Cosmochim. Acta* **1996**, *60*, 4811–4829. [CrossRef]
29. Podlesak, D.W.; Bowen, G.J.; O'Grady, S.; Cerling, T.E.; Ehleringer, J.R. δ2H and δ18O of human body water: A GIS model to distinguish residents from non-residents in the contiguous USA. *Isot. Environ. Health Stud.* **2012**, *48*, 259–279. [CrossRef]
30. Podlesak, D.W.; Torregrossa, A.M.; Ehleringer, J.R.; Dearing, M.D.; Passey, B.H.; Cerling, T.E. Turnover of oxygen and hydrogen isotopes in the body water, CO2, hair, and enamel of a small mammal. *Geochim. Cosmochim. Acta* **2008**, *72*, 19–35. [CrossRef]
31. Li, H.; Yu, C.; Wang, F.; Chang, S.J.; Yao, J.; Blake, R.E. Probing the metabolic water contribution to intracellular water using oxygen isotope ratios of PO4. *Proc. Natl. Acad. Sci. USA* **2016**, *113*, 5862–5867. [CrossRef]
32. Kreuzer-Martin, H.W.; Ehleringer, J.R.; Hegg, E.L. Oxygen isotopes indicate most intracellular water in log-phase Escherichia coli is derived from metabolism. *Proc. Natl. Acad. Sci. USA* **2005**, *102*, 17337–17341. [CrossRef]
33. Kreuzer-Martin, H.W.; Lott, M.J.; Ehleringer, J.R.; Hegg, E.L. Metabolic Processes Account for the Majority of the Intracellular Water in Log-Phase *Escherichia coli* Cells As Revealed by Hydrogen Isotopes. *Biochemistry* **2006**, *45*, 13622–13630. [CrossRef]
34. Wanders, R.J.A.; Waterham, H.R.; Ferdinandusse, S. Metabolic interplay between peroxisomes and other subcellular organelles including mitochondria and the endoplasmic reticulum. *Front. Cell Dev. Biol.* **2015**, *3*, 83. [CrossRef] [PubMed]
35. Schrader, M.; Fahimi, H.D. Peroxisomes and oxidative stress. *Biochim. Biophys. Acta* **2006**, *1763*, 1755–1766. [CrossRef] [PubMed]
36. Tanz, N.K.; Rossmann, A.; Schmidt, H.-L. Potentials and caveats with oxygen and sulfur stable isotope analyses in authenticity and origin checks of food and food commodities. *Food Control* **2015**, *48*, 143–150.
37. Yoshida, N.; Mizutani, Y. Preparation of carbon dioxide for oxygen-18 determination of water by use of a plastic syringe. *Anal. Chem.* **1986**, *58*, 1273–1275. [CrossRef]
38. Horita, J.; Ueda, A.; Mizukami, K.; Takatori, I. Automatic δD and δ18O analyses of multi-water samples using H2- and CO2-water equilibration methods with a common equilibration set-up. *Int. J. Radiat. Appl. Instrum. Part A. Appl. Radiat. Isot.* **1989**, *40*, 801–805. [CrossRef]
39. Schmidt, H.L.; Werner, R.A.; Roßmann, A. 18O Pattern and biosynthesis of natural plant products. *Phytochemistry* **2001**, *58*, 9–32. [CrossRef]
40. Estep, M.L.F.; Hoering, T.C. *The Stability of Organically Bonded Hydrogen Atoms in Microalgae Toward Isotopic Exchange with Water*; Carnegie Institution of Washington Year Book: Washington, DC, USA, 1979; pp. 652–655.
41. Kuribayashi, T.; Sugawara, M.; Sato, K.; Nabekura, Y.; Aoki, T.; Kano, N.; Joh, T.; Kaneoke, M. Stable Isotope Analysis of Hydrogen and Oxygen in a Traditional Japanese Alcoholic Beverage, Sake, from Niigata Prefecture in Japan and Other Countries. *Anal. Sci.* **2017**, *33*, 979–982. [CrossRef]
42. Mant, M.; Nagel, A.; Prowse, T. Investigating Residential History Using Stable Hydrogen and Oxygen Isotopes of Human Hair and Drinking Water. *J. Forensic Sci.* **2016**, *61*, 884–891. [CrossRef]
43. O'Grady, S.P.; Wende, A.R.; Remien, C.H.; Valenzuela, L.O.; Enright, L.E.; Chesson, L.A.; Abel, E.D.; Cerling, T.E.; Ehleringer, J.R. Aberrant Water Homeostasis Detected by Stable Isotope Analysis. *PLoS ONE* **2010**, *5*, e11699. [CrossRef]
44. Bowen, G.J.; Winter, D.A.; Spero, H.J.; Zierenberg, R.A.; Reeder, M.D.; Cerling, T.E.; Ehleringer, J.R. Stable hydrogen and oxygen isotope ratios of bottled waters of the world. *Rapid Commun. Mass Spectrom.* **2005**, *19*, 3442–3450. [CrossRef]
45. Dzhimak, S.S.; Basov, A.A.; Kopytov, G.F.; Kashaev, D.V.; Sokolov, M.E.; Artsybasheva, O.M.; Sharapov, K.S.; Baryshev, M.G. Application of NMR Spectroscopy to the Determination of Low Concentrations of Nonradioactive Isotopes in Liquid Media. *Russ. Phys. J.* **2015**, *58*, 923–929. [CrossRef]
46. Al-Basheer, W.; Al-Jalal, A.A.; Gasmi, K. Isotopic composition of bottled water in Saudi Arabia. *Isot. Environ. Health Stud.* **2017**, *54*, 1–7. [CrossRef] [PubMed]

47. Aleksandrov, R.A.; Laguntsov, N.I.; Kurchatov, I.M.; Sarychev, G.A.; Nechaev, I.A. Water Supply System with Light-Water Production Based on a Nuclear Desalination Complex. *At. Energy* **2018**, *124*, 398–402. [CrossRef]
48. Smirnov, A.Y.; Sulaberidze, A.G. Production of Water with Reduced Content of Deuterium for Water Supply System with Desalination Installation. *J. Physics: Conf. Ser.* **2018**, *1099*, 012035. [CrossRef]
49. Belkin, D.Y.; Selivanenko, I.L.; Rastunova, I.L.; Magomedbekov, E.P. Characteristics of the mass transfer of structured rolled ribbon-screw packings in isotope exchange columns during vacuum water distillation. *Theor. Found. Chem. Eng.* **2016**, *50*, 398–403.
50. Petriev, I.S.; Frolov, V.Y.; Bolotin, S.N.; Baryshev, M.G.; Kopytov, G.F. Kinetic Characteristics of Hydrogen Transfer Through Palladium-Modified Membrane. *Russ. Phys. J.* **2018**, *60*, 1611–1617. [CrossRef]
51. Yeh, H.M. Recovery of deuterium from water-isotopes in thermal diffusion columns connected in series. *Prog. Nucl. Energy* **2010**, *52*, 516–522. [CrossRef]
52. Gyöngyi, Z.; Budán, F.; Szabó, I.; Ember, I.; Kiss, I.; Krempels, K.; Somlyai, I.; Somlyai, G. Deuterium Depleted Water Effects on Survival of Lung Cancer Patients and Expression of Kras, Bcl2, and Myc Genes in Mouse Lung. *Nutr. Cancer* **2013**, *65*, 240–246. [CrossRef]
53. Avila, D.S.; Somlyai, G.; Somlyai, I.; Aschner, M. Anti-aging effects of deuterium depletion on Mn-induced toxicity in a C. elegans model. *Toxicol. Lett.* **2012**, *211*, 319–324. [CrossRef]
54. Olariu, L.; Petcu, M.; Tulcan, C.; Chis-Buiga, I.; Pup, M.; Florin, M.; Brudiu, I. *Deuterium Depleted Water–Antioxidant or Prooxidant*; Lucrari Stiintifice Medicina Veterinara: Timisoara, Romania, 2007.
55. Rehakova, R.; Klimentova, J.; Cebova, M.; Barta, A.; Matuskova, Z.; Labas, P.; Pechanova, O. Effect of deuterium-depleted water on selected cardiometabolic parameters in fructose-treated rats. *Physiol. Res.* **2016**, *65*, S401–S407.
56. Boros, L.G.; D'Agostino, D.P.; Katz, H.E.; Roth, J.P.; Meuillet, E.J.; Somlyai, G. Submolecular regulation of cell transformation by deuterium depleting water exchange reactions in the tricarboxylic acid substrate cycle. *Med. Hypotheses* **2016**, *87*, 69–74. [CrossRef] [PubMed]
57. Fisher-Wellman, K.H.; Lin, C.-T.; Ryan, T.E.; Reese, L.R.; Gilliam, L.A.A.; Cathey, B.L.; Lark, D.S.; Smith, C.D.; Muoio, D.M.; Neufer, P.D. Pyruvate dehydrogenase complex and nicotinamide nucleotide transhydrogenase constitute an energy consuming redox circuit. *Biochem. J.* **2015**, *467*, 271–280. [CrossRef] [PubMed]
58. Boros, L.; Lee, P.; Brandes, J.; Cascante, M.; Muscarella, P.; Schirmer, W.; Melvin, W.; Ellison, E. Nonoxidative pentose phosphate pathways and their direct role in ribose synthesis in tumors: Is cancer a disease of cellular glucose metabolism? *Med. Hypotheses* **1998**, *50*, 55–59. [CrossRef]
59. Billault, I.; Guiet, S.; Mabon, F.; Robins, R. Natural Deuterium Distribution in Long-Chain Fatty Acids Is Nonstatistical: A Site-Specific Study by Quantitative 2H NMR Spectroscopy. *Chem. Bio. Chem.* **2001**, *2*, 425–431. [CrossRef]
60. Boros, L.G.; Lee, W.N.P.; Cascante, M. Imatinib and Chronic-Phase Leukemias. *N. Engl. J. Med.* **2002**, *347*, 67–68. [CrossRef] [PubMed]
61. Somlyai, G.; Jancsó, G.; Jákli, G.; Vass, K.; Barna, B.; Lakics, V.; Gaál, T. Naturally occurring deuterium is essential for the normal growth rate of cells. *FEBS Lett.* **1993**, *317*, 1–4. [CrossRef]
62. Luo, A.L.; Zheng, Y.L.; Cong, F.S. Research progress of biological effects of deuterium-depleted water. *J. Shanghai Jiaotong Univ. (Med. Sci.)* **2018**, *38*, 467–471.
63. Syroeshkin, A.; Pleteneva, T.; Uspenskaya, E.; Zlatskiy, I.; Antipova, N.; Grebennikova, T.; Levitskaya, O. D/H control of chemical kinetics in water solutions under low deuterium concentrations. *Chem. Eng. J.* **2018**. [CrossRef]
64. Pedersen, L.G.; Bartolotti, L.; Li, L. Deuterium and its role in the machinery of evolution. *J. Theor. Biol.* **2006**, *238*, 914–918. [CrossRef]
65. Dzhimak, S.S.; Svidlov, A.A.; Basov, A.A.; Baryshev, M.G.; Drobotenko, M.I. The Effect of Single Deuterium Substitutions for Protium in a DNA Molecule on the Occurrence of Open States. *Biophysics* **2018**, *63*, 497–500. [CrossRef]
66. Dzhimak, S.S.; Drobotenko, M.I.; Basov, A.A.; Svidlov, A.A.; Fedulova, L.V.; Lyasota, O.M.; Baryshev, M.G. Mathematical Modeling of Open States in DNA Molecule Depending on the Deuterium Concentration in the Surrounding Liquid Media at Different Values of Hydrogen Bond Disruption Energy. *Dokl. Biochem. Biophys.* **2018**, *483*, 359–362. [CrossRef] [PubMed]

67. Fedulova, L.V.; Vasilevskaya, E.R.; Kotenkova, E.A.; Elkina, A.A.; Baryshev, M.G.; Lisitsyn, A.B. Influence of Different Polypeptides Fractions Derived from Sus Scrofa Immune Organs on the Rats Immunological Reactivity. *J. Pharm. Nutr. Sci.* **2017**, *7*, 35–40.
68. Vasilevskaya, E.R.; Akhremko, A.G. Proteomic study of pig's spleen. *Potravin. Slovak J. Food Sci.* **2019**, *13*, 314–317. [CrossRef]
69. Fedulova, L.; Elkina, A.; Vasilevskaya, E.; Barysheva, E. Identification of tissue-specific proteins of immunocompetent organs of Sus scrofa isolated in deuterium depleted medium. *Med. Sci.* **2018**, *22*, 509–513.
70. Sternberg, L.S.L.O. Oxygen stable isotope ratios of tree-ring cellulose: The next phase of understanding. *New Phytol.* **2009**, *181*, 553–562. [CrossRef]
71. Sternberg, L.S.L.; Vendramini Ellsworth, P.F. Divergent biochemical fractionation, not convergent temperature, explains cellulose oxygen isotope enrichment across latitudes. *PLoS ONE* **2011**, *6*, e28040. [CrossRef]
72. Waterhouse, J.S.; Cheng, S.; Juchelka, D.; Loader, N.J.; McCarroll, D.; Switsur, V.R.; Gautam, L. Position-specific measure-ment of oxygen isotope ratios in cellulose: Isotopic exchange during heterotrophic cellulose synthesis. *Geochim. Cosmochim. Acta* **2013**, *112*, 178–191. [CrossRef]
73. Zlatska, O.V.; Zubov, D.O.; Vasyliev, R.G.; Syroeshkin, A.V.; Zlatskiy, I.A.; Regeneration, M.C.I.B.L.I. Deuterium Effect on Proliferation and Clonogenic Potential of Human Dermal Fibroblasts In Vitro. *Probl. Cryobiol. Cryomedicine* **2018**, *28*, 049–053. [CrossRef]
74. Zlatska, A.; Gordiienko, I.; Vasyliev, R.; Zubov, D.; Gubar, O.; Rodnichenko, A.; Syroeshkin, A.; Zlatskiy, I. In Vitro Study of Deuterium Effect on Biological Properties of Human Cultured Adipose-Derived Stem Cells. *Sci. World J.* **2018**, *2018*, 1–10. [CrossRef]
75. Zlatskiy, I.A.; Zlatska, A.V.; Antipova, N.V.; Syroeshkin, A.V. Effect of deuterium on the morpho-functional characteristics of normal and cancer cells in vitro. *Trace Elem. Electrolytes* **2018**, *35*, 211–214. [CrossRef]
76. Dzhimak, S.S.; Basov, A.A.; Fedulova, L.V.; Didikin, A.S.; Bikov, I.M.; Arcybasheva, O.M.; Naumov, G.N.; Baryshev, M.G.; Fedulova, L. Correction of metabolic processes in rats during chronic endotoxicosis using isotope (D/H) exchange reactions. *Biol. Bull.* **2015**, *42*, 440–448. [CrossRef]
77. Chira, S.; Raduly, L.; Braicu, C.; Jurj, A.; Cojocneanu-Petric, R.; Pop, L.; Pileczki, V.; Ionescu, C.; Berindan-Neagoe, I. Premature senescence activation in DLD-1 colorectal cancer cells through adjuvant therapy to induce a miRNA profile modulating cellular death. *Exp. Ther. Med.* **2018**, *16*, 1241–1249. [CrossRef] [PubMed]
78. Basov, A.A.; Elkina, A.A.; Samkov, A.A.; Volchenko, N.N.; Moiseev, A.V.; Fedulova, L.V.; Baryshev, M.G.; Dzhimak, S.S. Influence of deuterium depleted water on the isotope D/H composition of liver tissue and morphological development of rats at different periods of ontogenesis. *Iran. Biomed. J.* **2019**, *23*, 129–141. [CrossRef]
79. Pomytkin, I.A.; Kolesova, O.E. Relationship between natural concentration of heavy water isotopologs and rate of H2O2 generation by mitochondria. *Bull. Exp. Biol. Med.* **2006**, *142*, 570–572. [CrossRef] [PubMed]
80. Wang, H.; Zhu, B.; He, Z.; Fu, H.; Dai, Z.; Huang, G.; Li, B.; Qin, D.; Zhang, X.; Tian, L.; et al. Deuterium-depleted water (DDW) inhibits the proliferation and migration of nasopharyngeal carcinoma cells in vitro. *Biomed. Pharmacother.* **2013**, *67*, 489–496. [CrossRef] [PubMed]
81. Tănase, C.; Boz, I.; Popa, V.I. Histo-anatomical aspects in maize (Zea mays l.) seedlings developing under influence of deuterium depleted water. Analele Ştiinţifice ale Universităţii „Al. I. Cuza" Iaşi, s. II a. *Biol. Veg.* **2014**, *60*, 5–10.
82. Petruş-Vancea, A. Cell ultrastructure and chlorophyll pigments in hyperhydric and non-hyperhydric Beta vulgaris var. Conditiva plantlets, treated with deuterium depleted water. *Plant Cell Tissue Organ Cult. (PCTOC)* **2018**, *135*, 13–21. [CrossRef]
83. Strekalova, T.; Evans, M.; Chernopiatko, A.; Couch, Y.; Costa-Nunes, J.P.; Cespuglio, R.; Chesson, L.; Vignisse, J.; Steinbusch, H.W.; Anthony, D.C.; et al. Deuterium content of water increases depression susceptibility: The potential role of a serotonin-related mechanism. *Behav. Brain Res.* **2015**, *277*, 237–244. [CrossRef]
84. Mladin, C.; Ciobica, A.; Lefter, R.; Popescu, A.; Bild, W. Deuterium depletion induces anxiolytic-like effects in rats. *Arch. Biol. Sci.* **2014**, *66*, 947–953. [CrossRef]
85. Mladin, C.; Ciobica, A.; Lefter, R.; Popescu, A.; Bild, W. Deuterium-depleted water has stimulating effects on long-term memory in rats. *Neurosci. Lett.* **2014**, *583*, 154–158. [CrossRef]

86. Kravtsov, A.A.; Kozin, S.V.; Vasilevskaya, E.R.; Elkina, A.A.; Fedulova, L.V.; Popov, K.A.; Malyshko, V.V.; Moiseev, A.V.; Shashkov, D.I.; Baryshev, M.G.; et al. Effect of Drinking Ration with Reduced Deuterium Content on Brain Tissue Prooxidant-Antioxidant Balance in Rats with Acute Hypoxia Model. *J. Pharm. Nutr. Sci.* **2018**, *8*, 42–51. [CrossRef]
87. Kozin, S.V.; Kravtsov, A.A.; Elkina, A.A.; Zlishcheva, E.I.; Barysheva, E.V.; Shurygina, L.V.; Moiseev, A.V.; Baryshev, M.G. Isotope Exchange of Deuterium for Protium in Rat Brain Tissues Changes Brain Tolerance to Hypoxia. *Biophysics* **2019**, *64*, 272–278. [CrossRef]
88. Dzhimak, S.S.; Fedulova, L.V.; Moiseev, A.V.; Basov, A.A. Change of 2H/1H ratio and adaptive potential in living systems under formation of isotope gradient. *J. Pharm. Nutr. Sci.* **2019**, *9*, 8–13.
89. Dzhimak, S.S.; Shikhliarova, A.I.; Zhukova, G.V.; Basov, A.A.; Kit, O.I.; Fedulova, L.V.; Kurkina, T.A.; Shirnina, E.A.; Protasova, T.P.; Baryshev, M.G.; et al. Some Systemic Effects of Deuterium Depleted Water on Presenile Female Rats. *Jundishapur J. Nat. Pharm. Prod.* **2018**, *13*, 83494. [CrossRef]
90. Dzhimak, S.S.; Basov, A.A.; Baryshev, M.G.; Dzhimak, S. Content of deuterium in biological fluids and organs: Influence of deuterium depleted water on D/H gradient and the process of adaptation. *Dokl. Biochem. Biophys.* **2015**, *465*, 370–373. [CrossRef]
91. Dzhimak, S.S.; Basov, A.A.; Fedulova, L.V.; Bykov, I.M.; Ivlev, V.A.; Melkonyan, K.I.; Timakov, A.A. Determination of deuterium concentration in biological liquids with the use of NMR-spectroscopy. *Aviakosmicheskaya Ekol. Meditsina (Russia)* **2016**, *50*, 42–47.
92. Sinyak, Y.E.; Grigoriev, A.I.; Skuratov, V.M.; Ivanova, S.M.; Pokrovsky, B.G. Fractionation of hydrogen stable isotopes in the human body. *Aviakosmicheskaya Ekol. Meditsina* **2006**, *40*, 38–41.
93. Dzhimak, S.S.; Basov, A.A.; Elkina, A.A.; Fedulova, L.V.; Kotenkova, E.A.; Vasilevskaya, E.R.; Lyasota, O.M.; Baryshev, M.G. Influence of deuterium-depleted water on hepatorenal toxicity. *Jundishapur J. Nat. Pharm. Prod.* **2018**, *13*, e69557. [CrossRef]
94. Abrosimova, A.N.; Rakov, D.V.; Siniak, E.I. [The "light" water effect on lenticular opacity development in mice after repeated low dose gamma-irradiation]. *Aerosp. Environ. Med.* **2009**, *43*, 29–32.
95. Rakov, D.V. [Alleviation of gamma-radiation damage by water with reduced deuterium and 18O content]. *Aerosp. Environ. Med.* **2007**, *41*, 36–39.
96. Editoiu, C.; Popescu, C.; Ispas, G.; Corneanu, G.C.; Zagnat, M.; Stefanescu, I. The effect of biologically active substances of Aralia Mandshurica and deuterium depleted water on the structure of spleen in Mus Muscullus. *Ann. RSCB* **2010**, *15*, 2012–2016.
97. Kulikova, E.I.; Kryuchkova, D.M.; Severyukhin, Y.S.; Gaevsky, V.N.; Ivanov, A.A. Radiomodifying properties of deuterium-depleted water with poor content of heavier isotopes of oxygen. *Aviakosmicheskaya Ekol. Meditsina* **2012**, *46*, 45–50.
98. Sinyak, Y.; Grigoriev, A.; Gaydadimov, V.; Gurieva, T.; Levinskih, M.; Pokrovskii, B. Deuterium-free water (1H2O) in complex life-support systems of long-term space missions. *Acta Astronaut.* **2003**, *52*, 575–580. [CrossRef]
99. Sinyak, Y.E.; Skuratov, V.M.; Gaidadymov, V.B.; Pokrovsky, B.G.; Grigoriev, A.I. Investigation into fractionating of hydrogen and oxygen stable isotopes aboard the international space station. *Aviakosmicheskaya Ekol. Meditsina* **2005**, *39*, 43–47.
100. Kotyk, A.; Dvořáková, M.; Koryta, J. Deuterons cannot replace protons in active transport processes in yeast. *FEBS Lett.* **1990**, *264*, 203–205. [CrossRef]
101. Hagag, N.; Lacal, J.C.; Graber, M.; Aaronson, S.; Viola, M.V. Microinjection of ras p21 induces a rapid rise in intracellular pH. *Mol. Cell. Biol.* **1987**, *7*, 1984–1988. [CrossRef] [PubMed]
102. Doppler, W.; Jaggi, R.; Groner, B. Induction of v-mos and activated Ha-ras oncogene expression in quiescent NIH 3T3 cells causes intracellular alkalinisation and cell-cycle progression. *Gene* **1987**, *54*, 147–153. [CrossRef]
103. Mooienaar, W.H. Ingezonden. *Annu. Rev. Physiol.* **1986**, *48*, 363–376. [CrossRef]
104. Wang, H.; Zhu, B.; Liu, C.; Fang, W.; Yang, H. [Deuterium-depleted water selectively inhibits nasopharyngeal carcinoma cell proliferation in vitro]. *Nan fang yi ke da xue xue bao = J. South. Med. Univ.* **2012**, *32*, 1394–1399.
105. Yavari, K.; Kooshesh, L. Deuterium Depleted Water Inhibits the Proliferation of Human MCF7 Breast Cancer Cell Lines by Inducing Cell Cycle Arrest. *Nutr. Cancer* **2019**, *71*, 1019–1029. [CrossRef]
106. Pop, A.; Balint, E.; Manolescu, N.; Stefanescu, I.; Militaru, M. The effect of deuterium depleted water administration on serum glycoproteins of cytostatics treated rats. *Roum. Biotechnol. Lett.* **2008**, *13*, 74–77.

107. Gyöngyi, Z.; Somlyai, G. Deuterium depletion can decrease the expression of C-myc Ha-ras and p53 gene in carcinogen-treated mice. *Vivo* **2000**, *14*, 437–439.
108. Soleyman-Jahi, S.; Zendehdel, K.; Akbarzadeh, K.; Haddadi, M.; Amanpour, S.; Muhammadnejad, S. In vitro assessment of antineoplastic effects of deuterium depleted water. *Asian Pac. J. Cancer Prev.* **2014**, *15*, 2179–2183. [CrossRef] [PubMed]
109. Perona, R.; Serrano, R. Increased pH and tumorigenicity of fibroblasts expressing a yeast proton pump. *Nature* **1988**, *334*, 438–440. [CrossRef] [PubMed]
110. Cong, F.S.; Zhang, Y.R.; Sheng, H.C.; Ao, Z.H.; Zhang, S.Y.; Wang, J.Y. Deuterium-depleted water inhibits human lung carcinoma cell growth by apoptosis. *Exp. Ther. Med.* **2010**, *1*, 277–283. [CrossRef] [PubMed]
111. Krempels, K.; Somlyai, I.; Somlyai, G.; Somlyai, I.; Somlyai, G. A Retrospective Evaluation of the Effects of Deuterium Depleted Water Consumption on 4 Patients with Brain Metastases from Lung Cancer. *Integr. Cancer Ther.* **2008**, *7*, 172–181. [CrossRef] [PubMed]
112. Kovács, A.; Guller, I.; Krempels, K.; Somlyai, I.; Jánosi, I.; Gyöngyi, Z.; Szabó, I.; Ember, I.; Somlyai, G. Deuterium Depletion May Delay the Progression of Prostate Cancer. *J. Cancer Ther.* **2011**, *2*, 548–556. [CrossRef]
113. Boros, L.G.; Collins, T.Q.; Somlyai, G. What to eat or what not to eat—that is still the question. *Neuro Oncol.* **2017**, *19*, 595–596. [CrossRef] [PubMed]
114. Rieger, J.; Steinbach, J.P. To diet or not to diet—That is still the question. *Neuro Oncol.* **2016**, *18*, 1035–1036. [CrossRef]
115. De Feyter, H.M.; Behar, K.L.; Rao, J.U.; Madden-Hennessey, K.; Ip, K.L.; Hyder, F.; Drewes, L.R.; Geschwind, J.F.; De Graaf, R.A.; Rothman, D.L. A ketogenic diet increases transport and oxidation of ketone bodies in RG2 and 9L gliomas without affecting tumor growth. *Neuro Oncol.* **2016**, *18*, 1079–1087. [CrossRef]
116. Fransen, M.; Lismont, C.; Walton, P. The Peroxisome-Mitochondria Connection: How and Why? *Int. J. Mol. Sci.* **2017**, *18*, 1126. [CrossRef] [PubMed]
117. Kotkina, I.T.; Titov, V.N.; Parkhimovich, R.M. The different notions about beta-oxidation of fatty acids in peroxisomes, peroxisomes and ketonic bodies. The diabetic, acidotic coma as an acute deficiency of acetyl-CoA and ATP. *Klin. Lab. Diagn.* **2014**, *3*, 14–23.
118. Zubarev, R.A. Role of Stable Isotopes in Life—Testing Isotopic Resonance Hypothesis. *Genom. Proteom. Bioinform.* **2011**, *9*, 15–20. [CrossRef]
119. Benton, C.R.; Holloway, G.P.; Campbell, S.E.; Yoshida, Y.; Tandon, N.N.; Glatz, J.F.; Luiken, J.J.; Spriet, L.L.; Bonen, A. Rosiglitazone increases fatty acid oxidation and fatty acid translocase (FAT/CD36) but not carnitine palmitoyltransferase I in rat muscle mitochondria. *J. Physiol.* **2008**, *586*, 1755–1766. [CrossRef] [PubMed]
120. Rasooli, A.; Fatemi, F.; Hajihosseini, R.; Vaziri, A.; Akbarzadeh, K.; Malayeri, M.R.M.; Dini, S.; Foroutanrad, M. Synergistic effects of deuterium depleted water and Mentha longifolia L. essential oils on sepsis-induced liver injuries through regulation of cyclooxygenase-2. *Pharm. Biol.* **2019**, *57*, 125–132. [CrossRef] [PubMed]
121. Lajos, R.; Braicu, C.; Jurj, A.; Chira, S.; Cojocneanu-Petric, R.; Pileczki, V.; Berindan-Neagoe, I. A miRNAs profile evolution of triple negative breast cancer cells in the presence of a possible adjuvant therapy and senescence inducer. *J. BUON* **2018**, *23*, 692–705.
122. Villanueva, G.L.; Mumma, M.; Novak, R.E.; Käufl, H.U.; Hartogh, P.; Encrenaz, T.; Tokunaga, A.; Khayat, A.; Smith, M.D. Strong water isotopic anomalies in the martian atmosphere: Probing current and ancient reservoirs. *Science* **2015**, *348*, 218–221. [CrossRef]

 © 2019 by the authors. Licensee MDPI, Basel, Switzerland. This article is an open access article distributed under the terms and conditions of the Creative Commons Attribution (CC BY) license (http://creativecommons.org/licenses/by/4.0/).

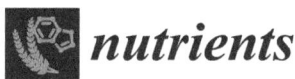

Article

High Hydration Factor in Older Hispanic-American Adults: Possible Implications for Accurate Body Composition Estimates

Rogelio González-Arellanes [1], Rene Urquidez-Romero [2], Alejandra Rodríguez-Tadeo [2], Julián Esparza-Romero [1], Rosa-Olivia Méndez-Estrada [1], Erik Ramírez-López [3], Alma-Elizabeth Robles-Sardin [1], Bertha-Isabel Pacheco-Moreno [1] and Heliodoro Alemán-Mateo [1,*]

[1] Centro de Investigación en Alimentación y Desarrollo, A.C. Coordinación de Nutrición. Carretera Gustavo Enrique Astiazarán Rosas #46, Col. La Victoria C.P. 83304, Hermosillo, Sonora, Mexico; rogelio.gonzalez@estudiantes.ciad.mx (R.G.-A.); julian@ciad.mx (J.E.-R.); romendez@ciad.mx (R.-O.M.-E.); melina@ciad.mx (A.-E.R.-S.); berthai@ciad.mx (B.-I.P.-M.)

[2] Universidad Autónoma de Ciudad Juárez. Instituto de Ciencias Biomédicas. Departamento de Ciencias de la Salud. Ave. Plutarco Elías Calles #1210, Col. Fovissste Chamizal C.P. 32310, Ciudad Juárez, Chihuahua, Mexico; rurquide@uacj.mx (R.U.-R.); alrodrig@uacj.mx (A.R.-T.)

[3] Universidad Autónoma de Nuevo León. Facultad de Salud Pública y Nutrición. Ave. Dr. Eduardo Aguirre Pequeño #905, Col. Mitras Centro C.P. 64460, Monterrey, Nuevo León, Mexico; erik.ramirezl@uanl.mx

* Correspondence: helio@ciad.mx; Tel./Fax: +52-(662)-280-0094

Received: 26 September 2019; Accepted: 12 November 2019; Published: 29 November 2019

Abstract: Age- and obesity-related body composition changes could influence the hydration factor (HF) and, as a result, body composition estimates derived from hydrometry. The aim of the present study was to compare the HF in older Hispanic-American adults to some published values. This cross-sectional study included a sample of 412 subjects, men and women, aged ≥60 years from northern Mexico. HF values were calculated based on the ratio of total body water-using the deuterium dilution technique-to fat-free mass, derived from the four-compartment model. The mean HF value for the total sample (0.748 ± 0.034) was statistically ($p \leq 0.01$) higher than the traditionally assumed value of 0.732 derived from chemical analysis, the "grand mean" value of 0.725 derived from in vivo methods, and the 0.734 value calculated for older French adults via the three-compartment model. The HF of the older women did not differ across the fat mass index categories, but in men the obese group was lower than the normal and excess fat groups. The hydration factor calculated for the total sample of older Hispanic-American people is higher than the HF values reported in the literature. Therefore, the indiscriminate use of these assumed values could produce inaccurate body composition estimates in older Hispanic-American people.

Keywords: aging; body composition; obesity; hydration factor and Hispanic Americans

1. Introduction

The demographic and epidemiological transition represents a huge challenge for governments and health and aging institutions worldwide, especially the double burden of malnutrition in several age groups, including older people [1,2]. Appropriate nutritional assessments of older people are necessary to improve medical and nutritional management and to design appropriate interventions. In this regard, accurate tools for assessing body composition in older people are key. Following Penchard and Azcue [3], fat-free mass (FFM) and fat mass (FM) are the most appropriate parameters for defining malnutrition. The most common methods used to assess body composition include such two-compartment (2C) models as hydrometry, among others. Specifically, this method calculates

FFM in kilograms (kg) based on the ratio of total body water (TBW) to the hydration factor value [4]. Subsequently, FM can be estimated by the difference in body weight, measured in kg, and FFM, also measured in kg. The hydration factor (HF) is the ratio of TBW in kg to FFM solids in kg, and its magnitude, according to chemical analyses, is around of 0.730 [4]. That HF value was obtained from ten human cadavers (seven males, three females) aged 25–67 years. The HF ranges in non-oedematous and oedematous corpses were 0.686–0.776 and 0.808–0.824, respectively [5–10]. New HF values obtained with two and three-compartment models have been reported. Ritz et al. [11] estimated a "grand mean" hydration factor of 0.725, compiled from data in several studies based on in vivo methods. Those researchers also found that the HF is similar between young ($n = 35$, 0.732 ± 0.024) and older subjects ($n = 68$, 0.734 ± 0.024).

In the field of body composition, a HF of 0.732 is generally accepted as a constant throughout the life-cycle, regardless of factors such as training level, obesity, age, gender, and ethnicity [12–14]. Regarding age, older subjects (60–69 years) had lower mean TBW values (35.4 liters) at the molecular level than adults (20–29 years; 39.1 liters) [15]; however, it seems that the HF estimated by in vivo methods is not affected by aging [11,16]. Obese subjects, meanwhile, could have a different HF than non-obese subjects, regardless of age and gender. Fuller et al. [17] found a low HF of 0.712 ± 0.016 with a range of 0.682–0.751 in obese adult women, whereas Das [18] found a high HF (0.756) in extremely obese men and women subjects, and Haroun et al. [19] reported a higher HF in obese children (0.763) than the mean value for non-obese children (0.737). Ritz et al. [20] reported a lower HF in obese adult women (0.733 ± 0.023) than in lean adult women (0.747 ± 0.022), although the HF was significantly higher (0.768 ± 0.012) in obese than lean adult men (0.740 ± 0.019). These results show that the behavior of the HF in conditions of obesity is not yet clear, and that our knowledge of aged and obese people in this regard is insufficient. If HF differs from the assumed value of 0.732 due to factors such as age, obesity, and ethnicity, then estimates of body composition may be affected and may lead to erroneous associations and misclassifications of people's nutritional status.

All the studies cited above [17–20] used the body mass index (BMI) to diagnose obesity, but this parameter is an unspecific marker of adiposity and, therefore, inaccurate for diagnosing obesity [21]. The fat mass index (FMI), in contrast, is a gender-specific measure of fat that is not confounded by lean tissue. Hence, it is one of the most accurate approaches available for diagnosing obesity [22]. In summary, the HF in obese older adults is still unknown. Therefore, the aims of the present study were to determine the HF in older Hispanic-American adults, and then compare it to some published values. Differences in the HF between obese and non-obese older Hispanic-American adults were also explored.

2. Materials and Methods

2.1. Subjects

This study included a sample of community-dwelling older (≥60 years) Hispanic-American adults from northern Mexico with stable body weight-by self-report-in the 3 months prior to the study. All subjects were apparently healthy and physically-independent according to Lawton and Brody's scale [23]. None were involved in sports activities. According to clinical assessment, all volunteers were free of severe oedema, medication, diseases, and metabolic disorders, such as cancer, diabetes, heart disease, and kidney or liver failure, that could have affected their hydration status and body composition. Subjects with well-controlled hypothyroidism and hypertension were included. All participants underwent an oral glucose tolerance test to confirm that they were free of type-2 diabetes and their specific gravity urine and haematocrit values indicated a good hydration status.

2.2. Design

A cross-sectional design was implemented. All volunteers were recruited from 2016–2019 in Hermosillo, Sonora; Ciudad Juárez, Chihuahua; and Monterrey, Nuevo León. The study protocol included two visits to the Body Composition Laboratories by all test subjects. During the first visit, potential volunteers underwent clinical and lab assessment to apply the inclusion and exclusion criteria. On the second, all the volunteers who met the inclusion criteria underwent anthropometric and body composition measurements. The study protocol was approved by the Ethics Committee of the Centro de Investigación en Alimentación y Desarrollo, AC (CE/008/2014), the Universidad Autónoma de Ciudad Juárez (CBE.ICB/023.10–14), and the Universidad Autónoma de Nuevo León (15-FaSPyN-SA-19). Volunteers received a full explanation of the protocol and signed the appropriate informed consent.

2.3. Anthropometry

All anthropometric variables were measured using a standard methodology [24]. Weight in kg was measured to the nearest 0.1 kg using an electronic scale (SECA 878, Germany, with the scale attached to the Bod-Pod System). Height in meters (m) was measured to the nearest 0.1 centimeter (cm) using a stadiometer (SECA 264, Germany). BMI was obtained from the weight in kg (SECA scale) divided by height-squared in m.

2.4. Body Composition and HF Measurements

In order to calculate the HF, fat-free mass was derived from the four-compartment (4C) model, which requires the following three independent measurements:

(1) Total body water. This is the major component of FFM. It was measured using deuterium oxide (D_2O, 99.8 atom percent, Lot. No. 14G-316, Cambridge Isotope Laboratories, Inc., USA) by two protocols. In one laboratory, D_2O was first measured by isotope ratio mass spectrometry (IRMS), though this was later replaced by a Fourier transform infrared spectrophotometer (FTIR; 8400S, Cat No. 206-72400-92, Shimadzu Corporation, USA). The FTIR technique was chosen because this equipment became available in the laboratory. It is important to note that the results of D_2O quantification in saliva samples by IRMS and FTIR did not differ [25]. TBW measurements were made in accordance with the International Atomic Energy Agency [14].

(2) Bone mineral content. The densest body composition component, or bone mineral content (BMC), was measured by dual-energy X-ray absorptiometry (DXA) using a General Electric Lunar DPX-MD+ at the Centro de Investigación en Alimentación y Desarrollo A.C., by the Lunar iDXA at the Universidad Autónoma de Nuevo León, and by Lunar prodigy advance at the Universidad Autónoma de Ciudad Juárez, following the previously published procedure [26] at each participating institution. Total body mineral mass (TBMM) was calculated using the following equation; $TBMM = BMC \times 1.279$, a factor that is an assumed value which represents the sum of osseous and cell mineral content [27]. For the present study, all DXA scans collected in each laboratory were edited by a trained staff member using LU43616ES©2015 GE Healthcare Lunar encore software. In addition, we ensured that BMC was measured in all obese and extremely obese subjects. The DXA equipment was calibrated daily in accordance with the manufacturer's guidelines before taking measurements.

(3) Body density. This variable was determined by the air displacement plethysmography technique using the Bod-Pod system (BodPod®Body Composition System, Life Measurement Instruments, Concord, CA, USA), following the protocol reported previously [26]. For the present study, total body volume (TBV) was corrected by thoracic gas volume (TGV), which was measured in most, but not all, subjects, since a few were unable to fulfil the requirements for measuring this factor. In those cases, the TGV predicted by the system was used to correct TBV, considering a determination coefficient of 0.96 between FM by the 4C model, and using the BD with TBV corrected by both measured and estimated TGV. The Bod-Pod system was calibrated daily in accordance with the manufacturer's guidelines.

First, these individual body composition components were used to obtain the corresponding fraction of each component to body weight, measured by the scale attached to the Bod-Pod System. The aqueous weight fraction (A) was obtained from the ratio of TBW in kg to body weight in kg, while the mineral weight fraction (M) was calculated from the following TBMM relations in kg/body weight in kg. After that, the body fractions, together with BD, were incorporated into Baumgartner's equation [27] to estimate the fat mass percentage, $\%FM = 205 \times \left(\frac{1.34}{BD} - 0.35(A) + 0.56(M) - 1\right)$ Subsequently, FM in kg was calculated with the following equation: $FM = \frac{\%FM \times weight}{100}$. Finally, FFM in kg was obtained from the differences between body weight in kg and FM in kg.

2.5. Hydration Factor

The HF was calculated as the ratio of TBW in kg, derived from the deuterium dilution technique, to FFM in kg, derived from the 4C model, such that $HF = \frac{TBW}{FFM}$.

2.6. Obesity Classification

In addition, the FMI was obtained using the 4C model. FM in kg derived from this model was divided by height-squared in m. Three classification ranges were obtained, as follows: Normal (3.0 to 6.0 kg/m² and 5.0 to 9.0 kg/m² for men and women, respectively), excess fat (>6.0 to 9.0 kg/m² and >9.0 to 13.0 kg/m² for men and women, respectively), and obesity (>9.0 kg/m² and >13.0 kg/m² for men and women, respectively) [22].

2.7. Statistical Analyses

The gender differences for several variables in the FMI categories were tested by a two-sample independent t-test. The differences for several variables within each gender across the FMI classification ranges were then tested by a one-way analysis of variance (ANOVA) with a post-hoc Tukey test ($p \leq 0.05$). The mean HF value obtained for the total sample, obese, and normal older subjects was compared to (i) the traditionally assumed value of 0.732, derived from chemical analyses [12]; (ii) the "grand mean" value of 0.725, derived from in vivo methods [11]; and (iii) the 0.734 value, derived from 68 healthy, non-obese, older French people [11] by separate analyses using the one-sample t-test. Significance was considered at a p-value ≤ 0.05. All analyses were run in the STATA/SE 12.0 statistical program (StataCorp LP, TX, USA).

3. Results

A total sample of 412 (265 women, 147 men) older Mexican subjects, aged 60–90 years, with BMIs in the range of 18.7–43.6 kg/m²-which corresponds to an FMI range of 3.6–24.7 kg/m²-were included. Based on the FMI ranges, 10.7%, 46.8%, and 42.5% subjects were classified as normal, with excess fat, and obese, respectively.

As expected, there was a difference between gender, regardless of FMI category, on some of the anthropometric variables analyzed by the two-sample independent t-test, as the men had significantly higher body weight and height than the women. FFM was also significantly higher in men than women ($p \leq 0.05$). In contrast, the mean FM and FMI values were higher in women than men ($p \leq 0.05$). According to the results of the ANOVA and post-hoc Tukey test, the differences in anthropometric and body composition variables within gender across the FMI categories shows that the mean values for body weight, BMI, FM, and FMI in the obesity category were higher than in the normal and excess fat category in both men and women (Table 1).

Regarding the HF, Figure 1 shows the correlation between FM and the components of the HF by Pearson's correlation test. It seems that in both genders there is a positive and moderate correlation ($p < 0.001$) between FM and TBW and FFM. However, the results in Table 1 show that a between-gender difference also appeared, as the mean HF value in men was lower than in women, though only in the obesity category. With respect to the behavior of the HF by FMI category, Table 1 shows that the mean HF value was lower in the men's obesity category than in the normal and excess fat categories. In the women's group, in contrast, the mean HF values were close across all FMI categories.

Table 1. Age, anthropometric, and body composition characteristics, and the FMI range classification assumed by gender.

Variable	Normal	Excess fat	Obesity	Total
Men				
Age, years	71.3 ± 5.5 [a]	67.9 ± 6.1 [a]	67.7 ± 5.8 [a]	68.3 ± 5.9
Weight, kg	60.1 ± 5.3 [a,*]	75.2 ± 9.5 [b,*]	85.7 ± 11.9 [c,*]	77.7 ± 13.1 *
Height, m	1.7 ± 0.04 [a,*]	1.7 ± 0.07 [a,*]	1.7 ± 0.06 [a,*]	1.7 ± 0.06 *
BMI, kg/m^2	21.8 ± 1.9 [a]	26.3 ± 2.1 [b]	29.7 ± 3.2 [c]	27.1 ± 3.7
FFM, kg	47.1 ± 5.3 [a,*]	53.1 ± 7.8 [b,*]	53.3 ± 7.7 [b,*]	52.4 ± 7.7 *
TBW, kg	35.7 ± 3.73 [a,*]	39.9 ± 6.0 [b,*]	39.3 ± 5.9 [b,*]	39.1 ± 5.8 *
FM, kg	13.8 ± 1.7 [a]	22.1 ± 2.9 [b]	32.4 ± 5.8 [c]	25.3 ± 7.9
FMI, kg/m^2	4.9 ± 0.7 [a]	7.7 ± 0.8 [b]	11.2 ± 1.6 [c]	8.8 ± 2.5
HF	0.759 ± 0.025 [a]	0.752 ± 0.027 [a]	0.737 ± 0.033 [b]	0.746 ± 0.030
Women				
Age, years	69.1 ± 8.3 [a]	67.9 ± 6.7 [a]	69.2 ± 6.4 [a]	68.5 ± 6.8
Weight, kg	55.2 ± 6.7 [a]	65.9 ± 7.5 [b]	77.5 ± 8.9 [c]	69.9 ± 10.8
Height, m	1.6 ± 0.07 [a]	1.5 ± 0.07 [a]	1.5 ± 0.06 [a]	1.6 ± 0.06
BMI, kg/m^2	22.9 ± 1.8 [a]	27.2 ± 2.1 [b,*]	32.4 ± 3.1 [c,*]	29.0 ± 4.1 *
FFM, kg	36.6 ± 5.1 [a]	38.3 ± 5.1 [a,b]	39.5 ± 4.6 [b]	38.6 ± 4.9
TBW, kg	27.2 ± 4.3 [a]	28.6 ± 4.2 [a,b]	29.7 ± 3.9 [b]	28.9 ± 4.1
FM, kg	18.7 ± 2.9 [a,*]	27.7 ± 3.6 [b,*]	37.9 ± 5.9 [c,*]	31.3 ± 7.9 *
FMI, kg/m^2	7.8 ± 1.0 [a,*]	11.4 ± 1.1 [b,*]	15.9 ± 2.3 [c,*]	12.9 ± 3.2 *
HF	0.743 ± 0.048 [a]	0.746 ± 0.033 [a]	0.753 ± 0.034 [a,*]	0.748 ± 0.035

BMI = body mass index, FFM = fat-free mass, TBW = total body water, FM = fat mass, FMI = fat mass index, HF = hydration factor. * $p < 0.05$ the between-gender comparison in each FMI category was tested by an two-sample independent t-test. [a,b,c] $p < 0.05$ the differences within each gender across the FMI classification ranges were tested by a one-way analysis of variance with a post-hoc Tukey test.

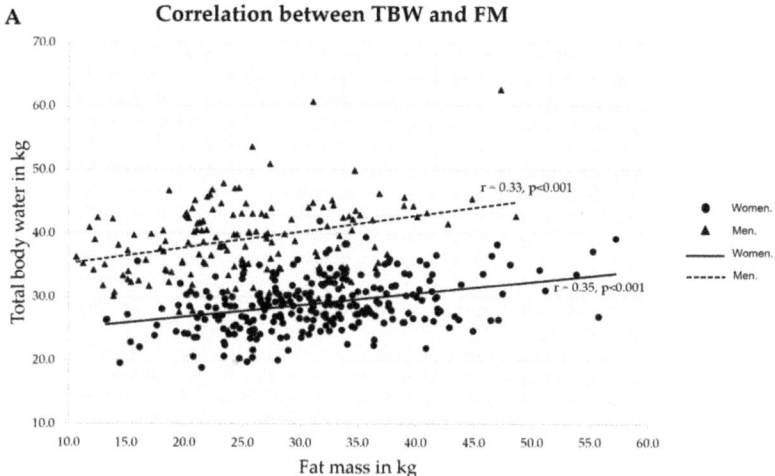

Figure 1. *Cont.*

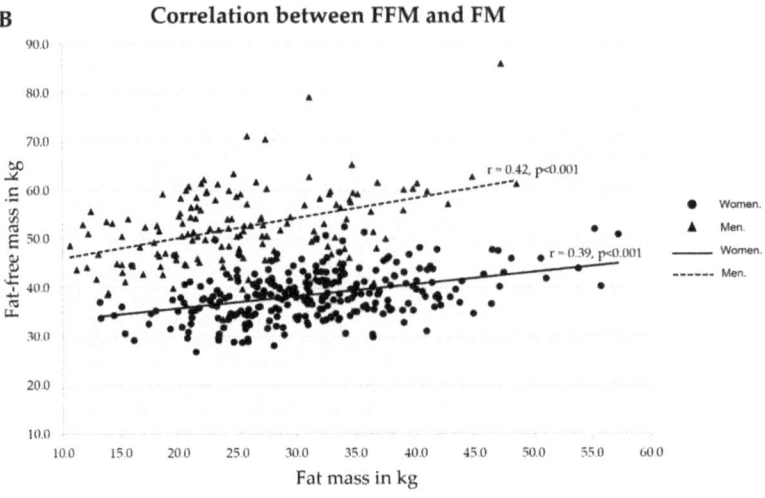

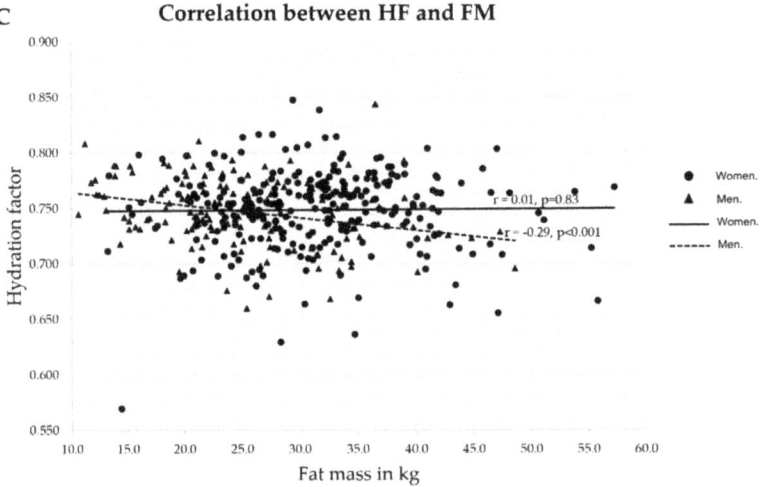

Figure 1. Correlation between total body water (**A**), fat-free mass (**B**), and hydration factor (**C**) to fat mass by gender.

Table 2 shows the results of the comparison between the HF calculated in this sample of older Hispanic-American adults to the values published in the literature (calculated mostly from Caucasian populations) by the one-sample t-test. The mean HF value for the total sample, i.e., for the normal, excess fat, and obesity categories together and separate, was statistically ($p \leq 0.01$) higher than the 0.732 value derived from chemical analyses, the "grand mean" value of 0.725 derived from in vivo methods, and the 0.734 value derived from older French adults using a multi-compartment model.

Table 2. Comparison of the mean hydration factor values in older non-Caucasian adults to several hydration factors cited in the literature.

FMI Category	Mean	0.732 Value from Chemical Analysis	0.725 Value from "Grand Mean"	0.734 Value from Older French Adults
Normal ($n = 44$)	0.750 ± 0.039	$p = 0.003$	$p \leq 0.001$	$p = 0.008$
Excess fat ($n = 193$)	0.748 ± 0.031	$p \leq 0.001$	$p \leq 0.001$	$p \leq 0.001$
Obesity ($n = 175$)	0.747 ± 0.035	$p \leq 0.001$	$p \leq 0.001$	$p \leq 0.001$
Total sample ($n = 412$)	0.748 ± 0.033	$p \leq 0.001$	$p \leq 0.001$	$p \leq 0.001$

FMI = fat mass index; comparison between mean hydration factor values and several hydration values cited in the literature by a one-sample t-test.

4. Discussion

This is the first study to assess the HF in a wide sample of older Hispanic-American adults with one of the most highly-recommended models for accurately determining fat mass and, hence, FFM; that is, the 4C model. This model considers the main molecular changes in body composition across the normal aging process, as well as obesity, bone mineral content, and TBW. In addition, TBW was assessed by the gold standard methodology using the deuterium dilution technique, following the recommended protocols. Therefore, the results for the HF estimated using these high-standard methodologies should raise awareness regarding the accuracy and precision of the hydrometric method for assessing body composition in older obese non-Caucasian subjects.

The accuracy of the hydrometric method primarily depends on obtaining an adequate value for the HF in order to estimate body composition, since these estimates could prove to be inaccurate if the assumed HF value differs from the "real" value [12]. Another often neglected contributing factor to hydrometric inaccuracy is the TBW determination. Unfortunately, variations in estimates of the HF value are common, likely due to differences among the methods used to measure both FFM and TBW. Two of the most important limitations of the chemical analysis of cadavers in terms of assessing hydration for the FFM is that the bodies (i) were analysed post-mortem, and (ii) that several subjects had suffered severe illnesses before death. Both factors could affect hydration status. Another significant limitation is the insensible water loss between the time of death and the performance of the chemical analysis [4].

Despite these limitations, the HF derived from the analysis of cadavers is one of the values that is most often used in the literature to estimate FFM. Our results clearly show a high HF for the total sample of older men and women subjects, compared to 0.732 (Table 2), which was independent of the FMI range classifications. We cannot, therefore, ignore the possible effect of the methods chosen. The HF calculated in the present study was consistently higher than the aforementioned 0.732 derived from chemical analysis, 0.725 derived from two-compartment model, and 0.734 values derived from three-compartment model. In addition, we cannot ignore a possible effect of ethnicity on the TBW and FFM variables. That older French ($n = 68$) subjects had a higher mean FFM in kg (46.1 ± 1.1) than our older Hispanic-American subjects (43.5 ± 8.9), though their mean TBW values in kg (33.9 ± 0.8 and 32.6 ± 6.8, respectively) were similar. Therefore, the ratio of TBW to FFM in older French adults is lower than in our older Hispanic-American adults. It should be noted that the effect of ethnicity on body composition in older people is well-recognized [28].

To speculate on the possible effect of methods on HF differences, we compared the HF calculated in the present study to values reported for older people using the 4C model to estimate FFM and TBW by deuterium dilution. Here, our HF results (0.748 ± 0.033) were similar to the mean HF values reported by Baumgartner et al. [27] (0.744) and Alemán-Mateo et al. [26] (0.752) for Caucasian and non-Caucasian older adults, respectively using Baumgartner's equation. In addition, using Baumgartner's equation, Goran et al. [29] found a higher value (0.747) of HF in older men, but not in women. In contrast, [30] using the 4C model, particularly Selinger's equation, Yee et al. found a higher value (0.761) in older women. It is important to clarify that these authors did not compare their results statistically against HF values reported in the literature. Considering these findings, it seems that there is only an effect of method and aging on the HF for the total sample assessed; however, additional studies of this kind are required in order to reach more general conclusions regarding the effect of methods and aging on the HF.

With respect to the influence of adiposity on the HF, existing evidence is limited and unclear, perhaps because this phenomenon could not be explained by certain physiological or biochemical mechanisms. Specifically, the mean HF value of the men in our obesity category (0.737 ± 0.033) was lower than for those in the normal category (0.759 ± 0.025), but similar to the 0.732 value (Table 1) derived from chemical analysis. According to our data, the mean TBW and FFM values of the men in the obesity category (39.3 ± 5.9 kg and 53.3 ± 7.7 kg, respectively) were higher than those of the normal category (35.7 ± 3.7 kg and 47.1 ± 5.3 kg, respectively). These differences in the mean TBW and FFM values led to a decrease in the HF (0.737 ± 0.033) values of the men in the obesity category compared to the HF values for those in the normal category (0.759 ± 0.025). In addition, the mean TBW and FFM values showed a different behaviour by gender across all FMI categories. In the women's group, mean TBW and FFM values were higher in the obesity than the normal category, though this did not affect HF values. In the men's group, we observed a slight decrease in TBW with a slight increase in FFM ($p > 0.05$) in the obesity category, compared to the excess fat category. These small changes decreased the HF values of the men in the obesity category.

Considering the present results, the hydrometric methods that assume a HF of 0.732 may be inadequate for obtaining accurate and precise body composition estimates in older Hispanic-American adults with a wide range of FMI. If we were to calculate the body composition in our sample using the hydrometric method and an HF of 0.732, we could overestimate the FFM and, therefore, underestimate the FM. For example, a subject with 70 kg of body weight and 31 kg of TBW would have an FFM (TBW/0.732) of 42.3 kg and an FM of 27.7 kg. However, applying our mean HF value of 0.748 decreased the FFM while increasing the FM by around 1 kg in both cases (FFM = 41.4 kg and FM = 28.6 kg). The inaccuracy of the hydrometric method due to the use of an erroneous HF value could appear in studies of other ethnic groups. Therefore, we highly recommend conducting studies designed to validate the hydrometric method in older adults from various ethnic groups.

5. Conclusions

The hydration factor in the total sample was higher than the classic value and the values calculated using in vivo methods in young Caucasian adults and older Caucasian people. However, other researchers using the 4C model in older adults have reported similar HF values, highlighting that older populations possibly have higher values of HF than young adult populations. The men in the obesity category in our study had a lower HF than those in the normal and excess fat categories, with a value similar to 0.732. Therefore, these assumed values may be inadequate for use with older Hispanic-American people in terms of accurately and precisely assessing body composition estimates.

Author Contributions: R.G.-A.: Responsible for the coordination of the field and laboratory studies in institution participants. Also, study design, data analysis, and the writing process. R.U.-R., A.R.-T., J.E.-R., R.-O.M.-E. and E.R.-L. contributed to the study design and critically reviewed the manuscript; A.-E.R.-S. was the adviser on deuterium determination by FTIR and critically reviewed the manuscript; B.-I.P.-M. contributed to the laboratory studies and critically reviewed the manuscript; H.A.-M. was the project leader and participated in study design, DXA measurements, the writing process, analysis, and interpretation.

Funding: The study was supported by CONACyT grant CB-2013-01/000000000221664.

Acknowledgments: The authors would like to thank all participants and their families, nursing homes and clubs for their collaboration, Mexico's National Science and Technology Council (CONACyT) for funding this study, and the CIAD, the UACJ, and the UANL, where the work was carried out. Thanks, as well, to all the students and technicians who helped develop the project: Karla Pimienta Ibarra, Karen Ochoa Esquer, Fernanda Navarro Moreno, Ricardo de Jesús Vega Sosa, Diego Javier Brambila López, Ariadna Tapia, Leticia Aizpuro Pérez, Itzel Nallely López Villa, Margarita Vázquez López, Jesús Donaldo Maytorena Salazar, José Manuel Munguía Figueroa, Angélica Castellanos Espinosa, Erik Morales Borbonio, Andrea Cereceres Aragón, Dulce María Velo Rey, Penelope Mónica Mendoza Viramontes, María Fernanda Orta, Israel Cañas García, Angélica Bugarín Noriega, Airam Reyes Castro, Rosa María Cabrera, José Antonio Ponce, Maribel Ramírez Torres, and Orlando Tortoledo.

Conflicts of Interest: The authors declare no conflict of interest.

References

1. Ng, M.; Fleming, T.; Robinson, M.; Thomson, B.; Graetz, N.; Margono, C.; Mullany, E.C.; Biryukov, S.; Abbafati, C.; Abera, S.F.; et al. Global, regional, and national prevalence of overweight and obesity in children and adults during 1980–2013: A systematic analysis for the global burden of disease study 2013. *Lancet* **2014**, *384*, 766–781. [CrossRef]
2. He, W.; Goodkind, D.; Kowal, P.R. *An Aging World: 2015*; U.S. Census Bureau: Washington, DC, USA, 2016.
3. Pencharz, P.B.; Azcue, M. Use of bioelectrical impedance analysis measurements in the clinical management of malnutrition. *Am. J. Clin. Nutr.* **1996**, *64*, 485S–488S. [CrossRef] [PubMed]
4. Wang, Z.; Deurenberg, P.; Wang, W.; Pietrobelli, A.; Baumgartner, R.N.; Heymsfield, S.B. Hydration of fat-free body mass: New physiological modeling approach. *Am. J. Physiol. Endocrinol. Metab.* **1999**, *276*, E995–E1003. [CrossRef] [PubMed]
5. Mitchell, H.H.; Hamilton, T.S.; Steggerda, F.R.; Bean, H.W. The chemical composition of the adult human body and its bearing on the biochemistry of growth. *J. Biol. Chem.* **1945**, *158*, 625–637.
6. Widdowson, E.M.; McCance, E.A.; Spray, C.M. The chemical composition of the human body. *Clin. Sci.* **1951**, *10*, 113–125. [PubMed]
7. Forbes, R.M.; Cooper, A.R.; Mitchell, H.H. The composition of the adult human body as determined by chemical analysis. *J. Biol. Chem.* **1953**, *203*, 359–366. [PubMed]
8. Forbes, G.B.; Lewis, A.M. Total sodium, potassium and chloride in adult man. *J. Clin. Investig.* **1956**, *35*, 596–600. [CrossRef] [PubMed]
9. Knight, G.S.; Beddoe, A.H.; Streat, S.J.; Hill, G.L. Body composition of two human cadavers by neutron activation and chemical analysis. *Am. J. Physiol.* **1986**, *250*, E179–E185. [CrossRef] [PubMed]
10. Moore, F.D. Determination of total body water and solids with isotopes. *Science* **1946**, *104*, 157–160. [CrossRef]
11. Ritz, P. Body water spaces and cellular hydration during healthy aging. *Ann. N. Y. Acad. Sci.* **2000**, *904*, 474–483. [CrossRef]
12. Sheng, H.-P.; Huggins, R.A. A review of body composition studies with emphasis on total body water and fat. *Am. J. Clin. Nutr.* **1979**, *32*, 630–647. [CrossRef] [PubMed]
13. Clarys, J.P.; Martin, A.D.; Marfell-Jones, M.J.; Janssens, V.; Caboor, D.; Drinkwater, D.T. Human body composition: A review of adult dissection data. *Am. J. Hum. Biol.* **1999**, *11*, 167–174. [CrossRef]
14. IAEA. *Introduction to Body Composition Assessment Using the Deuterium Dilution Technique with Analysis of Saliva Samples by Fourier Transform Infrared Spectrometry*; International Atomic Energy Agency: Vienna, Austria, 2013; Volume 12.
15. Cohn, S.H.; Vaswani, A.N.; Yasumura, S.; Yuen, K.; Ellis, K.J. Improved models for determination of body fat by in vivo neutron activation. *Am. J. Clin. Nutr.* **1984**, *40*, 255–259. [CrossRef] [PubMed]
16. Schoeller, D.A. Changes in total body water with age. *Am. J. Clin. Nutr.* **1989**, *50*, 1176–1181. [CrossRef]
17. Fuller, N.J.; Sawyer, M.B.; Elia, M. Comparative evaluation of body composition methods and predictions, and calculation of density and hydration fraction of fat-free mass, in obese women. *Int. J. Obes. Relat. Metab. Disord.* **1994**, *18*, 503.
18. Das, S.K. Body composition measurement in severe obesity. *Curr. Opin. Clin. Nutr. Metab. Care* **2005**, *8*, 602–606. [CrossRef]
19. Haroun, D.; Wells, J.C.K.; Williams, J.E.; Fuller, N.J.; Fewtrell, M.S.; Lawson, M.S. Composition of the fat-free mass in obese and nonobese children: Matched case–control analyses. *Int. J. Obes.* **2005**, *29*, 29–36. [CrossRef]
20. Ritz, P.; Vol, S.; Berrut, G.; Tack, I.; Arnaud, M.J.; Tichet, J. Influence of gender and body composition on hydration and body water spaces. *Clin. Nutr.* **2008**, *27*, 740–746. [CrossRef]
21. Romero-Corral, A.; Somers, V.K.; Sierra-Johnson, J.; Thomas, R.J.; Collazo-Clavell, M.L.; Korinek, J.; Allison, T.G.; Batsis, J.A.; Sert-Kuniyoshi, F.H.; Lopez-Jimenez, F. Accuracy of body mass index in diagnosing obesity in the adult general population. *Int. J. Obes.* **2008**, *32*, 959–966. [CrossRef]
22. Kelly, T.L.; Wilson, K.E.; Heymsfield, S.B. Dual energy X-ray absorptiometry body composition reference values from NHANES. *PLoS ONE* **2009**, *4*, e7038. [CrossRef]
23. Lawton, M.P.; Brody, E.M. Assessment of older people: Self-maintaining and instrumental activities of daily living. *Gerontologist* **1969**, *9*, 179–186. [CrossRef] [PubMed]

24. Marfell-Jones, M.J.; Stewart, A.D.; De Ridder, J.H. *International Standards for Anthropometric Assessment*; International Society for the Advancement of Kinanthropometry: Wellington, New Zealand, 2012.
25. Jennings, G.; Bluck, L.; Wright, A.; Elia, M. The use of infrared spectrophotometry for measuring body water spaces. *Clin. Chem.* **1999**, *45*, 1077–1081. [PubMed]
26. Aleman-Mateo, H.; Huerta, R.H.; Esparza-Romero, J.; Méndez, R.O.; Urquidez, R.; Valencia, M.E. Body composition by the four-compartment model: Validity of the BOD POD for assessing body fat in Mexican elderly. *Eur. J. Clin. Nutr.* **2007**, *61*, 830. [CrossRef] [PubMed]
27. Baumgartner, R.N.; Heymsfield, S.B.; Lichtman, S.; Wang, J.; Pierson, R.N., Jr. Body composition in elderly people: Effect of criterion estimates on predictive equations. *Am. J. Clin. Nutr.* **1991**, *53*, 1345–1353. [CrossRef]
28. Alemán-Mateo, H.; Lee, S.Y.; Javed, F.; Thornton, J.; Heymsfield, S.B.; Pierson, R.N.; Pi-Sunyer, F.X.; Wang, Z.M.; Wang, J.; Gallagher, D. Elderly Mexicans have less muscle and greater total and truncal fat compared to African-Americans and Caucasians with the same BMI. *J. Nutr. Health Aging* **2009**, *13*, 919–923. [CrossRef]
29. Goran, M.I.; Toth, M.J.; Poehlman, E.T. Assessment of research-based body composition techniques in healthy elderly men and women using the 4-compartment model as a criterion method. *Int. J. Obes. Relat. Metab. Disord.* **1998**, *22*, 135–142. [CrossRef]
30. Yee, A.J.; Fuerst, T.; Salamone, L.; Visser, M.; Dockrell, M.; Van Loan, M.; Kern, M. Calibration and validation of an air-displacement plethysmography method for estimating percentage body fat in an elderly population: A comparison among compartmental models. *Am. J. Clin. Nutr.* **2001**, *74*, 637–642. [CrossRef]

 © 2019 by the authors. Licensee MDPI, Basel, Switzerland. This article is an open access article distributed under the terms and conditions of the Creative Commons Attribution (CC BY) license (http://creativecommons.org/licenses/by/4.0/).

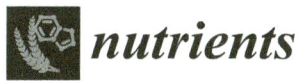

Review

Hydration Status and Cardiovascular Function

Joseph C. Watso * and William B. Farquhar

Department of Kinesiology and Applied Physiology, University of Delaware, Newark, DE 19713, USA
* Correspondence: JosephWatso@texashealth.org; Tel.: +1-214-345-4852

Received: 22 June 2019; Accepted: 8 August 2019; Published: 11 August 2019

Abstract: Hypohydration, defined as a state of low body water, increases thirst sensations, arginine vasopressin release, and elicits renin–angiotensin–aldosterone system activation to replenish intra- and extra-cellular fluid stores. Hypohydration impairs mental and physical performance, but new evidence suggests hypohydration may also have deleterious effects on cardiovascular health. This is alarming because cardiovascular disease is the leading cause of death in the United States. Observational studies have linked habitual low water intake with increased future risk for adverse cardiovascular events. While it is currently unclear how chronic reductions in water intake may predispose individuals to greater future risk for adverse cardiovascular events, there is evidence that acute hypohydration impairs vascular function and blood pressure (BP) regulation. Specifically, acute hypohydration may reduce endothelial function, increase sympathetic nervous system activity, and worsen orthostatic tolerance. Therefore, the purpose of this review is to present the currently available evidence linking acute hypohydration with altered vascular function and BP regulation.

Keywords: hypohydration; vascular function; sympathetic nervous system; blood pressure regulation

1. The Physiology of Hypohydration

Hypohydration is defined as a body water deficit caused by acute or chronic dehydration [1]. While extensive research has been conducted to identify the "elusive daily water requirement", well summarized by Armstrong and Johnson [2] within this special issue, acute hypohydration studies have provided important insight into the integrative physiology of water balance in humans. Human hypohydration can be elicited experimentally through the use of water restriction, prolonged exercise, heat stress, diuretic administration, or a combination of methods [3–31]. In response to hypohydration-induced reductions in plasma volume and increases in plasma sodium ([Na^+])/osmolality, the renin–angiotensin–aldosterone system becomes activated, thirst sensations increase, and arginine vasopressin (AVP, also referred to as anti-diuretic hormone) release increases [20,32–40]. A low extracellular fluid volume is sensed in the walls of the afferent arterioles proximal to the glomeruli and causes juxtaglomerular cells to secrete renin, which initiates a cascade culminating in increased circulating angiotensin II (Ang II) and aldosterone concentrations acting to increase [Na^+] and water retention. Central [Na^+] sensing, which may be distinct from osmo-sensing [41], occurs in circumventricular organs including the organum vasculosum of the lamina terminalis (OVLT) and subfornical organ (SFO) because both brain areas lack a complete blood–brain barrier (BBB) [42]. Specialized mechanical-stretch transient receptor potential vanilloid (TRPV) cation channels are one potential candidate thought to participate in osmo-sensing [43]. Nevertheless, these signals are communicated through neuronal projections to the median preoptic nucleus (MnPO) before activating thirst-promoting neurons in the paraventricular nucleus (PVN) of the hypothalamus via acid-sensing ion channel 1a (ASIC1a) by H^+ ions exported from Na_x-positive glial cells [44]. These signals are then 1) relayed to the lateral hypothalamus as well as the paraventricular hypothalamus and thalamus [45], and 2) stimulate AVP release from the posterior pituitary gland from upstream communication with the PVN and supraoptic nuclei [34,46]. Increased thirst sensations promote water intake [45,46]. Increased plasma [AVP] stimulate aquaporin-2-mediated water reabsorption from the luminal surface of renal collecting ducts to promote water retention [47]. Together, these integrated responses aim to restore body water homeostasis.

The following sections will discuss recent findings related to hypohydration and cardiovascular function. When applicable, we will mention the methods used to induce hypohydration (e.g., heat, exercise, fluid restriction, or diuretic) in humans because these methods have different side effects (e.g., diuretics promote iso-osmotic hypovolemia whereas heat stress promotes hyper-osmotic hypovolemia) [48]. Finally, for human hypohydration studies, we will report the resultant body mass deficit as the severity of hypohydration is defined as follows: mild hypohydration (1 to 5% body mass deficit), moderate hypohydration (5 to 10% body mass deficit), and severe hypohydration (>10% body mass deficit) [1].

2. Clinical Relevance

As early as 1933, insufficient body water stores were identified as a primary factor for heat exhaustion and fatigue, with scientists concluding, "Most people need the advice: Drink more water" [49]. Approximately a decade later, two scientists deprived themselves of water for over three days and became, "temperamental, hollow, and pale." Despite noting, "dry mouths, husky voices, and difficulty swallowing," the authors were, "never unbearably thirsty." While this prolonged fluid deprivation would now have major ethical concerns, this experiment serves as an early example of how a lack of fluid intake alone can elicit substantial (~5%) reductions in body mass and large (~10%) increases in plasma [Na$^+$] [9].

While one 2019 report acknowledges that the field has yet to agree on the biomarker(s) and cutoff(s) that define euhydration (optimal total body water content [1]), only 13 to 51% of individuals studied (depending on sex, age group, and disease status) met the authors hydration criteria [50]. Additionally, Americans are not meeting water intake recommendations [51], which is alarming as inadequate water intake is associated with obesity [52] and predicts greater future risk for developing cardiovascular disease [53], the leading cause of death in the United States [54]. Additionally, suboptimal water intake has been demonstrated to enhance serum- and glucocorticoid-inducible kinase 1 activity (SGK1), which participates in the pathophysiology of a number of disease states including hypertension, thrombosis, stroke, and cardiac fibrosis [55]. Further, there are data demonstrating a positive association between plasma [Na$^+$] and 10-year risk of coronary heart disease in participants from the Atherosclerosis Risk in Community (ARIC) Study [56]. Some [57–59] but not all [60] epidemiological evidence suggests an association between greater plasma [Na$^+$] and increased arterial blood pressure (BP).

While increasing age has been demonstrated to be associated with indices of reduced hydration status [61], the findings from one 2019 study suggest that increasing age is *not* associated with indices of reduced hydration status [50]. Nevertheless, there are several physiological reasons that old adults are less likely to have optimal hydration status including lower basal total body water [62], altered extracellular fluid sensing [63], blunted hormonal (e.g., AVP) responses [64,65], and impaired kidney function [66]. However, even within young healthy individuals, several investigations have provided evidence that acute hypohydration can significantly affect physiological function.

For example, there are well-appreciated deleterious effects of acute hypohydration including reduced exercise performance [3,4,10,12–14,16,67–88], worsened mood [18,89–91], impaired cognitive function [19–21,91,92], altered thermoregulatory function [73,74,80,82,84,87,93–108], and decreased glycemic regulation [11,109] (Figure 1). Chronic systemic hypohydration is a proposed pathogenic factor for hypertension, venous thromboembolism, fatal coronary heart disease, stroke [110]. However, there are relatively few randomized trials examining the effects of acute or chronic mild hypohydration on vascular function and BP regulation. Importantly, reduced vascular function [111–114], high resting BP (i.e., hypertension) [115], high BP variability [116–120], orthostatic intolerance [121,122], and exaggerated BP responses during exercise [123–127] are independent clinical predictors for adverse cardiovascular health outcomes. Thus, given the clinical relevance of this area of research, the purpose of this review is to present the currently available evidence on the effects of acute mild hypohydration on vascular function and BP regulation.

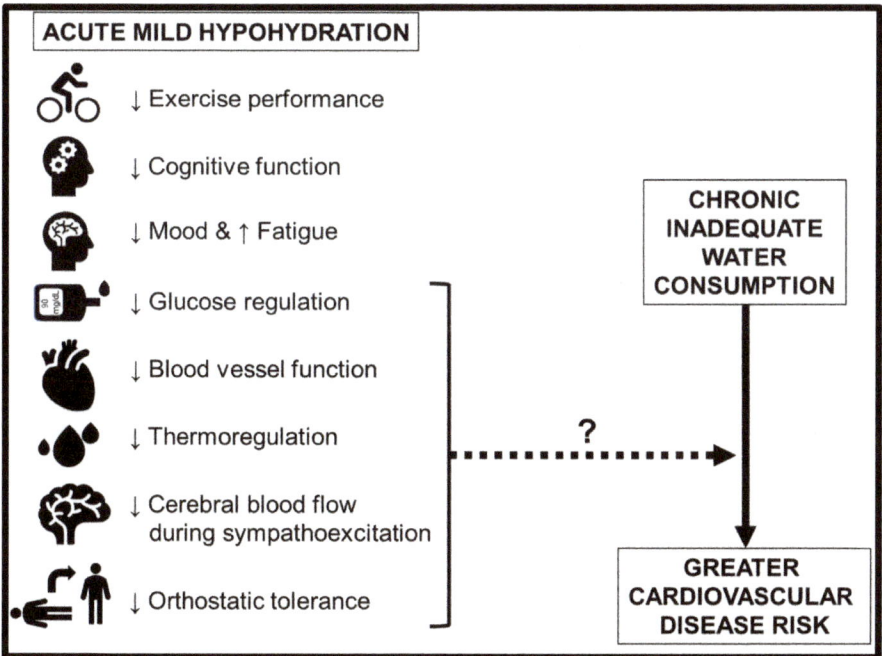

Figure 1. Summary of the physiological consequences of acute mild hypohydration in healthy humans. Further research is necessary to determine whether and how these acute effects influence the poor cardiovascular health outcomes associated with chronic inadequate water consumption. ↓, impaired or reduced; ↑, increased.

3. Vascular Health and Function

3.1. Inflammation

As discussed above, hypohydration is characterized by elevated plasma [Na^+]. Dmitrieva et al. [56] demonstrated that Human Primary Umbilical Endothelial Cells (HUVEC) exposed to media with increasing [NaCl] (several concentrations ranging from 270 to 380 mOsm/kg H_2O) for 4 days were found to have significant increases in the mRNA expression of several pro-inflammatory mediators including vascular cell adhesion molecule 1 (VCAM-1), endothelial-leukocyte adhesion molecule 1 (E-selectin), and monocyte chemoattractant protein 1 (MCP-1). The authors performed additional experiments in rodents to elucidate the effects of physiological increases in [Na^+] in vivo. Nine days of water restriction increased serum [Na^+] by ~5 mM without altering body mass and the increased mRNA expression of VCAM-1, E-selectin, and chemokine MCP-1 in several tissues (e.g., liver, spleen, kidney). Additionally, VCAM-1 protein expression was increased in endothelial cells of liver capillaries and coronary arteries. Because long-term inflammation could increase the risk for the development of atherosclerotic lesions, the authors performed a final experiment in mice. ApoE$^{-/-}$ mice were fed a Western diet for 7–9 weeks with water intake ad libitum or restricted. The authors demonstrated a greater development of atherosclerotic lesions in the aortic root and thicker walls of their coronary arteries in water-restricted mice, suggesting prolonged water restriction may contribute to unfavorable vascular health [56]. Costa et al. [128] sought to determine whether hypohydration worsened the inflammatory profile in healthy humans. In randomized crossover fashion, participants either maintained euhydration or had water restricted (hypohydration, ~3% reduction in body mass) while running at an ambient temperature (25 °C) on two separate occasions. The authors reported modest disturbances in gastrointestinal integrity and function as well as in-vitro neutrophil functional responses, but no effect on post-exercise total or differential leukocyte counts, endotoxemia, or cytokinemia following the hypohydration trial. The authors suggested that when taken together, this mild degree of hypohydration was insufficient to induce immune functional or cytokine responses of clinical significance [128]. While this human study was carried out with healthy endurance-trained adults, future studies investigating the influence of reduced water intake alone (i.e., not exercise induced) on the immune system in preclinical and clinical populations are warranted.

3.2. Endothelial Function

Endothelial dysfunction is a clinically significant marker of cardiovascular health [111,112,114]. There are cellular studies demonstrating that hypernatremia (high Na^+ concentrations in fluid) results in degradation of the endothelial glycocalyx, which may also contribute to impaired endothelial responsiveness to shear stress [129]. Arnaoutis et al. [27] sought to determine whether hypohydration impairs peripheral artery vasodilatory function in healthy young male adults. A ~2% reduction in body mass was achieved with 100 minutes of low-intensity (70% of maximal heart rate) walking in mild heat (31 °C) with a 500-mL water intake limit for the remainder of the day. Compared to the same perturbation without a water intake limit, participants demonstrated reduced flow-mediation dilation (FMD, an assessment of endothelial-dependent vasodilatory function) in the water-restricted state [27]. The authors acknowledge the limitation that blood viscosity was not assessed but could have been increased during hypohydration. This is relevant because some published data suggest blood viscosity does affect FMD values [130] but other data suggest that shear rate (blood velocity/vessel diameter) is a weaker correlate of FMD than shear stress (blood viscosity*blood velocity/vessel diameter) [131]. Nevertheless, shear stress was not different between conditions at baseline or during hyperemia [27]. Additionally, while it is unlikely that FMD values in the present study [27] were affected by exercise 24 hours prior [132], future investigations examining the effects of water restriction alone on endothelial function are warranted. Finally, these future studies should be carried out in both male and female adults.

3.3. Arterial Stiffness

Aortic stiffness expressed as aortic pulse wave velocity (PWV) is a strong predictor of future cardiovascular events and all-cause mortality [133]. One study examined whether hypohydration-induced via 24-hour fluid restriction or acute heat stress (49 °C water in perfused suit) affects PWV in healthy humans [26]. Caldwell et al. reported that 24-hour fluid restriction in young female adults elicited a ~1% reduction in body mass and reduced central, but not peripheral, PWV compared to the euhydrated control condition. In the same article, a cohort of young male adults underwent whole-body heating to increase rectal temperature +1.0 °C and had fluid intake restricted, resulting in a ~2% body mass loss relative to when participants repeated the whole-body heating on a separate occasion but ingested water to prevent body mass loss. Despite the presence of mild hypohydration in the water-restricted state, participants had similar reductions in peripheral PWV throughout heat stress regardless of condition. Finally, central PWV did not change during acute heat stress in either group [26]. These findings suggest that fluid restriction-induced hypohydration reduces central PWV and heat stress-induced hypohydration does not change central PWV. The authors purposefully designed the study to include homogenous groups because their pilot testing demonstrated large sex-related differences in resting PWV values that would have made the interpretation of findings much more difficult as biological sex could be as important of a factor for altering PWV as the technique used to elicit hypohydration [26]. Thus, it remains unclear whether fluid restriction in males or heat-stress and water restriction in females elicits similar responses.

3.4. Cutaneous Vascular Function

There is evidence that mild hypohydration (at either ~1% [22] or ~3% [23] body mass loss) impairs cutaneous vasodilation during exercise in the heat following fluid restriction in healthy male adults. More recent work suggests that hypohydration-induced reductions in skin blood flow are at least partially attributed to altered postsynaptic function in healthy young male adults. This hypothesis is supported by evidence that more methacholine chloride (an endothelium-dependent vasodilator) is required to achieve the drug concentration that provides half of the maximal response (EC_{50}) during hypohydration to ~2% body mass loss via exercise in the heat following fluid restriction compared to euhydration [25]. While only one [22] of these particular three studies examining vascular function [22,23,25] reported greater increases in body temperature in the hypohydrated state, several other studies have found hydration status to affect thermoregulatory function [73,74,80,82,84,87,93–108,134]. As a result, specific guidelines for hydration status have been set in certain populations, such as industrial workers in the heat [135], to minimize the potential for heat-stress and hypohydration-induced increases in cardiovascular strain and potential risk for adverse cardiovascular events. For further discussion on this topic, the reader is directed to several excellent reviews on the interactions between hydration and thermoregulation [70–72,103,136–138]. Additional work in this area is warranted, particularly studies that include female adults.

3.5. Circulating Factors

During hypohydration, elevated plasma [Ang II] elicits vasoconstriction in small arterioles to increase total peripheral resistance [139] and is thought to contribute to endothelial dysfunction [140]. Specifically, Ang II infusion elicits endothelial dysfunction in rodents [141–144] and stimulates NADPH oxidase (NOX)-mediated increases in reactive oxygen species (ROS) in smooth muscle cells from human resistance arterioles [145,146]. Further, data from rodent models suggest that hypohydration increases Ang II receptor density and affects neuronal nitric oxide synthase (nNOS) mRNA expression [147]. These data suggested that Ang II blockade may reduce oxidative stress and improve vascular function in humans. In support of this hypothesis, one study reported that Ang II blockade (candesartan) reduced oxidative stress and improved FMD in hypertensive adults [148]. More recent evidence suggests that Ang II blockade reduces inflammation and improves peripheral vascular function in healthy and clinical populations [149–153]. For an extended discussion on the effects of Ang II blockade on vascular function in hypertensive adults, the reader is directed to a recent review article on this topic [154].

Results from one rodent study suggest that increased plasma [AVP] during hypohydration contributes to the production of ROS, elicits cerebrovascular dysfunction (via reduced vasodilator function as assessed by increasing doses of acetylcholine (Ach)), and cognitive dysfunction as AVP receptor antagonist SR49059 prevents these changes following 48 hours of water deprivation in rodents [20]. Hypohydration has also been demonstrated to increase plasma [endothelin-1] in both rodents [155] and humans [156]. This could be problematic as greater plasma [endothelin-1] has been associated with reduced peripheral vasodilatory function [157,158]. Interestingly, the neocortical application of endothelin receptor type A (ET_AR) antagonist BQ123 ameliorates the cerebrovascular dysfunction induced by 48 hours of water deprivation in rodents [20]. Collectively, these data support a role for hypohydration influencing circulating factors that contribute to reduced blood vessel function.

3.6. Summary

There is a growing body of evidence that hypohydration induces inflammation, reduces endothelial function, and may affect measures of arterial stiffness in humans. Additionally, changes in several circulating factors during acute hypohydration may mediate changes in vascular function and BP regulation. The following sections will discuss the influence of acute hypohydration on cerebral blood flow regulation as well as BP regulation at rest, during orthostasis, and during exercise.

4. Cerebral Blood Flow Regulation

There are several reports of hypohydration being associated with worsened mood [18,89–91] and impaired cognitive function [19–21,91,92] that have prompted investigation into how acute hypohydration affects cerebral blood flow patterns. Tan et al. [87] had 10 male adults undergo magnetic resonance imaging (MRI) brain scans before running in ambient temperature (~25 °C) with a raincoat on to elicit a ~3% reduction in body mass on two occasions. Following exercise, participants either drank water to offset body mass loss or were restricted from fluid intake. During the second MRI brain scan 90 minutes after exercise, hypohydration produced reductions in total brain volume (total intracranial volume excluding ventricles) and increases in brain ventricular volume. However, there were no observed changes in global or regional brain perfusion, or functional activity of the brain during a motor-task based functional MRI (fMRI) scan during hypohydration [87]. Trangmar et al. [31] reported that incremental cycling exercise to exhaustion in the heat (35 °C) in 10 endurance-trained male adults elicited a ~3% reduction in body mass and lowered internal carotid and middle cerebral artery mean velocity (MCA_{vmean}) without affecting common carotid artery blood flow during exercise. However, when tested in the euhydrated state on a separate day, internal carotid and middle cerebral artery mean velocity and common carotid blood flow were preserved. This augmentation of hypohydration-induced decline in cerebral blood flow was reported to result from decreasing arterial carbon dioxide tension, which enhanced vasoconstrictor activity. Despite the reductions in cerebral blood flow, the cerebral metabolic rate for oxygen was maintained in the hypohydrated condition as a result of increased oxygen extraction [31]. Reductions in MCA_{vmean} and end-tidal carbon dioxide partial pressure ($P_{ET}CO_2$) have also been observed during a two-foot immersion cold pressor test in hypohydrated young male adults (~1% body mass loss via 24-hour fluid restriction) [159]. Together, these studies suggest that mild hypohydration in healthy young male adults is associated with alterations in cerebral blood flow regulation during acute sympathoexcitation (e.g., maximal exercise, the cold pressor test). Because hypohydration has been associated with reductions in cognitive function [19–21,92], more work in this area is warranted and future study designs should prioritize the inclusion of female adults.

5. Resting Cardiovascular Regulation

5.1. Sympathetic Nervous System

Aside from promoting thirst and stimulating renal water reabsorption, signals of high central [Na^+] are relayed to the rostral ventrolateral medulla (RVLM) and can affect BP through increases in sympathetic outflow [160–162]. During water deprivation in rats, blood hyperosmolality (i.e., elevated blood osmolality values) was found to influence sympathetic outflow and BP, independent of changes in plasma [AVP] and blood volume [163]. This is likely due to greater sensitivity of the PVN during times of blood hyperosmolality, demonstrated through studies using injections of γ-Aminobutyric acid (GABA) agonists and glutamate antagonists [32] and studies investigating changes to the intrinsic properties of RVLM neurons [160]. In support of these past reports, hypohydrated rats were found to have BP supported by PVN-driven increases in splanchnic sympathetic outflow that is not synchronized to changes in respiration or heart rate [161]. This is thought to occur from central hyperosmolality exciting discrete populations of neurons in the RVLM that increase sympathetic outflow and BP through the increased sensitivity of glutamate neurotransmission [162]. Importantly, alterations in sympathetic outflow and BP during central hyperosmolality are related to NaCl concentrations per se, as eqiu-osmotic sorbitol or mannitol does not produce the same OVLT neuronal discharge frequency [41]. Other animal studies suggest that activator protein-1 transcription factors are responsible for switching thoracic sympathetic outflow control from the hypothalamus to the commissural nucleus tractus solitarius (NTS) following water deprivation [164]. Blocking sympathetic outflow attenuates the BP elevations induced by high cerebrospinal fluid [Na^+] in rodents [162]. Nonetheless, potential sensing mechanisms for [Na^+] existing in the brain have been elucidated using rodent models [162,164–166]. A newly published study adds additional mechanistic insight, suggesting that Nax-positive glial cells in OVLT are activated by high [Na$^+$], leading to enhanced hydrogen and lactate through a monocarboxylate transporter to activate ASIC1a-positive OVLT neurons [43]. More recently, one study in rodents demonstrated that sympathetic blockade (via α1- and β1- adrenergic receptor antagonists) significantly attenuated the increases in resting BP following 48 hours of water deprivation [165]. Together, these studies have provided insight into the role of the sympathetic nervous system activation to support BP during hypohydration.

5.2. Circulating Factors

Reduced sympathetic baroreflex function is associated with hypertension [166] and reduced cardiac vagal baroreflex sensitivity is associated with increasing age [167,168]. Importantly, reductions in baroreflex function can increase (i.e., worsen) BP variability, which is associated with cardiovascular morbidities such as cerebral small vessel disease [169], increased carotid artery intima-media thickness [170], target organ damage [117,171], hypertensive status [172], and cardiovascular mortality [119,120]. However, to date, only one study has investigated the influence of hypohydration on BP variability [173]. This study reported that iso-osmotic hypovolemia via furosemide (no body mass data reported) did not change the power spectral density of mean BP, a measure of BP variability in the frequency domain. One study in humans administered exogenous Ang II and observed increases in muscle sympathetic nerve activity (MSNA) [174]. Rabbitts et al. [28] used a 24-hour water restriction model in healthy young adults to elicit increases in endogenous [Ang II]. While body mass data following the water restriction protocol were not reported, resting MSNA burst incidence was reportedly increased with no change in resting BP. Despite increased MSNA burst incidence, both sympathetic and cardiac vagal baroreflex sensitivity were unchanged following water restriction [28]. This finding that water restriction in humans does not alter arterial baroreflex sensitivity is consistent with one previous study in 48-hour water-deprived rabbits [175]. Interestingly, in the human study, the water restriction-mediated increase in MSNA burst incidence was attenuated after the administration of losartan (an angiotensin receptor blocker), suggesting elevated [Ang II] produced endogenously provoked increases in sympathetic outflow [28]. Another study investigating the effects of hypohydration (~2% body mass loss) on baroreflex function noted a tendency for lower sympathetic baroreflex gain following hypohydration induced by 90 minutes of acute aerobic exercise compared to exercise and intravenous rehydration 20–25 minutes later [176]. While insightful, these data could have potentially been influenced by the prior bout of exercise (collected about 45–60 minutes post exercise). Together, these studies also report conflicting results regarding the influence of hypohydration on arterial baroreflex function. Thus, additional research would provide helpful insight. Further, research investigating the influence of hypohydration on BP variability is warranted.

During hypohydration, elevations in plasma [AVP] (tightly linked to changes in plasma osmolality [17]) and [Ang II] contribute to the maintenance of BP through numerous mechanisms [32,35–37,40,175,177]. For example, hypohydration in rats has been demonstrated to increase plasma renin activity, even during renal denervation and adrenal demedullation, suggesting sympathoadrenomedullary-independent plasma renin activity release to support BP [37]. When plasma renin activity is increased during hypohydration, angiotensin type-1 receptors in the PVN and RVLM are thought to become more sensitive [32], suggesting the renin–angiotensin–aldosterone axis mediates alterations in BP control through interaction with central cardiovascular control centers (i.e., the RVLM). Excessive AVP release has been suggested to play a role in glucoregulatory health [178] and in the development of human hypertension [179]. For a general review on the influence of AVP in cardiovascular control, the reader is directed to a review by Liard [180].

During hypovolemia, AVP is released via actions of the forebrain and midbrain [181] and supports BP by increasing lumbar sympathetic outflow and heart rate [163], independent of the involvement of the subfornical organ [182]. AVP blockade following water deprivation causes a significant drop in BP, suggesting its actions are necessary for BP support during water deprivation (WD) [177,183]. Rodent models using intravenous AVP antagonism demonstrate attenuated pressor and bradycardic effects of α1-adrenergic receptor agonists (e.g., methoxamine, phenylephrine) [184]. AVP antagonism in dogs attenuates the depressor and tachycardic effects of systemic nitric oxide-mediated vasodilation (via sodium nitroprusside), with no additive effect of Ang II antagonism, suggesting AVP plays a primary role in BP control during hypotensive insults [185]. In agreement, one study in rats demonstrated that the administration of intravenous synthetic AVP increases BP following water deprivation [40]. Further, Aisenbrey et al. [40] demonstrated that AVP blockade in rats lowers BP via reductions in peripheral vascular resistance, and this occurs independent of cardiac or arterial baroreceptor input [186]. In contrast, one previous study in rats reported that after 24 or 48 hours of water deprivation, AVP did not significantly contribute to BP maintenance [187]. There is also evidence that AVP only has a minor influence on BP support following hypohydration in humans (2% body mass loss via 24-hour fluid restriction), as selective V1 receptor antagonist [d(CH2)5Tyr(ME)]AVP elicited only minor reductions in diastolic BP and cardiac preload [188]. Together, the conflicting results in the literature regarding the influence of Ang II and AVP on BP regulation during hypohydration suggests more investigation in this area is necessary. Finally, several studies that have been conducted regarding the influence of biological sex [189–198] and sex hormone fluctuations during the menstrual cycle in female adults [189,191–197] and BP regulation. These studies have provided important insight concerning the influence of sex and menstrual cycle-induced changes in blood volume on BP regulation, which is a prerequisite to studying the additional influence of hypohydration. In summary, several circulating factors appear to influence resting BP regulation and the discrepancies in findings may be related to species differences as well as the method and degree of hypovolemia/hypohydration.

6. Cardiovascular Regulation During Orthostatic Stress

Orthostatic stress in humans occurs during daily life when posture changes from the supine or seated positions to the standing position. Approximately 500 mL of blood pools in lower body venous circulation immediately upon changing from the supine to the upright position [199]. To maintain BP and adequate cerebral perfusion upon standing, the body relies on rapid baroreflex-mediated increases in heart rate and MSNA. Without appropriate mechanisms to regulate BP during standing, there is an increased risk of syncope (i.e., fainting), which can result in an injury. While estimates vary among epidemiological studies, it has been reported that approximately ~10% of the population is orthostatic intolerant, defined as having significant drops in systolic and/or diastolic BP upon standing [200]. As a result of the obvious health concerns of syncope and head injuries, there has been a great amount of investigations aimed to determine the internal (i.e., physiological) and external (i.e., ambient temperature) factors that contribute to orthostatic intolerance because it is associated with adverse cardiovascular health outcomes [121,122]. For more details regarding the prognosis and treatment of orthostatic intolerance, the reader is directed to the following review article [201].

Experimentally, head-up tilt testing and lower body negative pressure (LBNP) challenges are commonly used to assess the integrated physiological responses that occur during orthostatic stress. The common factor among standing, head-up tilt testing, and LBNP is progressive central hypovolemia and, for this reason, head-up tilt testing [202] and LBNP [203,204] are valid models for assessing orthostatic tolerance, and can be affected by hydration status [30]. There are detailed reviews available that discuss the clinical applications of head-up tilt testing [205] and LBNP [206].

Related to hypohydration, one study from 1990 used furosemide (iso-osmotic hypovolemia) to elicit a ~2% body mass loss in healthy male adults. These participants demonstrated increased gain in cardiopulmonary baroreflex during a head-up tilt testing challenge (i.e., larger increase in vascular resistance for a given decrease in central venous pressure) [207]. Later, Cheuvront et al. [208] demonstrated that moderate hypertonic hypohydration (~5% body mass loss via exercise in the heat (40 °C)) and mild isotonic hypohydration (~3% body mass loss via furosemide), but not mild hypertonic hypohydration (~3% body mass loss via exercise in the heat (40 °C)), significantly increased sit-to-stand-induced changes in heart rate in healthy male and female adults. Work that is more recent has indicated that in response to a head-up tilt challenge, iso-osmotic hypovolemia (~3% body mass loss via furosemide) modulates heart rate and hyperosmotic hypovolemia (~3% body mass loss via exercise in the heat (40 °C)) modulates both heart rate and MSNA to support BP in healthy male and female adults [6]. Iso-osmotic hypovolemia via aldosterone receptor antagonist spironolactone (Aldactone; no body mass loss data reported) in healthy young males has been demonstrated to augment changes in total MSNA and total peripheral resistance during orthostasis to compensate for plasma volume (16% reduction) contraction-induced decrements in stroke volume and cardiac output [29]. A later published analysis of these data demonstrated that MSNA burst amplitude but not MSNA burst frequency mediated the observed increases in MSNA total activity during LBNP [209]. These studies demonstrate that plasma volume deficits imposed by hypohydration (e.g., reductions in plasma volume and increases in plasma osmolality) elicit alterations in the complex integrative cardiovascular responses that occur during an orthostatic challenge. Given that orthostatic intolerance is more common in female adults [200] and this research concerning hypohydration and cardiovascular responses to orthostatic challenges has been completed in young male adults, additional work in female adults and older populations are warranted.

7. Cardiovascular Regulation During Exercise

Skeletal muscles require increased blood flow during exercise. Appropriate alterations in BP allow for increased blood flow to active skeletal muscle beds for the delivery of nutrients (e.g., oxygen) and for removal of metabolic byproducts (e.g., lactate). Augmented increases in BP during exercise is associated with greater future incidence of hypertension [124–126], as well as greater cardiovascular [123] and cardiometabolic [127] disease risk. Studies in rodents demonstrate that the hindbrain is responsible for mediating autonomic cardiovascular reflexes during hypovolemia to maintain BP [181]. Following 48 hours of water deprivation in rats, BP responses to unilateral RVLM microinjection of L-glutamate have been reported to be augmented, suggesting the increased sensitivity of RVLM neurons to excitatory amino acids during severe dehydration in rodents [210]. However, in our recent study, while 48 hours of WD in rodents increased resting lumbar sympathetic outflow and BP as previously reported in other studies [211], we did not observe water deprivation to change the responsiveness of sympathetic-regulatory neurons in the RVLM to the exogenous application of L-glutamate (sympathoexcitatory) or GABA (sympathoinhibitory) [212]. While the reasons for the discrepancies in findings between the former study [210] and our recent study [212] are unclear, we speculated that because injections were unilateral, intact compensatory contralateral pathways could have contributed to divergent observations. Nevertheless, additional work is warranted to provide insight into these autonomic cardiovascular responses following water deprivation.

In humans, moderate osmotic hypohydration (~5% body mass loss via cycling in the heat (35 °C)) has been demonstrated to attenuate the exercise-induced increases in BP, primarily by attenuating increases in cardiac output. One study in male adults demonstrated greater increases in heart rate and plasma [AVP] during exercise following mild hypohydration (3% body mass loss via cycling in the heat) versus 50 or 100% fluid replacement to offset body mass loss [134]. Additionally, these participants demonstrated accentuated increases in vascular resistance and plasma [norepinephrine], suggesting greater activation of the sympathetic nervous system during exercise in the hypohydrated state necessary to compensate for reductions in blood volume and pressure to maintain adequate skeletal muscle perfusion [5]. Recently, we sought to determine whether mild hypohydration affects sympathetic and BP responses during exercise pressor reflex activation. We found that very mild hypohydration (~0.5% body mass loss) did not affect MSNA or BP responses during static handgrip exercise in healthy young male and female adults [212]. While the observed changes in body mass were modest following voluntary reductions in water intake over three days concluded with a 16-hour water abstention period, key considerations in our study design were to elicit increases in serum [Na^+] and determine the resultant alterations in exercise pressor reflex function. Additionally, this study design allowed for a hypohydration stimulus in the absence of exercise, heat, and diuretic usage. It is possible that a combination of methods is required to produce more severe hypohydration and elicit alterations in exercise pressor reflex function.

8. Cardiovascular Regulation and Body Water Balance During Hypobaric Hypoxia

Acute hypobaric hypoxia (i.e., high-altitude) increases BP [213] and alters body water balance via fluid shifts and changes in hormonal control of body fluid and electrolytes [214–216]. The increases in BP during acute exposure to altitude is thought to occur through endothlin-1-mediated increases in heart rate and systemic sympathetic activation. With chronic altitude exposure, there is potential to develop chronic arterial and pulmonary hypertension, the mechanisms and evidence for which are discussed in depth by Riley et al. [213]. Specific to changes in body water balance, acute altitude exposure (3500 m for 12 days) elicits reductions in extracellular water and total body water [214]. In agreement with this observation, another study reported that during the first three days at an elevation of 5334 m, plasma volume and total body water were reduced, while plasma renin activity and serum [aldosterone] increased. As expected with these observations, sodium and potassium excretion were concomitantly reduced [216]. The findings from these previous studies are consistent with other work that demonstrated dehydration upon arrival to 4850 m was induced by fluid shifts to the interstitial space and produced rapid hemoconcentration (i.e., increases in hemoglobin concentrations and hematocrit values). The authors speculated that any further hemoconcentration observed during the climb from 4850 m to 7600m can be partially explained by stimulated erythropoiesis [215]. To summarize, acute hypobaric hypoxia elicits alterations in body water balance that produce unfavorable conditions for optimal physiological function. While extended discussion on strategies to mitigate the deleterious effects of altitude on physiological function is beyond the scope of this review article, the authors suggest a review [85] by Sawka and colleagues for more information on this topic.

9. Summary

Hypohydration is known to reduce mental and physical performance, and more recent evidence suggests hypohydration also impairs vascular function and cardiovascular regulation. Specifically, hypohydration has been demonstrated to impair cutaneous vascular function, reduce endothelial function, and alter BP regulation at rest during exercise and during orthostatic stress (Figure 1). Future studies examining the physiological effects of hypohydration in healthy female adults are warranted as most of the previous work has been completed within male adults. Additionally, studies determining the acute and chronic effects of hypohydration in preclinical populations, such as old adults and those with hypertension, are warranted.

10. Perspectives

Previous literature indicates that mild hypohydration impairs cognitive function, aerobic exercise performance, and thermoregulation. Here, we highlighted the negative implications of hypohydration on vascular function and cardiovascular regulation at rest and during various perturbations (e.g., orthostatic stress, exercise). While there is less consensus regarding more mild forms of hypohydration on these cardiovascular measures, there is strong evidence that mild-to-moderate hypohydration impairs several indices of cardiovascular function. Taken together, these studies indicate that acute reductions in water intake may negatively influence cardiovascular function in healthy young humans. These deleterious cardiovascular effects of mild hypohydration are more consistent during protocols that employ exercise, heat stress, and/or diuretic usage in addition to water restriction.

Author Contributions: J.C.W. generated and W.B.F. edited this manuscript.

Funding: This review was written while J.C.W. was supported by a University of Delaware Doctoral Fellowship and W.B.F. was supported by NIH R01 HL128388 & HL104106.

Acknowledgments: The authors would like to thank other members of Cardiovascular Physiology Research Laboratory at the University of Delaware for their critical evaluation and feedback for this review.

Conflicts of Interest: The authors declare no conflict of interest.

References

1. McDermott, B.P.; Anderson, S.A.; Armstrong, L.E.; Casa, D.J.; Cheuvront, S.N.; Cooper, L.; Kenney, W.L.; O'Connor, F.G.; Roberts, W.O. National Athletic Trainers' Association Position Statement: Fluid Replacement for the Physically Active. *J. Athl. Train.* **2017**, *52*, 877–895. [CrossRef] [PubMed]
2. Armstrong, L.E.; Johnson, E.C. Water Intake, Water Balance, and the Elusive Daily Water Requirement. *Nutrients* **2018**, *10*, 1928. [CrossRef] [PubMed]
3. Laitano, O.; Kalsi, K.K.; Pearson, J.; Lotlikar, M.; Reischak-Oliveira, A.; González-Alonso, J. Effects of graded exercise-induced dehydration and rehydration on circulatory markers of oxidative stress across the resting and exercising human leg. *Eur. J. Appl. Physiol.* **2012**, *112*, 1937–1944. [CrossRef] [PubMed]
4. González-Alonso, J.; Mora-Rodríguez, R.; Below, P.R.; Coyle, E.F. Dehydration markedly impairs cardiovascular function in hyperthermic endurance athletes during exercise. *J. Appl. Physiol.* **1997**, *82*, 1229–1236. [CrossRef] [PubMed]
5. González-Alonso, J.; Mora-Rodríguez, R.; Below, P.R.; Coyle, E.F. Dehydration reduces cardiac output and increases systemic and cutaneous vascular resistance during exercise. *J. Appl. Physiol.* **1995**, *79*, 1487–1496. [CrossRef] [PubMed]
6. Posch, A.M.; Luippold, A.J.; Mitchell, K.M.; Bradbury, K.E.; Kenefick, R.W.; Cheuvront, S.N.; Charkoudian, N. Sympathetic neural and hemodynamic responses to head-up tilt during iso-osmotic and hyper-osmotic hypovolemia. *J. Neurophysiol.* **2017**, *118*, 2232–2237. [CrossRef] [PubMed]
7. Armstrong, L.E.; Maresh, C.M.; Gabaree, C.V.; Hoffman, J.R.; Kavouras, S.A.; Kenefick, R.W.; Castellani, J.W.; Ahlquist, L.E. Thermal and circulatory responses during exercise: Effects of hypohydration, dehydration, and water intake. *J. Appl. Physiol.* **1997**, *82*, 2028–2035. [CrossRef] [PubMed]
8. Shore, A.C.; Markandu, N.D.; Sagnella, G.A.; Singer, D.R.; Forsling, M.L.; Buckley, M.G.; Sugden, A.L.; MacGregor, G.A. Endocrine and renal response to water loading and water restriction in normal man. *Clin. Sci.* **1988**, *75*, 171–177. [CrossRef]
9. Black, D.A.; McCance, R.A.; Young, W.F. A study of dehydration by means of balance experiments. *J. Physiol.* **1944**, *102*, 406–414. [CrossRef]
10. Adams, J.D.; Sekiguchi, Y.; Suh, H.; Seal, A.D.; Sprong, C.A.; Kirkland, T.W.; Kavouras, S.A. Dehydration Impairs Cycling Performance, Independently of Thirst: A Blinded Study. *Med. Sci. Sports Exerc.* **2018**. [CrossRef]
11. Johnson, E.C.; Bardis, C.N.; Jansen, L.T.; Adams, J.D.; Kirkland, T.W.; Kavouras, S.A. Reduced water intake deteriorates glucose regulation in patients with type 2 diabetes. *Nutr. Res.* **2017**, *43*, 25–32. [CrossRef]
12. Ganio, M.S.; Wingo, J.E.; Carrolll, C.E.; Thomas, M.K.; Cureton, K.J. Fluid ingestion attenuates the decline in VO2peak associated with cardiovascular drift. *Med. Sci. Sports Exerc.* **2006**, *38*, 901–909. [CrossRef]
13. James, L.J.; Moss, J.; Henry, J.; Papadopoulou, C.; Mears, S.A. Hypohydration impairs endurance performance: A blinded study. *Physiol. Rep.* **2017**, *5*. [CrossRef]
14. Nadel, E.R.; Fortney, S.M.; Wenger, C.B. Effect of hydration state of circulatory and thermal regulations. *J. Appl. Physiol. Respir. Environ. Exerc. Physiol.* **1980**, *49*, 715–721. [CrossRef]
15. Mack, G.W.; Weseman, C.A.; Langhans, G.W.; Scherzer, H.; Gillen, C.M.; Nadel, E.R. Body fluid balance in dehydrated healthy older men: Thirst and renal osmoregulation. *J. Appl. Physiol.* **1994**, *76*, 1615–1623. [CrossRef]
16. Fortney, S.M.; Wenger, C.B.; Bove, J.R.; Nadel, E.R. Effect of hyperosmolality on control of blood flow and sweating. *J. Appl. Physiol. Respir. Environ. Exerc. Physiol.* **1984**, *57*, 1688–1695. [CrossRef]
17. Stachenfeld, N.S.; DiPietro, L.; Nadel, E.R.; Mack, G.W. Mechanism of attenuated thirst in aging: Role of central volume receptors. *Am. J. Physiol.* **1997**, *272*, 148. [CrossRef]
18. Armstrong, L.E.; Ganio, M.S.; Casa, D.J.; Lee, E.C.; McDermott, B.P.; Klau, J.F.; Jimenez, L.; Le Bellego, L.; Chevillotte, E.; Lieberman, H.R. Mild dehydration affects mood in healthy young women. *J. Nutr.* **2012**, *142*, 382–388. [CrossRef]
19. Stachenfeld, N.S.; Leone, C.A.; Mitchell, E.S.; Freese, E.; Harkness, L. Water intake reverses dehydration associated impaired executive function in healthy young women. *Physiol. Behav.* **2017**, *185*, 103–111. [CrossRef]

20. Faraco, G.; Wijasa, T.S.; Park, L.; Moore, J.; Anrather, J.; Iadecola, C. Water deprivation induces neurovascular and cognitive dysfunction through vasopressin-induced oxidative stress. *J. Cereb. Blood Flow Metab.* **2014**, *34*, 852–860. [CrossRef]
21. Patsalos, O.C.; Thoma, V. Water supplementation after dehydration improves judgment and decision-making performance. *Psychol. Res.* **2019**. [CrossRef]
22. Kenney, W.L.; Tankersley, C.G.; Newswanger, D.L.; Hyde, D.E.; Puhl, S.M.; Turner, N.L. Age and hypohydration independently influence the peripheral vascular response to heat stress. *J. Appl. Physiol.* **1990**, *68*, 1902–1908. [CrossRef]
23. Fujii, N.; Honda, Y.; Hayashi, K.; Kondo, N.; Nishiyasu, T. Effect of hypohydration on hyperthermic hyperpnea and cutaneous vasodilation during exercise in men. *J. Appl. Physiol.* **2008**, *105*, 1509–1518. [CrossRef]
24. McNeely, B.D.; Meade, R.D.; Fujii, N.; Seely, A.J.E.; Sigal, R.J.; Kenny, G.P. Fluid replacement modulates oxidative stress- but not nitric oxide-mediated cutaneous vasodilation and sweating during prolonged exercise in the heat. *Am. J. Physiol. Regul. Integr. Comp. Physiol.* **2017**, *313*, R739. [CrossRef]
25. Tucker, M.A.; Six, A.; Moyen, N.E.; Satterfield, A.Z.; Ganio, M.S. Effect of hypohydration on postsynaptic cutaneous vasodilation and sweating in healthy men. *Am. J. Physiol. Regul. Integr. Comp. Physiol.* **2017**, *312*, R642. [CrossRef]
26. Caldwell, A.R.; Tucker, M.A.; Burchfield, J.; Moyen, N.E.; Satterfield, A.Z.; Six, A.; McDermott, B.P.; Mulvenon, S.W.; Ganio, M.S. Hydration status influences the measurement of arterial stiffness. *Clin. Physiol. Funct. Imaging.* **2018**, *38*, 447–454. [CrossRef]
27. Arnaoutis, G.; Kavouras, S.A.; Stratakis, N.; Likka, M.; Mitrakou, A.; Papamichael, C.; Sidossis, L.S.; Stamatelopoulos, K. The effect of hypohydration on endothelial function in young healthy adults. *Eur. J. Nutr.* **2017**, *56*, 1211–1217. [CrossRef]
28. Rabbitts, J.A.; Strom, N.A.; Sawyer, J.R.; Curry, T.B.; Dietz, N.M.; Roberts, S.K.; Kingsley-Berg, S.M.; Charkoudian, N. Influence of endogenous angiotensin II on control of sympathetic nerve activity in human dehydration. *J. Physiol.* **2009**, *587*, 5441–5449. [CrossRef]
29. Kimmerly, D.S.; Shoemaker, J.K. Hypovolemia and neurovascular control during orthostatic stress. *Am. J. Physiol. Heart Circ. Physiol.* **2002**, *282*, 645. [CrossRef]
30. Harrison, M.H.; Geelen, G.; Keil, L.C.; Wade, C.A.; Hill, L.C.; Kravik, S.E.; Greenleaf, J.E. Effect of hydration on plasma vasopressin, renin, and aldosterone responses to head-up tilt. *Aviat. Space Environ. Med.* **1986**, *57*, 420–425.
31. Trangmar, S.J.; Chiesa, S.T.; Stock, C.G.; Kalsi, K.K.; Secher, N.H.; González-Alonso, J. Dehydration affects cerebral blood flow but not its metabolic rate for oxygen during maximal exercise in trained humans. *J. Physiol.* **2014**, *592*, 3143–3160. [CrossRef]
32. Freeman, K.L.; Brooks, V.L. AT(1) and glutamatergic receptors in paraventricular nucleus support blood pressure during water deprivation. *Am. J. Physiol. Regul. Integr. Comp. Physiol.* **2007**, *292*, 1675. [CrossRef]
33. Phillips, P.A.; Rolls, B.J.; Ledingham, J.G.; Forsling, M.L.; Morton, J.J.; Crowe, M.J.; Wollner, L. Reduced thirst after water deprivation in healthy elderly men. *N Engl. J. Med.* **1984**, *311*, 753–759. [CrossRef]
34. Szinnai, G.; Morgenthaler, N.G.; Berneis, K.; Struck, J.; Müller, B.; Keller, U.; Christ-Crain, M. Changes in plasma copeptin, the c-terminal portion of arginine vasopressin during water deprivation and excess in healthy subjects. *J. Clin. Endocrinol. Metab.* **2007**, *92*, 3973–3978. [CrossRef]
35. Gregory, L.C.; Quillen, E.W.; Keil, L.C.; Chang, D.; Reid, I.A. Effect of vasopressin blockade on blood pressure during water deprivation in intact and baroreceptor-denervated conscious dogs. *Am. J. Physiol.* **1988**, *254*, 490. [CrossRef]
36. Schwartz, J.; Reid, I.A. Role of vasopressin in blood pressure regulation in conscious water-deprived dogs. *Am. J. Physiol.* **1983**, *244*, 74. [CrossRef]
37. Blair, M.L.; Woolf, P.D.; Felten, S.Y. Sympathetic activation cannot fully account for increased plasma renin levels during water deprivation. *Am. J. Physiol.* **1997**, *272*, 1197. [CrossRef]
38. Brooks, V.L.; Keil, L.C. Vasopressin and angiotensin II in reflex regulation of ACTH, glucocorticoids, and renin: Effect of water deprivation. *Am. J. Physiol.* **1992**, *263*, 762. [CrossRef]
39. Brooks, V.L.; Huhtala, T.A.; Silliman, T.L.; Engeland, W.C. Water deprivation and rat adrenal mRNAs for tyrosine hydroxylase and the norepinephrine transporter. *Am. J. Physiol.* **1997**, *272*, 1897. [CrossRef]

40. Aisenbrey, G.A.; Handelman, W.A.; Arnold, P.; Manning, M.; Schrier, R.W. Vascular effects of arginine vasopressin during fluid deprivation in the rat. *J. Clin. Invest.* **1981**, *67*, 961–968. [CrossRef]
41. Kinsman, B.J.; Browning, K.N.; Stocker, S.D. NaCl and osmolarity produce different responses in organum vasculosum of the lamina terminalis neurons, sympathetic nerve activity and blood pressure. *J. Physiol.* **2017**, *595*, 6187–6201. [CrossRef]
42. Duvernoy, H.M.; Risold, P. The circumventricular organs: An atlas of comparative anatomy and vascularization. *Brain Res. Rev.* **2007**, *56*, 119–147. [CrossRef]
43. Danziger, J.; Zeidel, M.L. Osmotic homeostasis. *Clin. J. Am. Soc. Nephrol.* **2015**, *10*, 852–862. [CrossRef]
44. Nomura, K.; Hiyama, T.Y.; Sakuta, H.; Matsuda, T.; Lin, C.; Kobayashi, K.; Kobayashi, K.; Kuwaki, T.; Takahashi, K.; Matsui, S.; et al. [Na+] Increases in Body Fluids Sensed by Central Nax Induce Sympathetically Mediated Blood Pressure Elevations via H+-Dependent Activation of ASIC1a. *Neuron* **2019**, *101*, 75. [CrossRef]
45. Leib, D.E.; Zimmerman, C.A.; Poormoghaddam, A.; Huey, E.L.; Ahn, J.S.; Lin, Y.; Tan, C.L.; Chen, Y.; Knight, Z.A. The Forebrain Thirst Circuit Drives Drinking through Negative Reinforcement. *Neuron* **2017**, *96*, 1281. [CrossRef]
46. Lowell, B.B. New Neuroscience of Homeostasis and Drives for Food, Water, and Salt. *N Engl. J. Med.* **2019**, *380*, 459–471. [CrossRef]
47. Deen, P.M.; Verdijk, M.A.; Knoers, N.V.; Wieringa, B.; Monnens, L.A.; van Os, C.H.; van Oost, B.A. Requirement of human renal water channel aquaporin-2 for vasopressin-dependent concentration of urine. *Science* **1994**, *264*, 92–95. [CrossRef]
48. Owen, J.A.; Fortes, M.B.; Rahman, S.U.; Jibani, M.; Walsh, N.P.; Oliver, S.J. Hydration Marker Diagnostic Accuracy to Identify Mild Intracellular and Extracellular Dehydration. *Int. J. Sport Nutr. Exerc. Metab.* **2019**, 1–23. [CrossRef]
49. Van Zwalenburg, C. Dehydration in Heat Exhaustion and in Fatigue. *Cal. West. Med.* **1933**, *38*, 354–358.
50. Stookey, J.D. Analysis of 2009–2012 Nutrition Health and Examination Survey (NHANES) Data to Estimate the Median Water Intake Associated with Meeting Hydration Criteria for Individuals Aged 12–80 in the US Population. *Nutrients* **2019**, *11*, 657. [CrossRef]
51. Drewnowski, A.; Rehm, C.D.; Constant, F. Water and beverage consumption among adults in the United States: Cross-sectional study using data from NHANES 2005-2010. *BMC Public Health* **2013**, *13*, 1068. [CrossRef]
52. Chang, T.; Ravi, N.; Plegue, M.A.; Sonneville, K.R.; Davis, M.M. Inadequate Hydration, BMI, and Obesity Among US Adults: NHANES 2009-2012. *Ann. Fam. Med.* **2016**, *14*, 320–324. [CrossRef]
53. Chan, J.; Knutsen, S.F.; Blix, G.G.; Lee, J.W.; Fraser, G.E. Water, other fluids, and fatal coronary heart disease: The Adventist Health Study. *Am. J. Epidemiol.* **2002**, *155*, 827–833. [CrossRef]
54. Xu, J.; Murphy, S.L.; Kochanek, K.D.; Bastian, B.; Arias, E. Deaths: Final Data for 2016. *Natl. Vital Stat. Rep.* **2018**, *67*, 1–76.
55. Lang, F.; Guelinckx, I.; Lemetais, G.; Melander, O. Two Liters a Day Keep the Doctor Away? Considerations on the Pathophysiology of Suboptimal Fluid Intake in the Common Population. *Kidney Blood Pres. Res.* **2017**, *42*, 483–494. [CrossRef]
56. Dmitrieva, N.I.; Burg, M.B. Elevated sodium and dehydration stimulate inflammatory signaling in endothelial cells and promote atherosclerosis. *PLoS ONE* **2015**, *10*, 1–22. [CrossRef]
57. Bulpitt, C.J.; Shipley, M.J.; Semmence, A. Blood pressure and plasma sodium and potassium. *Clin. Sci.* **1981**, *61*, 85s–87s. [CrossRef]
58. Komiya, I.; Yamada, T.; Takasu, N.; Asawa, T.; Akamine, H.; Yagi, N.; Nagasawa, Y.; Ohtsuka, H.; Miyahara, Y.; Sakai, H.; et al. An abnormal sodium metabolism in Japanese patients with essential hypertension, judged by serum sodium distribution, renal function and the renin-aldosterone system. *J. Hypertens.* **1997**, *15*, 65–72. [CrossRef]
59. Wannamethee, G.; Whincup, P.H.; Shaper, A.G.; Lever, A.F. Serum sodium concentration and risk of stroke in middle-aged males. *J. Hypertens.* **1994**, *12*, 971–979. [CrossRef]
60. Lago, R.M.; Pencina, M.J.; Wang, T.J.; Lanier, K.J.; D'Agostino, R.B.; Kannel, W.B.; Vasan, R.S. Interindividual variation in serum sodium and longitudinal blood pressure tracking in the Framingham Heart Study. *J. Hypertens.* **2008**, *26*, 2121–2125. [CrossRef]

61. Stookey, J.D. High Prevalence of Plasma Hypertonicity among Community-Dwelling Older Adults: Results from NHANES III. *J. Am. Diet. Assoc.* **2005**, *105*, 1231–1239. [CrossRef]
62. Davy, K.P.; Seals, D.R. Total blood volume in healthy young and older men. *J. Appl. Physiol.* **1994**, *76*, 2059–2062. [CrossRef]
63. Phillips, P.A.; Johnston, C.I.; Gray, L. Disturbed fluid and electrolyte homoeostasis following dehydration in elderly people. *Age Ageing* **1993**, *22*, S33. [CrossRef]
64. Phillips, P.A.; Bretherton, M.; Risvanis, J.; Casley, D.; Johnston, C.; Gray, L. Effects of drinking on thirst and vasopressin in dehydrated elderly men. *Am. J. Physiol.* **1993**, *264*, 877. [CrossRef]
65. Bevilacqua, M.; Norbiato, G.; Chebat, E.; Raggi, U.; Cavaiani, P.; Guzzetti, R.; Bertora, P. Osmotic and nonosmotic control of vasopressin release in the elderly: Effect of metoclopramide. *J. Clin. Endocrinol. Metab.* **1987**, *65*, 1243–1247. [CrossRef]
66. Crowe, M.J.; Forsling, M.L.; Rolls, B.J.; Phillips, P.A.; Ledingham, J.G.; Smith, R.F. Altered water excretion in healthy elderly men. *Age Ageing* **1987**, *16*, 285–293. [CrossRef]
67. Savoie, F.; Kenefick, R.; Ely, B.; Cheuvront, S.; Goulet, E. Effect of Hypohydration on Muscle Endurance, Strength, Anaerobic Power and Capacity and Vertical Jumping Ability: A Meta-Analysis. *Sports Med.* **2015**, *45*, 1207–1227. [CrossRef]
68. Adams, W.M.; Ferraro, E.M.; Huggins, R.A.; Casa, D.J. Influence of body mass loss on changes in heart rate during exercise in the heat: A systematic review. *J. Strength Cond Res.* **2014**, *28*, 2380–2389. [CrossRef]
69. Murray, B. Hydration and Physical Performance. *Am. Coll. Nutrition* **2007**, *26*, 542S. [CrossRef]
70. Sawka, M.N.; Cheuvront, S.N.; Kenefick, R.W. High skin temperature and hypohydration impair aerobic performance. *Exp. Physiol.* **2012**, *97*, 327–332. [CrossRef]
71. Sawka, M.N.; Francesconi, R.P.; Young, A.J.; Pandolf, K.B. Influence of hydration level and body fluids on exercise performance in the heat. *JAMA* **1984**, *252*, 1165–1169. [CrossRef]
72. Sawka, M.N. Physiological consequences of hypohydration: Exercise performance and thermoregulation. *Med. Sci. Sports Exerc.* **1992**, *24*, 657–670. [CrossRef]
73. Roy, B.D.; Green, H.J.; Burnett, M.E. Prolonged exercise following diuretic-induced hypohydration: Effects on cardiovascular and thermal strain. *Can. J. Physiol. Pharmacol.* **2000**, *78*, 541–547. [CrossRef]
74. Cheung, S.S.; McLellan, T.M. Influence of short-term aerobic training and hydration status on tolerance during uncompensable heat stress. *Eur. J. Appl. Physiol. Occup. Physiol.* **1998**, *78*, 50–58. [CrossRef]
75. Hayes, L.D.; Morse, C.I. The effects of progressive dehydration on strength and power: Is there a dose response? *Eur. J. Appl. Physiol.* **2010**, *108*, 701–707. [CrossRef]
76. McLellan, T.M.; Cheung, S.S.; Latzka, W.A.; Sawka, M.N.; Pandolf, K.B.; Millard, C.E.; Withey, W.R. Effects of dehydration, hypohydration, and hyperhydration on tolerance during uncompensable heat stress. *Can. J. Appl. Physiol.* **1999**, *24*, 349–361. [CrossRef]
77. Maughan, R.J. Impact of mild dehydration on wellness and on exercise performance. *Eur. J. Clin. Nutr.* **2003**, *57*, 19. [CrossRef]
78. Cheuvront, S.N.; Carter, R.; Castellani, J.W.; Sawka, M.N. Hypohydration impairs endurance exercise performance in temperate but not cold air. *J. Appl. Physiol.* **2005**, *99*, 1972–1976. [CrossRef]
79. MacLeod, H.; Sunderland, C. Previous-day hypohydration impairs skill performance in elite female field hockey players. *Scand J. Med. Sci. Sports* **2012**, *22*, 430–438. [CrossRef]
80. Kenefick, R.W.; Cheuvront, S.N.; Palombo, L.J.; Ely, B.R.; Sawka, M.N. Skin temperature modifies the impact of hypohydration on aerobic performance. *J. Appl. Physiol.* **2010**, *109*, 79–86. [CrossRef]
81. Montain, S.J.; Sawka, M.N.; Latzka, W.A.; Valeri, C.R. Thermal and cardiovascular strain from hypohydration: Influence of exercise intensity. *Int. J. Sports Med.* **1998**, *19*, 87–91. [CrossRef]
82. Merry, T.L.; Ainslie, P.N.; Cotter, J.D. Effects of aerobic fitness on hypohydration-induced physiological strain and exercise impairment. *Acta Physiol.* **2010**, *198*, 179–190. [CrossRef]
83. Bardis, C.N.; Kavouras, S.A.; Arnaoutis, G.; Panagiotakos, D.B.; Sidossis, L.S. Mild dehydration and cycling performance during 5-kilometer hill climbing. *J. Athl. Train.* **2013**, *48*, 741–747. [CrossRef]
84. Bardis, C.N.; Kavouras, S.A.; Kosti, L.; Markousi, M.; Sidossis, L.S. Mild hypohydration decreases cycling performance in the heat. *Med. Sci. Sports Exerc.* **2013**, *45*, 1782–1789. [CrossRef]
85. Sawka, M.N.; Cheuvront, S.N.; Kenefick, R.W. Hypohydration and Human Performance: Impact of Environment and Physiological Mechanisms. *Sports Med.* **2015**, *45*, 51. [CrossRef]

86. Judelson, D.A.; Maresh, C.M.; Farrell, M.J.; Yamamoto, L.M.; Armstrong, L.E.; Kraemer, W.J.; Volek, J.S.; Spiering, B.A.; Casa, D.J.; Anderson, J.M. Effect of hydration state on strength, power, and resistance exercise performance. *Med. Sci. Sports Exerc.* **2007**, *39*, 1817–1824. [CrossRef]
87. Tan, X.R.; Low, I.C.C.; Stephenson, M.C.; Kok, T.; Nolte, H.W.; Soong, T.W.; Lee, J.K.W. Altered Brain Structure with Preserved Cortical Motor Activity Following Exertional Hypohydration: A MRI study. *J. Appl. Physiol.* **2019**. [CrossRef]
88. Gamble, A.S.; Bigg, J.L.; Vermeulen, T.F.; Boville, S.M.; Eskedjian, G.S.; Jannas-Vela, S.; Whitfield, J.; Palmer, M.S.; Spriet, L.L. Estimated Sweat Loss, Fluid and CHO Intake, and Sodium Balance of Male Major Junior, AHL, and NHL Players During On-Ice Practices. *Int. J. Sport Nutr. Exerc. Metab.* **2019**, 1–25. [CrossRef]
89. Ely, B.R.; Sollanek, K.J.; Cheuvront, S.N.; Lieberman, H.R.; Kenefick, R.W. Hypohydration and acute thermal stress affect mood state but not cognition or dynamic postural balance. *Eur. J. Appl. Physiol.* **2013**, *113*, 1027–1034. [CrossRef]
90. Moyen, N.E.; Ganio, M.S.; Wiersma, L.D.; Kavouras, S.A.; Gray, M.; McDermott, B.P.; Adams, J.D.; Binns, A.P.; Judelson, D.A.; McKenzie, A.L.; et al. Hydration status affects mood state and pain sensation during ultra-endurance cycling. *J. Sports Sci.* **2015**, *33*, 1962–1969. [CrossRef]
91. Zhang, N.; Du, S.M.; Zhang, J.F.; Ma, G.S. Effects of Dehydration and Rehydration on Cognitive Performance and Mood among Male College Students in Cangzhou, China: A Self-Controlled Trial. *Int. J. Environ. Res. Public Health* **2019**, *16*, 1891. [CrossRef]
92. Benton, D.; Jenkins, K.T.; Watkins, H.T.; Young, H.A. Minor degree of hypohydration adversely influences cognition: A mediator analysis. *Am. J. Clin. Nutr.* **2016**, *104*, 603–612. [CrossRef]
93. Greenleaf, J.E.; Castle, B.L. Exercise temperature regulation in man during hypohydration and hyperhydration. *J. Appl. Physiol.* **1971**, *30*, 847–853. [CrossRef]
94. Candas, V.; Libert, J.P.; Brandenberger, G.; Sagot, J.C.; Kahn, J.M. Thermal and circulatory responses during prolonged exercise at different levels of hydration. *J. Physiol. (Paris)* **1988**, *83*, 11–18.
95. Cadarette, B.S.; Sawka, M.N.; Toner, M.M.; Pandolf, K.B. Aerobic fitness and the hypohydration response to exercise-heat stress. *Aviat. Space Environ. Med.* **1984**, *55*, 507–512.
96. Sawka, M.N.; Gonzalez, R.R.; Young, A.J.; Muza, S.R.; Pandolf, K.B.; Latzka, W.A.; Dennis, R.C.; Valeri, C.R. Polycythemia and hydration: Effects on thermoregulation and blood volume during exercise-heat stress. *Am. J. Physiol.* **1988**, *255*, 456. [CrossRef]
97. Montain, S.J.; Latzka, W.A.; Sawka, M.N. Control of thermoregulatory sweating is altered by hydration level and exercise intensity. *J. Appl. Physiol.* **1995**, *79*, 1434–1439. [CrossRef]
98. Buono, M.J.; Wall, A.J. Effect of hypohydration on core temperature during exercise in temperate and hot environments. *Eur. J. Physiol.* **2000**, *440*, 476–480. [CrossRef]
99. Meade, R.D.; Notley, S.R.; D'Souza, A.W.; Dervis, S.; Boulay, P.; Sigal, R.J.; Kenny, G.P. Interactive effects of age and hydration state on human thermoregulatory function during exercise in hot-dry conditions. *Acta Physiol.* **2018**, e13226. [CrossRef]
100. Kenefick, R.W.; Sollanek, K.J.; Charkoudian, N.; Sawka, M.N. Impact of skin temperature and hydration on plasma volume responses during exercise. *J. Appl. Physiol.* **2014**, *117*, 413–420. [CrossRef]
101. Raines, J.; Snow, R.; Nichols, D.; Aisbett, B. Fluid intake, hydration, work physiology of wildfire fighters working in the heat over consecutive days. *Ann. Occup. Hyg.* **2015**, *59*, 554–565.
102. Horowitz, M.; Kaspler, P.; Simon, E.; Gerstberger, R. Heat acclimation and hypohydration: Involvement of central angiotensin II receptors in thermoregulation. *Am. J. Physiol.* **1999**, *277*, 47. [CrossRef]
103. Sawka, M.N.; Latzka, W.A.; Matott, R.P.; Montain, S.J. Hydration effects on temperature regulation. *Int. J. Sports Med.* **1998**, *19*, 108. [CrossRef]
104. Sawka, M.N.; Young, A.J.; Francesconi, R.P.; Muza, S.R.; Pandolf, K.B. Thermoregulatory and blood responses during exercise at graded hypohydration levels. *J. Appl. Physiol.* **1985**, *59*, 1394–1401. [CrossRef]
105. Moyen, N.E.; Burchfield, J.M.; Butts, C.L.; Glenn, J.M.; Tucker, M.A.; Treece, K.; Smith, A.J.; McDermott, B.P.; Ganio, M.S. Effects of obesity and mild hypohydration on local sweating and cutaneous vascular responses during passive heat stress in females. *Appl. Physiol. Nutr. Metab.* **2016**, *41*, 879–887. [CrossRef]
106. Tokizawa, K.; Yasuhara, S.; Nakamura, M.; Uchida, Y.; Crawshaw, L.I.; Nagashima, K. Mild hypohydration induced by exercise in the heat attenuates autonomic thermoregulatory responses to the heat, but not thermal pleasantness in humans. *Physiol. Behav.* **2010**, *100*, 340–345. [CrossRef]

107. Ikegawa, S.; Kamijo, Y.; Okazaki, K.; Masuki, S.; Okada, Y.; Nose, H. Effects of hypohydration on thermoregulation during exercise before and after 5-day aerobic training in a warm environment in young men. *J. Appl. Physiol.* **2011**, *110*, 972–980. [CrossRef]
108. Tucker, M.A.; Caldwell, A.R.; Butts, C.L.; Robinson, F.B.; Reynebeau, H.C.; Kavouras, S.A.; McDermott, B.P.; Washington, T.A.; Turner, R.C.; Ganio, M.S. Effect of hypohydration on thermoregulatory responses in men with low and high body fat exercising in the heat. *J. Appl. Physiol.* **2017**, *122*, 142–152. [CrossRef]
109. Roussel, R.; Fezeu, L.; Bouby, N.; Balkau, B.; Lantieri, O.; Alhenc-Gelas, F.; Marre, M.; Bankir, L. Low water intake and risk for new-onset hyperglycemia. *Diabetes Care* **2011**, *34*, 2551–2554. [CrossRef]
110. Manz, F. Hydration and Disease. *J. Am. Coll Nutr.* **2007**, *26*, 541S. [CrossRef]
111. Yeboah, J.; Folsom, A.R.; Burke, G.L.; Johnson, C.; Polak, J.F.; Post, W.; Lima, J.A.; Crouse, J.R.; Herrington, D.M. Predictive value of brachial flow-mediated dilation for incident cardiovascular events in a population-based study: The multi-ethnic study of atherosclerosis. *Circulation* **2009**, *120*, 502–509. [CrossRef]
112. Yeboah, J.; Crouse, J.R.; Hsu, F.; Burke, G.L.; Herrington, D.M. Brachial flow-mediated dilation predicts incident cardiovascular events in older adults: The Cardiovascular Health Study. *Circulation* **2007**, *115*, 2390–2397. [CrossRef]
113. Lind, L.; Berglund, L.; Larsson, A.; Sundström, J. Endothelial function in resistance and conduit arteries and 5-year risk of cardiovascular disease. *Circulation* **2011**, *123*, 1545–1551. [CrossRef]
114. Widlansky, M.E.; Gokce, N.; Keaney, J.F.; Vita, J.A. The clinical implications of endothelial dysfunction. *J. Am. Coll. Cardiol.* **2003**, *42*, 1149–1160. [CrossRef]
115. Benjamin, E.J.; Muntner, P.; Alonso, A.; Bittencourt, M.S.; Callaway, C.W.; Carson, A.P.; Chamberlain, A.M.; Chang, A.R.; Cheng, S.; Das, S.R.; et al. Heart Disease and Stroke Statistics-2019 Update: A Report From the American Heart Association. *Circulation* **2019**, *139*, e56–e528. [CrossRef]
116. Parati, G.; Pomidossi, G.; Albini, F.; Malaspina, D.; Mancia, G. Relationship of 24-hour blood pressure mean and variability to severity of target-organ damage in hypertension. *J. Hypertens.* **1987**, *5*, 93–98. [CrossRef]
117. Tatasciore, A.; Renda, G.; Zimarino, M.; Soccio, M.; Bilo, G.; Parati, G.; Schillaci, G.; De Caterina, R. Awake systolic blood pressure variability correlates with target-organ damage in hypertensive subjects. *Hypertension* **2007**, *50*, 325–332. [CrossRef]
118. Veloudi, P.; Blizzard, C.L.; Head, G.A.; Abhayaratna, W.P.; Stowasser, M.; Sharman, J.E. Blood Pressure Variability and Prediction of Target Organ Damage in Patients with Uncomplicated Hypertension. *Am. J. Hypertens* **2016**, *29*, 1046–1054. [CrossRef]
119. Mancia, G.; Bombelli, M.; Facchetti, R.; Madotto, F.; Corrao, G.; Trevano, F.Q.; Grassi, G.; Sega, R. Long-term prognostic value of blood pressure variability in the general population: Results of the Pressioni Arteriose Monitorate e Loro Associazioni Study. *Hypertension* **2007**, *49*, 1265–1270. [CrossRef]
120. Pringle, E.; Phillips, C.; Thijs, L.; Davidson, C.; Staessen, J.A.; de Leeuw, P.W.; Jaaskivi, M.; Nachev, C.; Parati, G.; O'Brien, E.T.; et al. Systolic blood pressure variability as a risk factor for stroke and cardiovascular mortality in the elderly hypertensive population. *J. Hypertens.* **2003**, *21*, 2251–2257. [CrossRef]
121. Fleg, J.L.; Evans, G.W.; Margolis, K.L.; Barzilay, J.; Basile, J.N.; Bigger, J.T.; Cutler, J.A.; Grimm, R.; Pedley, C.; Peterson, K.; et al. Orthostatic Hypotension in the ACCORD (Action to Control Cardiovascular Risk in Diabetes) Blood Pressure Trial: Prevalence, Incidence, and Prognostic Significance. *Hypertension* **2016**, *68*, 888–895. [CrossRef]
122. Veronese, N.; De Rui, M.; Bolzetta, F.; Zambon, S.; Corti, M.C.; Baggio, G.; Toffanello, E.D.; Maggi, S.; Crepaldi, G.; Perissinotto, E.; et al. Orthostatic Changes in Blood Pressure and Mortality in the Elderly: The Pro.V.A Study. *Am. J. Hypertens.* **2015**, *28*, 1248–1256. [CrossRef]
123. Tzemos, N.; Lim, P.O.; Mackenzie, I.S.; MacDonald, T.M. Exaggerated Exercise Blood Pressure Response and Future Cardiovascular Disease. *J. Clin. Hyper.* **2015**, *17*, 837–844. [CrossRef]
124. Miyai, N.; Arita, M.; Miyashita, K.; Morioka, I.; Shiraishi, T.; Nishio, I. Blood pressure response to heart rate during exercise test and risk of future hypertension. *Hypertension* **2002**, *39*, 761–766. [CrossRef]
125. Matthews, K.A.; Woodall, K.L.; Allen, M.T. Cardiovascular reactivity to stress predicts future blood pressure status. *Hypertension* **1993**, *22*, 479–485. [CrossRef]
126. Schultz, M.G.; Otahal, P.; Picone, D.S.; Sharman, J.E. Clinical Relevance of Exaggerated Exercise Blood Pressure. *J. Am. Coll. Cardiol.* **2015**, *66*, 1843–1845. [CrossRef]

127. Côté, C.E.; Rhéaume, C.; Poirier, P.; Després, J.P.; Alméras, N. Deteriorated Cardiometabolic Risk Profile in Individuals with Excessive Blood Pressure Response to Submaximal Exercise. *Am. J. Hypertens.* **2019**. [CrossRef]
128. Costa, R.J.S.; Camoes-Costa, V.; Snipe, R.M.J.; Dixon, D.; Russo, I.; Huschtscha, Z. The impact of exercise-induced hypohydration on gastrointestinal integrity, function, symptoms, and systemic endotoxin and inflammatory profile. *J. Appl. Physiol.* **2019**. [CrossRef]
129. Martin, J.V.; Liberati, D.M.; Diebel, L.N. Excess sodium is deleterious on endothelial and glycocalyx barrier function: A microfluidic study. *J. Trauma Acute Care Surg.* **2018**, *85*, 128–134. [CrossRef]
130. Tremblay, J.C.; Hoiland, R.L.; Howe, C.A.; Coombs, G.B.; Vizcardo-Galindo, G.A.; Figueroa-Mujíca, R.J.; Bermudez, D.; Gibbons, T.D.; Stacey, B.S.; Bailey, D.M.; et al. Global REACH 2018: High Blood Viscosity and Hemoglobin Concentration Contribute to Reduced Flow-Mediated Dilation in High-Altitude Excessive Erythrocytosis. *Hypertension* **2019**, *73*, 1327–1335. [CrossRef]
131. Parkhurst, K.L.; Lin, H.; Devan, A.E.; Barnes, J.N.; Tarumi, T.; Tanaka, H. Contribution of blood viscosity in the assessment of flow-mediated dilation and arterial stiffness. *Vasc. Med.* **2012**, *17*, 231–234. [CrossRef]
132. Rognmo, O.; Bjørnstad, T.H.; Kahrs, C.; Tjønna, A.E.; Bye, A.; Haram, P.M.; Stølen, T.; Slørdahl, S.A.; Wisløff, U. Endothelial function in highly endurance-trained men: Effects of acute exercise. *J. Strength Cond. Res.* **2008**, *22*, 535–542. [CrossRef]
133. Vlachopoulos, C.; Aznaouridis, K.; Stefanadis, C. Prediction of cardiovascular events and all-cause mortality with arterial stiffness: A systematic review and meta-analysis. *J. Am. Coll. Cardiol.* **2010**, *55*, 1318–1327. [CrossRef]
134. McConell, G.K.; Burge, C.M.; Skinner, S.L.; Hargreaves, M. Influence of ingested fluid volume on physiological responses during prolonged exercise. *Acta Physiol. Scand.* **1997**, *160*, 149–156. [CrossRef]
135. Brake, D.J.; Bates, G.P. Fluid losses and hydration status of industrial workers under thermal stress working extended shifts. *Occup. Environ. Med.* **2003**, *60*, 90–96. [CrossRef]
136. Senay, L.C. Temperature regulation and hypohydration: A singular view. *J. Appl. Physiol. Respir. Environ. Exerc. Physiol.* **1979**, *47*, 1–7. [CrossRef]
137. Sawka, M.N.; Montain, S.J.; Latzka, W.A. Hydration effects on thermoregulation and performance in the heat. *Comp. Biochem. Physiol. Part. A Mol. Integr. Physiol.* **2001**, *128*, 679–690. [CrossRef]
138. Kenefick, R.W.; Cheuvront, S.N. Physiological adjustments to hypohydration: Impact on thermoregulation. *Auton. Neurosci.* **2016**, *196*, 47–51. [CrossRef]
139. Hall, J.E. *Guyton and Hall Textbook of Medical Physiology*, 13th ed.; Elsevier: Amsterdam, The Nederland, 2016.
140. Endemann, D.H.; Schiffrin, E.L. Endothelial dysfunction. *J. Am. Soc. Nephrol.* **2004**, *15*, 1983–1992. [CrossRef]
141. Diep, Q.N.; Amiri, F.; Touyz, R.M.; Cohn, J.S.; Endemann, D.; Neves, M.F.; Schiffrin, E.L. PPARalpha activator effects on Ang II-induced vascular oxidative stress and inflammation. *Hypertension* **2002**, *40*, 866–871. [CrossRef]
142. Diep, Q.N.; El Mabrouk, M.; Cohn, J.S.; Endemann, D.; Amiri, F.; Virdis, A.; Neves, M.F.; Schiffrin, E.L. Structure, endothelial function, cell growth, and inflammation in blood vessels of angiotensin II-infused rats: Role of peroxisome proliferator-activated receptor-gamma. *Circulation* **2002**, *105*, 2296–2302. [CrossRef]
143. Rajagopalan, S.; Kurz, S.; Münzel, T.; Tarpey, M.; Freeman, B.A.; Griendling, K.K.; Harrison, D.G. Angiotensin II-mediated hypertension in the rat increases vascular superoxide production via membrane NADH/NADPH oxidase activation. Contribution to alterations of vasomotor tone. *J. Clin. Invest.* **1996**, *97*, 1916–1923. [CrossRef]
144. Robinson, A.T.; Fancher, I.S.; Sudhahar, V.; Bian, J.T.; Cook, M.D.; Mahmoud, A.M.; Ali, M.M.; Ushio-Fukai, M.; Brown, M.D.; Fukai, T.; et al. Short-term regular aerobic exercise reduces oxidative stress produced by acute in the adipose microvasculature. *Am. J. Physiol. Heart Circ. Physiol.* **2017**, *312*, H906. [CrossRef]
145. Touyz, R.M.; Schiffrin, E.L. Ang II-stimulated superoxide production is mediated via phospholipase D in human vascular smooth muscle cells. *Hypertension* **1999**, *34*, 976–982. [CrossRef]
146. Touyz, R.M.; Chen, X.; Tabet, F.; Yao, G.; He, G.; Quinn, M.T.; Pagano, P.J.; Schiffrin, E.L. Expression of a functionally active gp91phox-containing neutrophil-type NAD(P)H oxidase in smooth muscle cells from human resistance arteries: Regulation by angiotensin II. *Circ. Res.* **2002**, *90*, 1205–1213. [CrossRef]
147. Schwimmer, H.; Gerstberger, R.; Horowitz, M. Nitric oxide and angiotensin II: Neuromodulation of thermoregulation during combined heat and hypohydration stress. *Brain Res.* **2004**, *1006*, 177–189. [CrossRef]

148. Koh, K.K.; Ahn, J.Y.; Han, S.H.; Kim, D.S.; Jin, D.K.; Kim, H.S.; Shin, M.; Ahn, T.H.; Choi, I.S.; Shin, E.K. Pleiotropic effects of angiotensin II receptor blocker in hypertensive patients. *J. Am. Coll. Cardiol.* **2003**, *42*, 905–910. [CrossRef]
149. Willemsen, J.M.; Westerink, J.W.; Dallinga-Thie, G.M.; van Zonneveld, A.; Gaillard, C.A.; Rabelink, T.J.; de Koning Eelco, J.P. Angiotensin II type 1 receptor blockade improves hyperglycemia-induced endothelial dysfunction and reduces proinflammatory cytokine release from leukocytes. *J. Cardiovasc. Pharmacol.* **2007**, *49*, 6–12. [CrossRef]
150. Preumont, N.; Unger, P.; Goldman, S.; Berkenboom, G. Effect of long-term angiotensin II type I receptor antagonism on peripheral and coronary vasomotion. *Cardiovasc. Drugs Ther.* **2004**, *18*, 197–202. [CrossRef]
151. Bellien, J.; Iacob, M.; Eltchaninoff, H.; Bourkaib, R.; Thuillez, C.; Joannides, R. AT1 receptor blockade prevents the decrease in conduit artery flow-mediated dilatation during NOS inhibition in humans. *Clin. Sci.* **2007**, *112*, 393–401. [CrossRef]
152. Warnholtz, A.; Ostad, M.A.; Heitzer, T.; Thuneke, F.; Fröhlich, M.; Tschentscher, P.; Schwedhelm, E.; Böger, R.; Meinertz, T.; Munzel, T. AT1-receptor blockade with irbesartan improves peripheral but not coronary endothelial dysfunction in patients with stable coronary artery disease. *Atherosclerosis* **2007**, *194*, 439–445. [CrossRef]
153. Watanabe, Y.; Kikuchi, T.; Mitsuhashi, T.; Kimura, H.; Tsuchida, Y.; Otsuka, K. Administration of angiotensin receptor II blockade improves vascular function, urinary albumin excretion, and left ventricular hypertrophy in low-risk essential hypertensive patients receiving antihypertensive treatment with calcium channel blockers. *Clin. Exp. Hypertens.* **2013**, *35*, 87–94. [CrossRef]
154. Mizuno, Y.; Jacob, R.F.; Mason, R.P. Effects of calcium channel and renin-angiotensin system blockade on intravascular and neurohormonal mechanisms of hypertensive vascular disease. *Am. J. Hypertens.* **2008**, *21*, 1076–1085. [CrossRef]
155. Płonowski, A.; Szymańska-Debińska, T.; Radzikowska, M.; Baranowska, B.; Woźniewicz, B. Are mu-opioid receptors involved in the control of endothelin-1 release from the pituitary gland in normal and dehydrated rats? *Regul. Pept.* **1997**, *69*, 89–94. [CrossRef]
156. Maeda, S.; Miyauchi, T.; Waku, T.; Koda, Y.; Kono, I.; Goto, K.; Matsuda, M. Plasma endothelin-1 level in athletes after exercise in a hot environment: Exercise-induced dehydration contributes to increases in plasma endothelin-1. *Life Sci.* **1996**, *58*, 1259–1268. [CrossRef]
157. Bellien, J.; Iacob, M.; Monteil, C.; Rémy-Jouet, I.; Roche, C.; Duflot, T.; Vendeville, C.; Gutierrez, L.; Thuillez, C.; Richard, V.; et al. Physiological role of endothelin-1 in flow-mediated vasodilatation in humans and impact of cardiovascular risk factors. *J. Hypertens* **2017**, *35*, 1204–1212. [CrossRef]
158. Nishiyama, S.K.; Zhao, J.; Wray, D.W.; Richardson, R.S. Vascular function and endothelin-1: Tipping the balance between vasodilation and vasoconstriction. *J. Appl. Physiol.* **2017**, *122*, 354–360. [CrossRef]
159. Perry, B.G.; Bear, T.L.K.; Lucas, S.J.E.; Mündel, T. Mild dehydration modifies the cerebrovascular response to the cold pressor test. *Exp. Physiol.* **2016**, *101*, 135–142. [CrossRef]
160. Adams, J.M.; McCarthy, J.J.; Stocker, S.D. Excess dietary salt alters angiotensinergic regulation of neurons in the rostral ventrolateral medulla. *Hypertension* **2008**, *52*, 932–937. [CrossRef]
161. Holbein, W.W.; Bardgett, M.E.; Toney, G.M. Blood pressure is maintained during dehydration by hypothalamic paraventricular nucleus-driven tonic sympathetic nerve activity. *J. Physiol.* **2014**, *592*, 3783–3799. [CrossRef]
162. Stocker, S.D.; Lang, S.M.; Simmonds, S.S.; Wenner, M.M.; Farquhar, W.B. Cerebrospinal Fluid Hypernatremia Elevates Sympathetic Nerve Activity and Blood Pressure via the Rostral Ventrolateral Medulla. *Hypertension* **2015**, *66*, 1184–1190. [CrossRef]
163. Scrogin, K.E.; Grygielko, E.T.; Brooks, V.L. Osmolality: A physiological long-term regulator of lumbar sympathetic nerve activity and arterial pressure. *Am. J. Physiol.* **1999**, *276*, 1579. [CrossRef]
164. Colombari, D.S.A.; Colombari, E.; Freiria-Oliveira, A.H.; Antunes, V.R.; Yao, S.T.; Hindmarch, C.; Ferguson, A.V.; Fry, M.; Murphy, D.; Paton, J.F.R. Switching control of sympathetic activity from forebrain to hindbrain in chronic dehydration. *J. Physiol.* **2011**, *589*, 4457–4471. [CrossRef]
165. Veitenheimer, B.J.; Engeland, W.C.; Guzman, P.A.; Fink, G.D.; Osborn, J.W. Effect of global and regional sympathetic blockade on arterial pressure during water deprivation in conscious rats. *Am. J. Physiol. Heart Circ. Physiol.* **2012**, *303*, 1022. [CrossRef]

166. Grassi, G.; Seravalle, G.; Brambilla, G.; Pini, C.; Alimento, M.; Facchetti, R.; Spaziani, D.; Cuspidi, C.; Mancia, G. Marked sympathetic activation and baroreflex dysfunction in true resistant hypertension. *Int. J. Cardiol.* **2014**, *177*, 1020–1025. [CrossRef]
167. James, M.A.; Robinson, T.G.; Panerai, R.B.; Potter, J.F. Arterial baroreceptor-cardiac reflex sensitivity in the elderly. *Hypertension* **1996**, *28*, 953–960. [CrossRef]
168. Ebert, T.J.; Morgan, B.J.; Barney, J.A.; Denahan, T.; Smith, J.J. Effects of aging on baroreflex regulation of sympathetic activity in humans. *Am. J. Physiol.* **1992**, *263*, 798. [CrossRef]
169. Filomena, J.; Riba-Llena, I.; Vinyoles, E.; Tovar, J.L.; Mundet, X.; Castane, X.; Vilar, A.; Lopez-Rueda, A.; Jimenez-Balado, J.; Cartanya, A.; et al. ISSYS Investigators Short-Term Blood Pressure Variability Relates to the Presence of Subclinical Brain Small Vessel Disease in Primary Hypertension. *Hypertension* **2015**, *66*, 634–640. [CrossRef]
170. Mancia, G.; Parati, G.; Hennig, M.; Flatau, B.; Omboni, S.; Glavina, F.; Costa, B.; Scherz, R.; Bond, G.; Zanchetti, A. Relation between blood pressure variability and carotid artery damage in hypertension: Baseline data from the European Lacidipine Study on Atherosclerosis (ELSA). *J. Hypertens.* **2001**, *19*, 1981–1989. [CrossRef]
171. Madden, J.M.; O'Flynn, A.M.; Dolan, E.; Fitzgerald, A.P.; Kearney, P.M. Short-term blood pressure variability over 24 h and target organ damage in middle-aged men and women. *J. Hum. Hypertens.* **2015**, *29*, 719–725. [CrossRef]
172. Palatini, P.; Penzo, M.; Racioppa, A.; Zugno, E.; Guzzardi, G.; Anaclerio, M.; Pessina, A.C. Clinical relevance of nighttime blood pressure and of daytime blood pressure variability. *Arch. Intern. Med.* **1992**, *152*, 1855–1860. [CrossRef]
173. Ogawa, Y.; Iwasaki, K.; Aoki, K.; Saitoh, T.; Kato, J.; Ogawa, S. Dynamic cerebral autoregulation after mild dehydration to simulate microgravity effects. *Aviat. Space Environ. Med.* **2009**, *80*, 443–447. [CrossRef]
174. Matsukawa, T.; Gotoh, E.; Minamisawa, K.; Kihara, M.; Ueda, S.; Shionoiri, H.; Ishii, M. Effects of intravenous infusions of angiotensin II on muscle sympathetic nerve activity in humans. *Am. J. Physiol.* **1991**, *261*, 690. [CrossRef]
175. Trapani, A.J.; Undesser, K.P.; Keeton, T.K.; Bishop, V.S. Neurohumoral interactions in conscious dehydrated rabbit. *Am. J. Physiol.* **1988**, *254*, 338. [CrossRef]
176. Charkoudian, N.; Halliwill, J.R.; Morgan, B.J.; Eisenach, J.H.; Joyner, M.J. Influences of hydration on post-exercise cardiovascular control in humans. *J. Physiol.* **2003**, *552*, 635–644. [CrossRef]
177. Andrews, C.E., Jr.; Brenner, B.M. Relative contributions of arginine vasopressin and angiotensin II to maintenance of systemic arterial pressure in the anesthetized water-deprived rat. *Circ. Res.* **1981**, *48*, 254–258. [CrossRef]
178. Carroll, H.A.; James, L.J. Hydration, Arginine Vasopressin, and Glucoregulatory Health in Humans: A Critical Perspective. *Nutrients* **2019**, *11*, 1201. [CrossRef]
179. Johnston, C. Vasopressin in Circulatory Control and Hypertension. *J. Hyper.* **1985**, *3*, 557–569. [CrossRef]
180. Liard, J.F. Vasopressin in cardiovascular control: Role of circulating vasopressin. *Clin. Sci.* **1984**, *67*, 473–481. [CrossRef]
181. Flynn, F.W.; Stricker, E.M. Hypovolemia stimulates intraoral intake of water and NaCl solution in intact rats but not in chronic decerebrate rats. *Physiol. Behav.* **2003**, *80*, 281–287. [CrossRef]
182. Collister, J.P.; Nahey, D.B.; Hendel, M.D.; Brooks, V.L. Roles of the subfornical organ and area postrema in arterial pressure increases induced by 48-h water deprivation in normal rats. *Physiol. Rep.* **2014**, *2*, e00191. [CrossRef]
183. Tyagi, M.G.; Thomas, M. Enhanced cardiovascular reactivity to desmopressin in water-restricted rats: Facilitatory role of immunosuppression. *Methods Find. Exp. Clin. Pharmacol.* **1999**, *21*, 619–624.
184. Hiwatari, M.; Johnston, C.I. Involvement of vasopressin in the cardiovascular effects of intracerebroventricularly administered alpha 1-adrenoceptor agonists in the conscious rat. *J. Hyper.* **1985**, *3*, 613. [CrossRef]
185. Brooks, V.L. Vasopressin and ANG II in the control of ACTH secretion and arterial and atrial pressures. *Am. J. Physiol.* **1989**, *256*, 339. [CrossRef]
186. Schreihofer, A.M.; Stricker, E.M.; Sved, A.F. Chronic nucleus tractus solitarius lesions do not prevent hypovolemia-induced vasopressin secretion in rats. *Am. J. Physiol.* **1994**, *267*, 965. [CrossRef]

187. Fejes-Tóth, G.; Náray-Fejes-Tóth, A.; Ratge, D. Evidence against role of antidiuretic hormone in support of blood pressure during dehydration. *Am. J. Physiol.* **1985**, *249*. [CrossRef]
188. Huch, K.M.; Wall, B.M.; Mangold, T.A.; Bobal, M.A.; Cooke, C.R. Hemodynamic response to vasopressin in dehydrated human subjects. *J. Investig. Med.* **1998**, *46*, 312–318.
189. Wenner, M.M.; Stachenfeld, N.S. Blood pressure and water regulation: Understanding sex hormone effects within and between men and women. *J. Physiol.* **2012**, *590*, 5949–5961. [CrossRef]
190. Stachenfeld, N.S.; Silva, C.; Keefe, D.L.; Kokoszka, C.A.; Nadel, E.R. Effects of oral contraceptives on body fluid regulation. *J. Appl. Physiol.* **1999**, *87*, 1016–1025. [CrossRef]
191. Minson, C.T.; Halliwill, J.R.; Young, T.M.; Joyner, M.J. Influence of the menstrual cycle on sympathetic activity, baroreflex sensitivity, and vascular transduction in young women. *Circulation* **2000**, *101*, 862–868. [CrossRef]
192. Carter, J.R.; Lawrence, J.E.; Klein, J.C. Menstrual cycle alters sympathetic neural responses to orthostatic stress in young, eumenorrheic women. *Am. J. Physiol. Endocrinol. Metab.* **2009**, *297*, 85. [CrossRef]
193. Fu, Q.; Okazaki, K.; Shibata, S.; Shook, R.P.; VanGunday, T.B.; Galbreath, M.M.; Reelick, M.F.; Levine, B.D. Menstrual cycle effects on sympathetic neural responses to upright tilt. *J. Physiol.* **2009**, *587*, 2019–2031. [CrossRef]
194. Baker, S.E.; Limberg, J.K.; Ranadive, S.M.; Joyner, M.J. Neurovascular control of blood pressure is influenced by aging, sex, and sex hormones. *Am. J. Physiol. Regul. Integr. Comp. Physiol.* **2016**, *311*, R1275. [CrossRef]
195. Harvey, R.E.; Hart, E.C.; Charkoudian, N.; Curry, T.B.; Carter, J.R.; Fu, Q.; Minson, C.T.; Joyner, M.J.; Barnes, J.N. Oral Contraceptive Use, Muscle Sympathetic Nerve Activity, and Systemic Hemodynamics in Young Women. *Hypertension* **2015**, *66*, 590–597. [CrossRef]
196. Claydon, V.E.; Younis, N.R.; Hainsworth, R. Phase of the menstrual cycle does not affect orthostatic tolerance in healthy women. *Clin. Auton. Res.* **2006**, *16*, 98–104. [CrossRef]
197. Lawrence, J.E.; Ray, C.A.; Carter, J.R. Vestibulosympathetic reflex during the early follicular and midluteal phases of the menstrual cycle. *Am. J. Physiol. Endocrinol. Metab.* **2008**, *294*, 1046. [CrossRef]
198. Robinson, A.T.; Babcock, M.C.; Watso, J.C.; Brian, M.S.; Migdal, K.U.; Wenner, M.M.; Farquhar, W.B. Relation between resting sympathetic outflow & vasoconstrictor responses to sympathetic nerve bursts: Sex differences in healthy young adults. *Am. J. Physiol. Regul. Integr. Comp. Physiol.* **2019**. [CrossRef]
199. Thompson, W.O.; Thompson, P.K.; Dailey, M.E. The Effect of Posture upon the Composition and Volume of the Blood in Man. *J. Clin. Invest.* **1928**, *5*, 573–604. [CrossRef]
200. Fedorowski, A.; Burri, P.; Melander, O. Orthostatic hypotension in genetically related hypertensive and normotensive individuals. *J. Hypertens.* **2009**, *27*, 976–982. [CrossRef]
201. Ricci, F.; De Caterina, R.; Fedorowski, A. Orthostatic Hypotension: Epidemiology, Prognosis, and Treatment. *J. Am. Coll. Cardiol.* **2015**, *66*, 848–860. [CrossRef]
202. Sheldon, R.S.; Grubb, B.P.; Olshansky, B.; Shen, W.; Calkins, H.; Brignole, M.; Raj, S.R.; Krahn, A.D.; Morillo, C.A.; Stewart, J.M.; et al. 2015 heart rhythm society expert consensus statement on the diagnosis and treatment of postural tachycardia syndrome, inappropriate sinus tachycardia, and vasovagal syncope. *Heart Rhythm.* **2015**, *12*. [CrossRef]
203. Cooke, W.H.; Ryan, K.L.; Convertino, V.A. Lower body negative pressure as a model to study progression to acute hemorrhagic shock in humans. *J. Appl. Physiol.* **2004**, *96*, 1249–1261. [CrossRef]
204. Hinojosa-Laborde, C.; Shade, R.E.; Muniz, G.W.; Bauer, C.; Goei, K.A.; Pidcoke, H.F.; Chung, K.K.; Cap, A.P.; Convertino, V.A. Validation of lower body negative pressure as an experimental model of hemorrhage. *J. Appl. Physiol.* **2014**, *116*, 406–415. [CrossRef]
205. Cheshire, W.P.; Goldstein, D.S. Autonomic uprising: The tilt table test in autonomic medicine. *Clin. Auton. Res.* **2019**, *29*, 215–230. [CrossRef]
206. Goswami, N.; Blaber, A.P.; Hinghofer-Szalkay, H.; Convertino, V.A. Lower Body Negative Pressure: Physiological Effects, Applications, and Implementation. *Physiol. Rev.* **2019**, *99*, 807–851. [CrossRef]
207. Thompson, C.A.; Tatro, D.L.; Ludwig, D.A.; Convertino, V.A. Baroreflex responses to acute changes in blood volume in humans. *Am. J. Physiol.* **1990**, *259*, 792. [CrossRef]
208. Cheuvront, S.N.; Ely, B.R.; Kenefick, R.W.; Buller, M.J.; Charkoudian, N.; Sawka, M.N. Hydration assessment using the cardiovascular response to standing. *Eur. J. Appl. Physiol.* **2012**, *112*, 4081–4089. [CrossRef]
209. Kimmerly, D.S.; Shoemaker, J.K. Hypovolemia and MSNA discharge patterns: Assessing and interpreting sympathetic responses. *Am. J. Physiol. Heart Circ. Physiol.* **2003**, *284*, 1198. [CrossRef]

210. Brooks, V.L.; Freeman, K.L.; Clow, K.A. Excitatory amino acids in rostral ventrolateral medulla support blood pressure during water deprivation in rats. *Am. J. Physiol. Heart Circ. Physiol.* **2004**, *286*, 1642. [CrossRef]
211. Brooks, V.L.; Qi, Y.; O'Donaughy, T.L. Increased osmolality of conscious water-deprived rats supports arterial pressure and sympathetic activity via a brain action. *Am. J. Physiol. Regul. Integr. Comp. Physiol.* **2005**, *288*, 1248. [CrossRef]
212. Watso, J.C.; Babcock, M.C.; Robinson, A.T.; Migdal, K.U.; Wenner, M.M.; Stocker, S.D.; Farquhar, W.B. Water deprivation does not augment sympathetic or pressor responses to sciatic afferent nerve stimulation in rats or to static exercise in humans. *J. Appl. Physiol.* **2019**. [CrossRef]
213. Riley, C.J.; Gavin, M. Physiological Changes to the Cardiovascular System at High Altitude and Its Effects on Cardiovascular Disease. *High Alt. Med. Biol.* **2017**, *18*, 102–113. [CrossRef]
214. Jain, S.C.; Bardhan, J.; Swamy, Y.V.; Krishna, B.; Nayar, H.S. Body fluid compartments in humans during acute high-altitude exposure. *Aviat. Space Environ. Med.* **19809**, *51*, 234–236.
215. annheimer, M.; Fusch, C.; Boning, D.; Thomas, A.; Engelhardt, M.; Schmidt, R. Changes of hematocrit and hemoglobin concentration in the cold Himalayan environment in dependence on total body fluid. *Sleep Breath.* **2010**, *14*, 193–199. [CrossRef]
216. Frayser, R.; Rennie, I.D.; Gray, G.W.; Houston, C.S. Hormonal and electrolyte response to exposure to 17,500 ft. *J. Appl. Physiol.* **1975**, *38*, 636–642. [CrossRef]

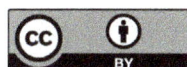

© 2019 by the authors. Licensee MDPI, Basel, Switzerland. This article is an open access article distributed under the terms and conditions of the Creative Commons Attribution (CC BY) license (http://creativecommons.org/licenses/by/4.0/).

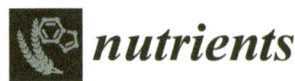

Article

Osmolality of Commercially Available Oral Rehydration Solutions: Impact of Brand, Storage Time, and Temperature

Kurt J. Sollanek [1],*, Robert W. Kenefick [2] and Samuel N. Cheuvront [3]

1. Department of Kinesiology, Sonoma State University, Rohnert Park, CA 94928, USA
2. Sports Science Consulting, LLC, Hopkinton, MA 01748, USA
3. Sports Science Synergy, LLC, Franklin, MA 02038, USA
* Correspondence: sollanek@sonoma.edu

Received: 7 April 2019; Accepted: 27 June 2019; Published: 29 June 2019

Abstract: Oral rehydration solutions (ORS) are specifically formulated with an osmolality to optimize fluid absorption. However, it is unclear how many ORS products comply with current World Health Organization (WHO) osmolality guidelines and the osmotic shelf-life stability is not known. Therefore, the purpose of this investigation was to examine the within and between ORS product osmolality variation in both pre-mixed and reconstituted powders. Additionally, the osmotic stability was examined over time. The osmolality of five different pre-mixed solutions and six powdered ORS products were measured. Pre-mixed solutions were stored at room temperatures and elevated temperatures (31 °C) for two months to examine osmotic shelf stability. Results demonstrated that only one pre-mixed ORS product was in compliance with the current guidelines both before and after the prolonged storage. Five of the six powdered ORS products were in compliance with minimal inter-packet variation observed within the given formulations. This investigation demonstrates that many commercially available pre-mixed ORS products do not currently adhere to the WHO recommended osmolality guidelines. Additionally, due to the presence of particular sugars and possibly other ingredients, the shelf-life stability of osmolality for certain ORS products may be questioned. These findings should be carefully considered in the design of future ORS products.

Keywords: oral rehydration therapy; dehydration; rehydration; euhydration; electrolytes

1. Introduction

Dehydration stemming from cholera and non-cholera (e.g., viruses, etc.) sources is a major cause of hospitalization and even mortality in many parts of the developed and less-developed world [1,2]. Key advances were made in the 1960s with the identification of electrolyte losses in diarrhea and the subsequent improvements seen in patients following administration of solutions containing glucose and electrolyte for oral rehydration known as oral rehydration therapy (ORT) [3–5]. Although these oral rehydration solutions (ORS) were successful in treating dehydration, the physiological mechanisms involving fluid absorption were not fully established until many years later, with the identification of the sodium–glucose transporters and many other dynamic mechanisms related to net fluid absorption [6–11]. Since these initial findings, many variations of the ORS have been created in an attempt to optimize efficacy [12,13].

Initially, the World Health Organization (WHO) and the United Nations Children's Fund (UNICEF) advocated for an ORS with specific amounts of electrolytes and a slightly hypertonic osmolality of 311 mmol/kg [5]. However, this solution lacked broad usage due to gastrointestinal upset, nausea, and concerns about hypernatremia [14]. Additionally, this solution did not appear to significantly reduce stool output [13]. Consequently, the WHO and UNICEF revised their recommended formulation advocating for an ORS with a reduced electrolyte content and a corresponding lower osmolality of 245 mmol/kg [15]. In addition, studies of luminal perfusion indicate that beverages should be hypotonic with an osmolality range of 200 to 260 mmol/kg, which has been shown to facilitate the greatest rate of net fluid absorption [16].

It is important to note that many commercial ORS formulations are available and are sold as either pre-mixed solutions or in powdered form. However, it is unclear how many commercially available ORS products meet the 245 mmol/kg (200–260 mmol/kg) recommendation since beverage osmolality is not required for nutrition labeling; hence, there is a need for independent verification of WHO ORS osmolality compliance. The shelf-life stability of beverage osmolality is also not known. However, the solid-state stability of ORS powder is ingredient and environment dependent [17]. For example, pre-mixed liquid ORS can be sent to underdeveloped areas that lack clean water [18] and subsequently expose these products to prolonged storage with high environmental temperatures [19]. These conditions could increase beverage osmolality due to temperature-dependent sugar hydrolysis reactions depending on the sugars and other product ingredients [20].

Based upon the aforementioned questions, the current investigation was designed to answer the following: 1) What is the baseline osmolality and variability within commercial pre-mixed ORS? 2) what is the baseline osmolality and variability within commercial powdered ORS after reconstitution? and 3) what is the impact of the storage time and temperature on the osmolality of pre-mixed ORS?

2. Materials and Methods

2.1. Drink and Drink Preparations

Commercially available ORS were obtained from online retailers and local stores. The current investigation examined four different pre-mixed ORS, one pre-mixed sports drink, and six powdered ORS. The following pre-mixed drinks were analyzed: Pedialyte® Classic mixed fruit flavor (Abbott Laboratories, Columbus, OH, USA), Pediatric Oral Electrolyte Solution fruit flavor (Up & Up, Target Brand, Minneapolis, MN, USA), Speedlyte® wild orange flavor (Einsof Biohealth, Dover, DE, USA), and enterade® AD ORS orange flavor (Entrinsic Health Solutions, Inc, Norwood, MA, USA). Gatorade® orange flavor (Pepsico, Chicago, IL, USA) was tested as a representative sports drink, since these are commonly used [21] or recommended [22] in the treatment of diarrhea, despite no marketing claims for this use. Product ingredients are listed in Table A1 (Appendix A). Lastly, six ORS powders were assessed: Hydralyte™ orange flavor (Hydralyte LLC, Thomastown, Victoria, Australia), Ceralyte® 70 lemon flavor (Cera Products Inc., Hilton Head Island, SC. USA), Dioralyte™ citrus flavor (Sanofi, Guildford, Surrey, UK), Dioralyte™ Relief raspberry flavor (Sanofi, Guildford, Surrey, UK), DripDrop® lemon flavor (DripDrop Hydration PBC, Oakland, CA, USA), and TRIORAL Oral rehydration salts natural flavor (Trifecta Pharmaceuticals, Ft. Lauderdale, FL, USA).

2.2. Study Overview

The current investigation was comprised of three separate studies. The first study tested the baseline osmolality and variation of pre-mixed ORS products. To accomplish the first study, three new bottles of each pre-mixed ORS were opened and the osmolality was immediately assessed. This allowed us to examine the variability that was present due to manufacturing (inter-bottle variability). Within each beverage product type, the products had the same expiration date.

The second study assessed the baseline osmolality and variation within carefully reconstituted ORS powders. All powdered ORS varieties were prepared with room temperature distilled water (Market Pantry, Target Brand, Minneapolis, MN, USA) according to the respective manufacturers' instructions. Three separate packets of each ORS were individually prepared and sampled to assess inter-packet variability and all three packets had the same expiration date. The dry powder from each packet was carefully diluted with the appropriate volumes of fluid using a calibrated scale. To enhance uniformity during drink preparation, each combination of powder and water was set to mix on the same Cimarec® magnetic stirring plate (Barnstead/Thermolyne, Dueuque, IA, USA) at an equivalent speed for precisely 5 min. Immediately thereafter, samples were pipetted into sampling cuvettes for osmolality assessment.

The third study examined the impact of storage time and temperature on beverage osmolality in the pre-mixed products. Details for this part of the investigation are depicted in Figure 1. At time point #0 (baseline), one new bottle of each pre-mixed ORS was opened and the osmolality was immediately assessed. The originally opened baseline bottle was then dispensed in 5 mL aliquots into 4 individual plastic centrifuge tubes (BIPPE, TS15; polypropylene). Subsequently, 2 tubes were stored at room temperature (~19 °C) and 2 tubes were stored at an elevated temperature (~31 °C) in a laboratory incubator. One tube from each beverage stored at room temperature and the elevated temperature was assessed 1 month later (time point #1) and 2 months later (time point #2) to determine the impact of storage time and temperature on osmolality measures.

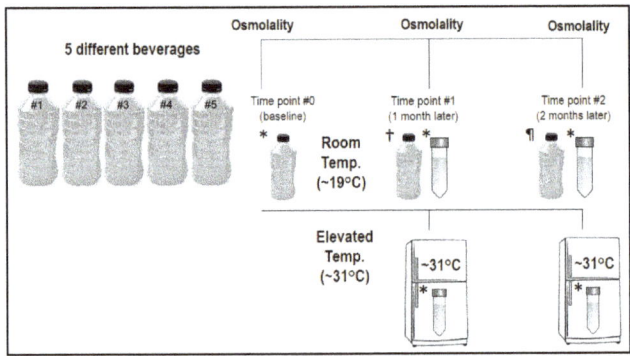

Figure 1. Schematic outlining the study methodologies for the third experiment; see text for further details. * The baseline bottle was aliquoted and subsequently stored for sampling at each time point. †,¶ A new bottle of each test beverage was also sampled at each time point.

Additionally, at time points #1 and #2, a new pre-mixed bottle of each ORS was opened and assessed. These unopened bottles were stored concurrently with the tubes at room temperature during the ensuing months. Within each beverage type, all three bottles sampled had the same expiration date. Our rationale for measuring a freshly opened bottle of each beverage during the two different time points was to assess whether our method of storing beverages in centrifuge tubes qualitatively altered the beverages; hence, the fresh bottles served as an internal control.

2.3. Osmometry

The main variable assessed in the current investigations was osmolality. Every beverage had at a minimum, osmometry performed in triplicate using a 250 µL sample on a freezing point depression device (Advanced® Instruments 3250, Norwood, MA, USA). Importantly, recent work from our laboratory demonstrated that the use of larger sample volumes for osmolality measures gives greater uniformity in the values obtained and is less influenced by the sample composition [23,24]. When the triplicate intra-sample measures differed by ≤3 mmol/kg (~1%), the median value was used. If the triplicate intra-sample measures differed by >3 mmol/kg, two additional samples were measured and the median value was used [25]. The accuracy of the osmometer was confirmed at the start and completion of each testing session by assaying a known reference solution (Clinitrol™ 290, Advanced Instruments, Norwood, MA, USA) that listed an osmolality within the desired range of anticipated values. Reference solution measurements during all testing sessions were within the normal limits of the osmometer. Lastly, for all investigations, beverages were equilibrated to standard laboratory temperatures (~21 °C) prior to assessment.

2.4. Water Content

The percent of water in each pre-mixed beverage was ascertained using the thermogravimetric method based upon previously establish protocols in biological samples [26,27]. Briefly, 2 mL of each beverage was carefully weighed in an evaporation dish. Dishes were then heated over an open flame until visible moisture was gone (~2 min). Subsequently, dishes were placed in an electric oven (110 °C) for 10 mins for further desiccation. Dishes were cooled to room temperature before a final weight was obtained. The percentage of water content was calculated from the wet and dry weight.

2.5. Statistics and Data Presentation

Standard statistics (e.g., mean, median, SD, percent coefficient of variation [%CV]) were calculated using Microsoft Excel® 2016. All graphs were completed with the use of a computerized statistical software package (GraphPad Prism® version 6 for Windows). Freshly sampled beverage osmolality values and samples subjected to storage were considered compliant and stable, respectively, if they fell within the 200 to 260 mmol/kg range [15,16]; those above or below the range were considered non-compliant.

3. Results

3.1. Pre-Mixed ORS Variability

The results from the first investigation—examining the baseline osmolality values and variability of pre-mixed ORS—are shown in Figure 2a. Three bottles of each ORS were assessed to derive the variability that exists within a given formulation. Many of the beverages (enterade, Speedlyte, Pediatric Oral Electrolyte Solution) had no variation between bottles (0% coefficient of variation (CV)). Gatorade and Pedialyte had minimal variation with 0.17% and 0.18% CV, respectively. Lastly, the water content of the pre-mixed solutions was experimentally determined: Gatorade, 96%; Speedlyte, 97%; Pedialyte, 98%; Up & Up, 98%; and enterade, 99% water.

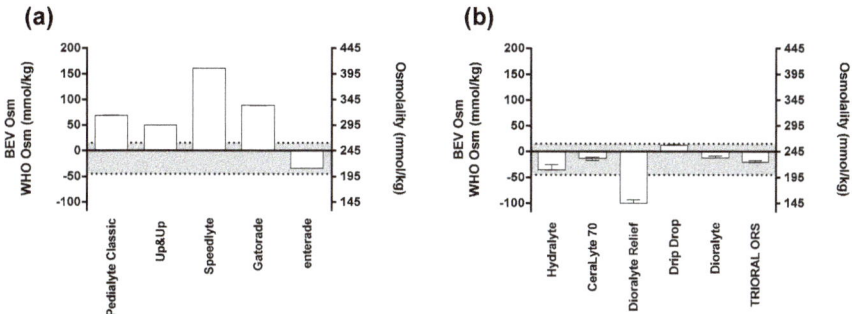

Figure 2. Beverage osmolality for: (**a**) pre-mixed solutions; and, (**b**) reconstituted powders. The left y-axis denotes the difference between beverage and WHO-UNICEF osmolality; the right y-axis denotes the absolute beverage osmolality. Each bar represents the median value for the three bottles tested. The variation plotted represents the range. The horizontal dotted lines denote the optimal range for beverage osmolality (200–260 mmol/kg; see text for details).

Additionally, as shown in Figure 2a, a demarcation was placed between 200 and 260 mmol/kg to represent the osmolality range where the greatest rate of net fluid absorption occurred [16]. Of note, enterade was the only pre-mixed beverage that was within this standard at baseline. It is also important to note that many beverages at baseline were in excess of the original osmolality recommendation from the WHO (311 mmol/kg): Pedialyte Classic, ~313 mmol/kg; Gatorade, ~334 mmol/kg; and Speedlyte, ~406 mmol/kg.

3.2. Powdered ORS Variability

The results from the second investigation, examining the baseline osmolality values and variability of carefully reconstituted powdered ORS, are shown in Figure 2b. Three packets of powdered ORS were carefully reconstituted using distilled water according to each of the different manufacturer's instructions. Immediately after the beverages were reconstituted, the osmolality was assessed to derive the variability that exists within and between the given formulations. Our results demonstrate that greater variation exists within the powdered forms compared to the pre-mixed solutions. The following is a list of the products sampled with their % CV, presented in order of their variation from lowest to highest: Drip Drop (0.45%), TRIORAL ORS (0.92%), Dioralyte original (0.99%), CeraLyte 70 (1.32%), Dioralyte Relief (2.74%), and Hydralyte (2.86%). In a similar fashion to the first investigation, Figure 2b denotes an optimal beverage osmolality range between 200 and 260 mmol/kg [16]. Of the six powdered ORS tested, only one (Dioralyte Relief; ~145 mmol/kg) had an osmolality outside of this range.

3.3. Impact of Time and Temperature

The results from the third investigation, examining the impact of time and temperature on osmolality, are displayed in Figure 3. Figure 3a depicts the changes in pre-mixed ORS that occurred when the beverages were stored at room temperature in their original unopened package (i.e., "fresh bottles"). As expected, there was minimal change between baseline (0 days) and the 30- and 60-day samples. Figure 3b shows the data from the originally opened bottle, which was sampled at baseline and then pipetted into centrifuge tubes for subsequent storage at room temperature. These results closely mirror Figure 3a; thus, demonstrating that the storage of aliquots in centrifuge tubes did not inadvertently alter the osmolality. Lastly, Figure 3c shows the impact of storing beverages at elevated temperatures (~31 °C) [19]. These data demonstrate that many of the beverages had dramatic increases in osmolality during two months of storage at 31 °C. Of note, enterade demonstrated the lowest change from baseline (Δ 19 mmol/kg), while Speedlyte (Δ 89 mmol/kg) and Gatorade (Δ 108 mmol/kg) demonstrated the largest changes from baseline after 60 days in the hot temperatures.

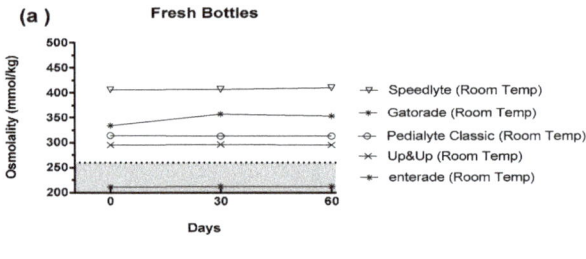

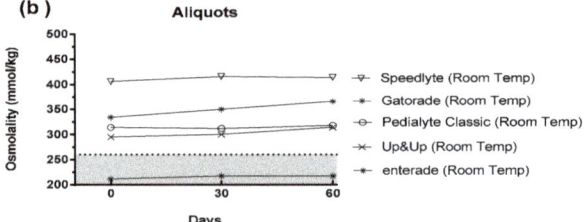

Figure 3. *Cont.*

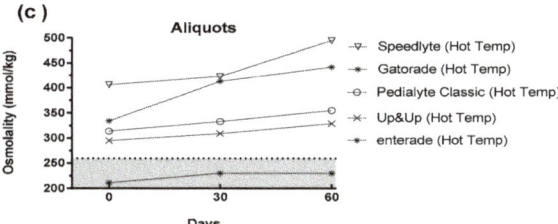

Figure 3. Impact of time and storage conditions on the osmolality of various pre-mixed oral rehydration solutions [ORS] for: (**a**) freshly opened bottles stored at room temperature; (**b**) beverage aliquots stored at room temperature; and, and (**c**) beverage aliquots stored at elevated temperatures. The shaded area denotes the optimal range for beverage osmolality (200–260 mmol/kg; see text for details).

Lastly, the same range for optimal beverage osmolality (200–260 mmol/kg) was placed in Figure 3 [16]. As previously shown, enterade was the only beverage that demonstrated osmolality values within this range at baseline and following room temperature storage. More importantly, enterade was still within this range even after 60 days at elevated temperatures.

4. Discussion

The present results demonstrate the following: 1) enterade was the only premixed ORS product that had baseline osmolality values between 200 and 260 mmol/kg and it stayed within this range after two months of storage at 31 °C; 2) some beverages, such as sports drinks and Speedlyte, had very high osmolality values at baseline and demonstrated robust increases during prolonged storage; and 3) little variation existed within premixed or powdered ORS products.

The World Health Organization (WHO) and the United Nations Children's Fund (UNICEF) currently recommend a reduced osmolality of 245 mmol/kg in their ORS formulations, which is a drop from the previous 311 mmol/kg recommendation [15]. The reductions in osmolality and electrolyte levels were a result of reported gastrointestinal upset, nausea, concerns about hypernatremia with the higher osmolality solution, and lack of reduced stool output [13,14]. It is important to note that research in healthy volunteers has demonstrated a range of hypotonic beverage osmolalities (200–260 mmol/kg) for optimal net intestinal fluid absorption [16] that includes the 245 mmol/kg recommended value in the treatment of diarrhea [14]. Since osmolality is not required on nutrition labeling, one aim of the current investigation was to independently verify which commercially available products are in compliance with these recommendations. Our results demonstrate high compliance with powdered ORS products since five of the six products analyzed fell within the desired range. However, of the five pre-mixed formulations tested, only one product (enterade) had an osmolality within the recommended range. These results call into question the overall ingredient composition within these products.

A range of osmolality values for pre-mixed products was obtained at baseline in the current studies; ranging from a low of 211 mmol/kg (enterade) to a high of 406 mmol/kg (Speedlyte). Our results fall in-line with other limited data-sets demonstrating a wide range of osmolality values for ORS products [28]. Of note, many of the products tested had electrolyte values lower than those recommended by the WHO/UNICEF, and yet still had osmolality values in excess of the original osmolality recommendation of 311 mmol/kg. The main contributing factor to these elevated osmolality values appears to be the high sugar concentrations and the types of sugar used. For example, Gatorade was tested as a representative sports drink and the osmolality value was found to be ~334 mmol/kg, which aligns with other published values for Gatorade [29,30]. The main sugar used in many sports drinks is table sugar (i.e., sucrose), which is a disaccharide. Over time, sucrose (and other more complex sugars) can hydrolyze into their monosaccharide components [31] and increase the overall osmolality of the solution, a process that is exacerbated by storage in warm conditions [19,20]. Indeed, Gatorade demonstrated the highest absolute change in osmolality after 2 months in the heat (Δ 108 mmol/kg compared to baseline). Our results mirror what others have found in that osmolality may be strongly influenced by the quantity and quality of carbohydrates used (e.g., monosaccharides, disaccharides, polysaccharides, etc.) [29,32]. Other ingredients, such as artificial sweeteners and flavoring agents, may also be heat unstable. For example, the osmolality of Pedialyte Classic increased by 41 mmol/kg after 60 days in warm storage despite containing only dextrose (hydrolysis resistant). However, it also contained sucralose and acesulfame potassium, the effects of which are unknown with respect to osmolality.

The beverage with the highest baseline osmolality was Speedlyte. Presently, a paucity of published data exists on this product. Speedlyte contains multiple forms of sugar and a unique electrolyte formulation where the electrolytes are encapsulated in liposomes (i.e., microelectrolytes technology™). Importantly, the manufacturers claim that the osmolality of this product is 188 mmol/kg [33]; however, over the course of this entire investigation, five separate bottles of this product were assayed and the osmolality values ranged from 406 to 410 mmol/kg. Moreover, this product demonstrated the second highest absolute changes in osmolality (Δ 90 mmol/kg increase compared to baseline) after 2 months at high temperatures. Although it is possible that the presence of liposomes (solids) in the sample might have spuriously elevated the osmolality measured by freezing point depression, the large sample volume (250 µL) should have minimized this potential [23,24]. For example, the water content of Speedlyte (97% water) was similar to the other commercial beverages tested (96–99% water); liposomes could have only contributed between 0.1% and 1.0% to the total [33]. In contrast, whole blood (~80% water), which contains considerable solids, can still have its osmolality accurately measured by freezing point depression when using a 250 µL volume [24]. In addition, similar outcomes were observed using a vapor pressure osmometer (data not shown). These results raise interesting and unresolved questions about liposome technology for use in ORS.

The WHO currently recommends that a small amount of glucose should be added in an ORS to capitalize on sodium–glucose transporters that facilitate fluid movement [15]. enterade was the only product tested that does not contain glucose but instead contains electrolytes and amino acids to leverage amino acid coupled transporters that also facilitate fluid absorption [34]. It is interesting to note recent findings that small amounts of glucose (less than 1 millimolar) in a solution stimulates chloride secretion and as a consequence may reduce fluid absorption and may exacerbate diarrhea [35–37]. Furthermore, based upon the fact that the glucose-free product demonstrated the smallest change in osmolality over time, the degree to which glucose should be included in an ORS formulation may be questioned. The results of the current investigation have important implications for when these beverages are shipped and stored in locations where high ambient temperatures may be present, such as low-income countries with tropical climates [18,19].

The powdered versions of the ORS appeared to show better compliance with the recommended osmolality guidelines [15,16], but these powdered products can have their own limitations. For example, previous research has stressed that these products should be prepared extemporaneously to prevent alterations in product components over time [17]. However, if ORS needs to be used in areas without potable water, these beverages will not safely be reconstituted and will not be stable enough for storage. Lastly, some of the powdered ORS products contain components (e.g., rice powers) that have reduced solubility and thus alter the osmolality within these products (e.g., Dioralyte Relief) after reconstitution; thus, creating larger potential variation in measured osmolality values.

In summary, this investigation demonstrated that many commercially available pre-mixed ORS products currently do not adhere to recommended osmolality guidelines. Additionally, due to the high sugar content of some products used to treat diarrhea, their osmotic shelf-life stability may be questioned, especially when stored in the warm but ecologically valid environments. As the osmolality of ORS is important for optimal fluid absorption and patient acceptance (e.g., stomach upset), the findings of this study should be carefully considered in the design of future ORS products.

Author Contributions: Conceptualization, K.J.S., R.W.K., and S.N.C.; methodology, K.J.S., R.W.K., and S.N.C.; formal analysis, K.J.S., investigation, K.J.S.; data curation, K.J.S., writing—original draft preparation, K.J.S., R.W.K., and S.N.C.; writing—review and editing, K.J.S., R.W.K., and S.N.C.; funding acquisition, K.J.S.,

Funding: This research was funded by Entrinsic Health Solutions, Inc (EHS). Enterade® product was donated by EHS.

Acknowledgments: The authors would like to thank Jennifer Whiles-Lillig, (Sonoma State University) for her insights and support that allowed this work to be completed.

Conflicts of Interest: S.N.C. and R.W.K. are paid consultants to EHS and contributed to the research study concept and design, writing, and editing of the manuscript.

Appendix A

Table A1. Listing of ingredients for each premixed beverage tested.

Beverage Name	Ingredients
Pedialyte® Classic mixed (fruit flavor)	Water, Dextrose. Less than 2% of: Citric Acid, Natural & Artificial Flavor, Potassium Citrate, Salt, Sodium Citrate, Sucralose, Acesulfame Potassium, Zinc Gluconate, and Yellow 6.
Pediatric Oral Electrolyte Solution (fruit flavor)	Water, Dextrose, Citric Acid, Potassium Citrate, Sodium Chloride, Sodium Citrate, Acesulfame Potassium, Zinc Gluconate, Natural & Artificial Fruit Flavor, Sucralose, FD&C Yellow #6.
Speedlyte® (wild orange flavor)	Purified water; Less than 2% of: Dextrose, Sucrose, Liposomal Salt [Citrate, Chloride, Sodium, Potassium, Soy Lecithin, Xanthan Gum], Citric Acid, Sodium Benzoate, Stevia Extract, Monk Fruit, Beta Carotene, Rose Anthocyanin, Methylparaben, Sodium Metabisulfite, Natural Flavor.
enterade®AD ORS (orange flavor)	Water, Amino Acid Blend (L-Valine, L-Aspartic Acid, L-Serine, L-Isoleucine, L-Threonine, L-Lysine, L-Glycine, L-Tyrosine), sodium chloride, potassium citrate, trisodium citrate, natural flavor, magnesium citrate, calcium chloride, stevia.
Gatorade® (orange flavor)	Water, Sugar, Dextrose, Citric Acid, Salt, Sodium Citrate, Monopotassium Phosphate, Gum Arabic, Natural Flavor, Sucrose Acetate Isobutyrate, Glycerol Ester of Rosin, Yellow 6

References

1. King, C.K.; Glass, R.; Bresee, J.S.; Duggan, C. Managing acute gastroenteritis among children: Oral rehydration, maintenance, and nutritional therapy. *MMWR. Recomm. Rep.* **2003**, *52*, 1–16. [PubMed]
2. Kosek, M.; Bern, C.; Guerrant, R.L. The global burden of diarrhoeal disease, as estimated from studies published between 1992 and 2000. *Bull. World Health Organ.* **2003**, *81*, 197–204. [PubMed]
3. Farthing, M.J. Oral rehydration: An evolving solution. *J. Pediatr. Gastroenterol. Nutr.* **2002**, *34* (Suppl. 1), S64–67. [CrossRef] [PubMed]
4. Nalin, D.R.; Cash, R.A. 50 years of oral rehydration therapy: The solution is still simple. *Lancet* **2018**, *392*, 536–538. [CrossRef]
5. Hirschhorn, N. The treatment of acute diarrhea in children. An historical and physiological perspective. *Am. J. Clin. Nutr.* **1980**, *33*, 637–663. [CrossRef]
6. Banks, M.R.; Farthing, M.J. Fluid and electrolyte transport in the small intestine. *Curr. Opin. Gastroenterol.* **2002**, *18*, 176–181. [CrossRef]
7. Crane, R.K. Hypothesis for mechanism of intestinal active transport of sugars. *Fed. Proc.* **1962**, *21*, 891–895.
8. Curran, P.F. Coupling between transport processes in intestine. *Physiologist* **1968**, *11*, 3–23.
9. Fordtran, J.S.; Rector, F.C., Jr.; Carter, N.W. The mechanisms of sodium absorption in the human small intestine. *J. Clin. Invest.* **1968**, *47*, 884–900. [CrossRef]
10. Schultz, S.G.; Zalusky, R. Ion transport in isolated rabbit ileum. I. Short-circuit current and Na fluxes. *J. Gen. Physiol.* **1964**, *47*, 567–584. [CrossRef]
11. Schultz, S.G.; Zalusky, R. Ion transport in isolated rabbit ileum. II. The interaction between active sodium and active sugar transport. *J. Gen. Physiol.* **1964**, *47*, 1043–1059. [CrossRef] [PubMed]

12. Atia, A.N.; Buchman, A.L. Oral rehydration solutions in non-cholera diarrhea: A review. *Am. J. Gastroenterol.* **2009**, *104*, 2596–2604, quiz 2605. [CrossRef] [PubMed]
13. Impact of glycine-containing ORS solutions on stool output and duration of diarrhoea: A meta-analysis of seven clinical trials. The International Study Group on Improved ORS. *Bull. World Health Organ.* **1991**, *69*, 541–548.
14. Duggan, C.; Fontaine, O.; Pierce, N.F.; Glass, R.I.; Mahalanabis, D.; Alam, N.H.; Bhan, M.K.; Santosham, M. Scientific rationale for a change in the composition of oral rehydration solution. *JAMA* **2004**, *291*, 2628–2631. [CrossRef] [PubMed]
15. WHO. Reduced Osmolarity Oral Rehydration Salts (ORS) Formulation: A Report from a Meeting of Expert Jointly Organised by UNICEF and WHO: UNICEF House, New York, USA, July 18, 2001. Available online: https://apps.who.int/iris/handle/10665/67322 (accessed on 7 April 2019).
16. Leiper, J.B. Fate of ingested fluids: Factors affecting gastric emptying and intestinal absorption of beverages in humans. *Nutr. Rev.* **2015**, *73 Suppl. 2*, 57–72. [CrossRef]
17. Izgu, E.; Baykara, T. The solid state stability of oral rehydration salts. *J. Clin. Hosp. Pharm.* **1981**, *6*, 135–144. [CrossRef] [PubMed]
18. WHO. *Climate Change and Human Health: Risk and Responses*; WHO: Geneva, Switzerland, 2003.
19. Mora, C.; Dousset, B.; Caldwell, I.R.; Powell, F.E.; Geronimo, R.C.; Bielecki, C.R.; Counsell, C.W.; Dietrich, B.S.; Johnston, E.T.; Louis, L.V.; et al. Global risk of deadly heat. *Nat. Clim. Chang.* **2017**, *7*, 501. [CrossRef]
20. Goldberg, R.N.; Tewari, Y.B.; Ahluwalia, J.C. Thermodynamics of the hydrolysis of sucrose. *J. Bio. Chem.* **1989**, *264*, 9901–9904.
21. Pantenburg, B.; Ochoa, T.J.; Ecker, L.; Ruiz, J. Use of Commercially Available Oral Rehydration Solutions in Lima, Peru. *Am. J. Trop. Med. Hyg.* **2012**, *86*, 922–924. [CrossRef]
22. Rao, S.S.; Summers, R.W.; Rao, G.R.; Ramana, S.; Devi, U.; Zimmerman, B.; Pratap, B.C. Oral rehydration for viral gastroenteritis in adults: A randomized, controlled trial of 3 solutions. *JPEN J. Parenter. Enteral. Nutr.* **2006**, *30*, 433–439. [CrossRef]
23. Sollanek, K.J.; Kenefick, R.W.; Cheuvront, S.N. Importance of sample volume to the measurement and interpretation of plasma osmolality. *J. Clin. Lab. Anal.* **2019**, *33*, e22727. [CrossRef] [PubMed]
24. Cheuvront, S.N.; Kenefick, R.W.; Heavens, K.R.; Spitz, M.G. A comparison of whole blood and plasma osmolality and osmolarity. *J. Clin. Lab. Anal.* **2014**, *28*, 368–373. [CrossRef]
25. Bohnen, N.; Terwel, D.; Markerink, M.; Ten Haaf, J.A.; Jolles, J. Pitfalls in the measurement of plasma osmolality pertinent to research in vasopressin and water metabolism. *Clin. Chem.* **1992**, *38*, 2278–2280.
26. Plaisier, A.; Maingay-de Groof, F.; Mast-Harwig, R.; Kalkman, P.M.; Wulkan, R.W.; Verwers, R.; Neele, M.; Hop, W.C.; Groeneweg, M. Plasma water as a diagnostic tool in the assessment of dehydration in children with acute gastroenteritis. *Eur. J. Pediatr.* **2010**, *169*, 883–886. [CrossRef] [PubMed]
27. Eisenman, A.J.; Mackenzie, L.B.; Peters, J.P. Protein and water of serum and cells of human blood, with a note on the measurement of red blood cell volume. *J. Biol. Chem.* **1936**, *116*, 33–45.
28. Al-Ramahi, R.; Zaid, A.; Hussein, A.; Yaseen, A.; Abdallah, K.; Odeh, M. Evaluation of mothers' practice in the treatment of children diarrhea and measurement of the osmolality and PH of some oral rehydration solutions and carbonated beverages. *An-Najah Univ. J. Res. (N. Sc.)* **2016**, *30*, 269–282.
29. Mettler, S.; Rusch, C.; Colombani, P.C. Osmolality and pH of sport and other drinks available in Switzerland. *Schweiz. Z. Med. Traumatol.* **2006**, *54*, 92.
30. Wesley, J.F. Osmolality—A novel and sensitive tool for detection of tampering of beverages adulterated with ethanol, γ-butyrolactone, and 1,4-butanediol, and for detection of dilution-tampered demerol syringes. *Microgram J.* **2003**, 8–17.
31. Clarke, M.A. Technological value of sucrose in food products. In *Sucrose: Properties and Applications*; Mathlouthi, M., Reiser, P., Eds.; Springer: Boston, MA, USA, 1995.
32. Hofman, D.L.; van Buul, V.J.; Brouns, F.J. Nutrition, Health, and Regulatory Aspects of Digestible Maltodextrins. *Crit. Rev. Food Sci. Nutr.* **2016**, *56*, 2091–2100. [CrossRef] [PubMed]
33. Nicastro, A.; Barbarini, A.L.; Souss, G.M. Liposomal Rehydration Salt Formulation and Associated Method of Use. U.S. Patent 15/797,031, 22 February 2018.
34. Yin, L.; Gupta, R.; Vaught, L.; Grosche, A.; Okunieff, P.; Vidyasagar, S. An amino acid-based oral rehydration solution (AA-ORS) enhanced intestinal epithelial proliferation in mice exposed to radiation. *Sci. Rep.* **2016**, *6*, 37220. [CrossRef] [PubMed]

35. Yin, L.; Vijaygopal, P.; MacGregor, G.G.; Menon, R.; Ranganathan, P.; Prabhakaran, S.; Zhang, L.; Zhang, M.; Binder, H.J.; Okunieff, P.; et al. Glucose stimulates calcium-activated chloride secretion in small intestinal cells. *Am. J. Physiol. Cell Physiol.* **2014**, *306*, C687–C696. [CrossRef] [PubMed]
36. Yin, L.; Menon, R.; Gupta, R.; Vaught, L.; Okunieff, P.; Vidyasagar, S. Glucose enhances rotavirus enterotoxin-induced intestinal chloride secretion. *Pflugers Arch.* **2017**, *469*, 1093–1105. [CrossRef] [PubMed]
37. Hodges, K.; Gill, R. Infectious diarrhea: Cellular and molecular mechanisms. *Gut Microbes* **2010**, *1*, 4–21. [CrossRef] [PubMed]

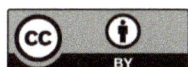

© 2019 by the authors. Licensee MDPI, Basel, Switzerland. This article is an open access article distributed under the terms and conditions of the Creative Commons Attribution (CC BY) license (http://creativecommons.org/licenses/by/4.0/).

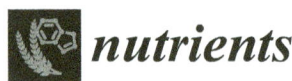

Review

The Potential for Renal Injury Elicited by Physical Work in the Heat

Zachary J. Schlader [1,2,*], David Hostler [1], Mark D. Parker [3,4], Riana R. Pryor [1], James W. Lohr [5], Blair D. Johnson [1] and Christopher L. Chapman [1]

1. Center for Research and Education in Special Environments, Department of Exercise and Nutrition Sciences, University at Buffalo, Buffalo, NY 14214, USA
2. Department of Kinesiology, School of Public Health, Indiana University, Bloomington, IN 47405, USA
3. Department of Physiology and Biophysics, Jacobs School of Medicine and Biomedical Sciences, University at Buffalo, Buffalo, NY 14214, USA
4. Department of Ophthalmology, Jacobs School of Medicine and Biomedical Sciences, University at Buffalo, Buffalo, NY 14214, USA
5. Department of Medicine, Jacobs School of Medicine and Biomedical Sciences, University at Buffalo, Buffalo, NY 14214, USA
* Correspondence: zschlade@indiana.edu; Tel.: +001-812-855-6953

Received: 20 June 2019; Accepted: 22 August 2019; Published: 4 September 2019

Abstract: An epidemic of chronic kidney disease (CKD) is occurring in laborers who undertake physical work in hot conditions. Rodent data indicate that heat exposure causes kidney injury, and when this injury is regularly repeated it can elicit CKD. Studies in humans demonstrate that a single bout of exercise in the heat increases biomarkers of acute kidney injury (AKI). Elevations in AKI biomarkers in this context likely reflect an increased susceptibility of the kidneys to AKI. Data largely derived from animal models indicate that the mechanism(s) by which exercise in the heat may increase the risk of AKI is multifactorial. For instance, heat-related reductions in renal blood flow may provoke heterogenous intrarenal blood flow. This can promote localized ischemia, hypoxemia and ATP depletion in renal tubular cells, which could be exacerbated by increased sodium reabsorption. Heightened fructokinase pathway activity likely exacerbates ATP depletion occurring secondary to intrarenal fructose production and hyperuricemia. Collectively, these responses can promote inflammation and oxidative stress, thereby increasing the risk of AKI. Equivalent mechanistic evidence in humans is lacking. Such an understanding could inform the development of countermeasures to safeguard the renal health of laborers who regularly engage in physical work in hot environments.

Keywords: acute kidney injury; chronic kidney disease; heat stress; dehydration; exercise

1. Background

An epidemic of chronic kidney disease of unknown etiology (CKDu) is occurring in laborers who undertake physical work outdoors in hot conditions [1,2]. This disease was first described in 2002, when nephropathy was identified in a disproportionate number of young Central American sugarcane workers [3]. Thereafter, people in other occupations [4–6] and in other regions of the world [1,7,8] have been diagnosed with what appears to be the same disease, although there is some heterogeneity in the clinical signs, symptoms, and likely etiology [1,2]. The effects of CKDu are devastating. For instance, the Pan American Health Organization estimates that CKDu caused more than 60,000 deaths in Central America from 1997 to 2013, with 41% of these deaths occurring in people younger than 60 y of age [9]. Furthermore, the World Health Organization estimates that ~15% of workers in endemic areas are at risk of developing CKDu [10]. This estimate was recently corroborated in a meta-analysis by Flouris et al. [11]. Thus, there is an urgent need to identify effective strategies to mitigate the risk of CKDu.

The development of countermeasures for CKDu requires an understanding of the etiology of the disease. Unfortunately, the etiology underlying the development of CKDu is largely unknown [12]. Patients diagnosed with CKDu usually present with an asymptomatic rise in serum creatinine and low grade proteinuria [4,5]. Renal biopsies show interstitial fibrosis, low grade inflammation, tubular atrophy, and glomerulosclerosis with signs of ischemia [13]. The two hallmarks of CKDu are that it is not associated with traditional risk factors of chronic kidney disease (CKD) (e.g., advanced age, diabetes, hypertension) and that it is more common in laborers regularly exposed to hot environments [7,14–16]. There may also be a contributing role for toxin exposures (e.g., agrochemicals, heavy metals or infectious agents) [14,17] and/or the use of agents with nephrotoxic side effects (e.g., nonsteroidal anti-inflammatory drugs (NSAIDs)) [18,19]. However, convincing evidence supporting these factors as being primary in the etiology of CKDu is lacking [2,20,21]. Thus, it has been suggested that heat may be the key occupational exposure contributing to the development of CKDu [7,14,22]. This is supported by data indicating a higher prevalence of CKDu in agriculture workers exposed to hotter climates compared to those working in cooler climates, despite otherwise enduring the same occupational conditions [4,6]. As a result, it has been proposed that CKDu is a form of 'heat stress nephropathy', the risk of which could worsen with climate change [7,16,23]. That said, it is important to note that while factors associated with engaging in physical work in the heat are likely to play an important role, the etiology of CKDu is mostly unknown and may be multifaceted [7,24,25].

One leading etiological hypothesis for CKDu is that physical work (i.e., exercise) in the heat, which leads to heat strain (i.e., increased core body temperature) and dehydration (i.e., a hypovolemic–hyperosmotic state caused by the loss of body water due to sweating combined with inadequate fluid intake), causes acute kidney injury (AKI) [2,7,15,16,26–28]. This heat-related AKI is probably transient in nature [29–32], which is clinically defined as lasting <3 days [33]. Nevertheless, it has been proposed that multiple transient AKI exposures can manifest as nephropathy, affecting the renal tubules and glomeruli [7,15,16,27].

Subclinical rhabdomyolysis (i.e., muscle injury), which may occur during (or after) unaccustomed intense or prolonged exercise [34], is often proposed to contribute to heat-related AKI and CKDu [7,14,35]. This is supported by human data demonstrating that the presence of muscle damage increases the risk of AKI during exercise in the heat [36]. These data were recently corroborated in a rodent model of repeated heat exposure, which demonstrated that experimental rhabdomyolysis worsened heat-induced kidney injury [37]. That said, epidemiological data obtained from Guatemalan sugarcane workers indicate that the presence of rhabdomyolysis is not associated with cross-shift declines in kidney function [26], suggesting that the contribution of rhabdomyolysis to progressive reductions in kidney function in this population is likely small. This can be explained by the adaptation of skeletal muscle to become more resistant to damage after the initial injurious exercise [38]. Thus, while the first few days of unaccustomed intense physical work in the heat may induce subclinical rhabdomyolysis, the subsequent muscle damage incurred by manual laborers on a daily basis is probably small. Therefore, the contribution of subclinical rhabdomyolysis to heat-related AKI and CKDu is likely minimal.

It is important to note that there is currently no direct support for recurrent heat-related AKI in the etiology of CKDu [39]. For instance, to our knowledge a dose–response relation between the frequency and severity of heat-related AKI and the subsequent development of CKD has never been experimentally examined in rodent models nor explored in epidemiological studies. That said, in the absence of heat exposure, data from pre-clinical models indicate that AKI can result in renal tubular remodeling [40,41], which can lead to long-term impairments in kidney function, the defining characteristic of CKD [40,42–46]. More recently, these findings have been extended to instances of combined heat exposure and dehydration. For instance, rodents develop nephropathy with intermittent, repeated passive (i.e., resting) heat exposure without access to fluids over 4–5 weeks [47–49]. Importantly, these animals demonstrate evidence of kidney injury, which is consistent with the recurrent heat-related AKI hypothesis [47–49]. These data are corroborated by workplace data demonstrating increases in biomarkers of AKI both across a work shift and across the harvest season [31,32,50–55]. Notably, the working conditions during these periods are conducive to increased heat strain, dehydration, and reductions in kidney function [31,32,50–55]. Whether the observed increases in AKI biomarkers translate to an increased risk of CKD is unclear [56]. That said, epidemiological evidence clearly indicates that the frequency and severity of non-heat-related AKI is associated with the incidence and severity of CKD [57–61]. For instance, a single episode of relatively mild (Stage 1) AKI results in a 43% increased risk of developing advanced stage CKD within one year [57]. Furthermore, even a single episode of transient AKI that lasted ≤2 days is associated with a ~2-fold increased risk of death [62] and a 1.4-fold increased risk of developing CKD [57]. Thus, it is generally accepted that an increased frequency, severity, and/or duration of AKI elevates the risk of developing CKD [63,64], although this remains a topic of debate that requires additional exploration [44,63–65]. Against this background, the etiology of CKDu may be better understood by investigating the pathophysiology of the increased risk of AKI in humans exercising in the heat. This latter point is particularly important. For instance, experimentally manipulating CKDu risk in humans is unethical. However, quantification of the risk of AKI in humans may be readily accomplished when studies are carefully designed to ensure the risk of AKI is short lasting and completely resolved between experimental periods.

Despite the proposed relation between heat exposure and CKDu, the effects of heat strain and dehydration elicited by exercise in the heat on kidney health and the risk of AKI in humans is largely unexplored. We believe that this is likely because changes in kidney function induced by heat strain, exercise, and/or dehydration are believed to be physiological in nature, clinically benign, and completely reversed with recovery [17]. Emerging evidence, however, calls this dogma into question [2,14,16,36,47,51,54,66–70]. Therefore, the purpose of this narrative review is to present evidence that exercise in the heat may increase the risk of developing AKI in humans. In doing so, we will also address how the risk of AKI can be examined in humans and we will discuss some of the potential mechanisms underlying this risk. A focus will be placed on human subjects research, but data from non-human animals will be included where necessary. Several important knowledge gaps will also be presented. Filling these knowledge voids is vital to identifying strategies to mitigate the risk of AKI and CKDu in workers who regularly engage in physical work in hot environments.

2. Acute Kidney Injury

AKI refers to a clinical condition characterized by a rapid (i.e., occurring within ≤7 days) reduction in kidney function [71]. AKI can be further categorized as transient (i.e., lasting <3 days) or sustained (i.e., lasting ≥ 3 days) [33]. AKI is often reversible, but can be fatal both in the acute setting and in relation to an increased risk of CKD, which is defined as a gradual loss of kidney function that persists for >90 days [72]. Clinically, the presence and the severity of AKI is diagnosed via criteria established by international working groups such as the Acute Kidney Injury Network (AKIN) [73], the Acute Dialysis Quality Initiative (ADQI) [74], and Kidney Disease: Improving Global Outcomes (KDIGO) [71,75], amongst others. The criteria for identifying and categorizing the severity AKI differs slightly between these working groups. However, the common denominator for classifying AKI among these working groups is an acute reduction in kidney function. Changes in kidney function are often quantified via changes in glomerular filtration rate (GFR), which is widely accepted as the best overall index of kidney function in both health and disease [71], and the rate of urine production (aka: urine flow rate). Precise measurements of GFR can be cumbersome, impractical and/or costly. Thus, GFR is often estimated from the clearance of endogenous creatinine from the circulation [76]. Creatinine is formed from muscle creatine and released into the blood at a relatively constant rate provided there are no changes in muscle mass or muscle damage during the period of observation. Importantly, creatinine is not reabsorbed along the nephron tubule lumen. Correcting urinary creatinine excretion rate for serum creatinine (a systemic variable that could also influence urinary creatinine excretion) provides an accurate measure of GFR [76]. Thus, creatinine clearance is a function of urine flow rate and serum and urinary creatinine concentrations at any given time and can be calculated as:

$$GFR \approx Clearance_{Creatinine} = \frac{[Creatinine]_{urine} \times Urine\ flow\ rate}{[Creatinine]_{serum}}$$

where: GFR is glomerular filtration rate, $Clearance_{Creatinine}$ is creatinine clearance, $[Creatinine]_{urine}$ is the urinary concentration of creatinine, $Urine\ flow\ rate$ is the volume of urine produced per unit time, and $[Creatinine]_{serum}$ is the serum concentration of creatinine.

Precise assessment of urine flow rate can be difficult in ambulatory or free-living settings. Therefore, GFR is often further estimated based upon serum creatinine and equations incorporating corrections for age, sex, race and body size, thereby eliminating the need for urine collection [76]. As a result, a spot assessment of serum creatinine is often part of routine medical practice for assessment of kidney function [77]. It is also important to note that there is growing support for a spot assessment of circulating cystatin C as a marker of kidney function [78]. Cystatin C is produced at a stable rate by all cells within the body and freely filtered by the glomeruli. The potential benefit of using cystatin C is that changes in cystatin C during dynamic fluctuations in kidney function may occur much earlier than changes in serum creatinine [79]. In theory, this could provide for more rapid diagnoses of AKI [78]. Importantly, to our knowledge, cystatin C has never been used to quantify kidney function during exercise in the heat. Moreover, despite evidence that cystatin C may provide useful information, the clinical practice guidelines for the diagnosis and classification of the severity of AKI are currently based on acute changes in serum creatinine and/or absolute urine flow rate (Table 1).

The underlying basis for the AKI guidelines is the relation between serum creatinine and kidney function, and that rapid decreases in kidney function define AKI. A limitation regarding the use of changes in kidney function as diagnostic criteria for AKI (whether quantified via changes in serum creatinine, urine flow rate, or cystatin C), is that GFR is often acutely reduced as a result of an integrated physiological response (i.e., conditions extrinsic to the kidneys). This is often referred to as prerenal AKI [80], whereby increases in serum creatinine (and/or reductions in urine flow rate) may satisfy the definition of AKI, but these reductions in kidney function are due to neural, hormonal, and/or hemodynamic responses upstream of the kidneys. For example, GFR and urine flow rate are decreased during dehydration [81,82]. This is likely due to reductions in renal blood flow [83,84] caused by increases in renal sympathetic nerve activity [85,86], vasopressin release [87], and activation of the renin–angiotensin–aldosterone system [88]. These are normal and healthy physiological responses that promote fluid conservation [89]. Thus, increases in serum creatinine, which are normally reflective of a reduction in GFR, may not always be indicative of kidney injury during dehydration [80]. Because of this, it is often recommended that the creatinine and/or urine flow rate-based diagnostic criteria for AKI be used only after an optimal state of hydration has been achieved [73]. However, an optimal hydration state is ill-defined given that no single variable truly captures body fluid status [90].

Given the limitations of kidney function-derived AKI diagnoses, a rapidly growing body of literature aiming to identify biomarkers of AKI has emerged [91]. The goal of these biomarkers is to identify those individuals at risk of developing AKI before any reductions in kidney function occur [92–95]. It has recently been reported that over the past 10 years there have been 3300 scientific publications and hundreds of AKI biomarkers investigated [91]. The validity and clinical utility of many of these biomarkers remains to be determined, even for well-studied AKI biomarkers [91,96]. However, when combined with standard indices of kidney function, measurement of AKI biomarkers may provide unique information regarding interactions between changes in kidney function and the potential for AKI [96,97]. In the following, we will introduce a few promising AKI biomarkers, with an emphasis on those that have been used in experimental human subjects research, particularly as it relates to exercise, dehydration, and/or heat strain, or that demonstrate potential for use in laboratory-based (i.e., not clinical settings) human subjects studies. An in-depth overview of AKI biomarkers is outside of the scope of this review. Thus, to the interested reader we recommend a number of more comprehensive reviews addressing the pathophysiological bases and clinical performance of AKI biomarkers [92–95].

Table 1. Clinical criteria for identifying acute kidney injury and staging the severity of injury.

	Criteria	
	Serum Creatinine	Urine Output
Acute Kidney Injury Network (AKIN) Classification		
Stage 1	Increase ≥0.3 mg/dL (≥26.5 µmol/L) OR increase ≥1.5–2.0-fold from baseline	<0.5 mL/kg/h for 6 h
Stage 2	Increase >2.0–3.0-fold from baseline	<0.5 mL/kg/h for 12 h
Stage 3	Increase >3.0-fold from baseline OR serum creatinine ≥4.0 mg/dL (≥354 µmol/L) with an acute increase of ≥0.5 mg/dL (44 µmol/L) OR need for renal replacement therapy	<0.3 mL/kg/h for 24 h OR anuria for 12 h OR need for renal replacement therapy
Kidney Disease: Improving Global Outcomes (KDIGO) Classification		
Stage 1	Increase ≥0.3 mg/dL (≥26.5 µmol/L) OR 1.5–1.9 times baseline	<0.5 mL/kg/h for 6-12 h
Stage 2	2.0–2.9 times baseline	<0.5 mL/kg/h for 12 h
Stage 3	3.0 times baseline OR increase in serum creatinine to ≥4.0 mg/dL (≥354 µmol/L) OR need for renal replacement therapy OR in patients <18 years old a decrease in eGFR to <35 mL/min/1.73 m²	<0.3 mL/kg/h for 24 h OR anuria for 12 h
Acute Dialysis Quality Initiative (ADQI): Risk, Injury, Failure, Loss of Kidney Function and End-Stage Kidney Disease (RIFLE) Classification		
Risk	1.5-fold increase OR GFR decrease >25% from baseline	<0.5 mL/kg/h for 6-12 h
Injury	2.0-fold increase OR GFR decrease >50% from baseline	<0.5 mL/kg/h for 12 h
Failure	3.0-fold increase OR GFR decrease >75% from baseline OR serum creatinine ≥4.0 mg/dL (≥354 µmol/L) with an acute increase of ≥0.5 mg/dL (44 µmol/L)	<0.3 mL/gk/h for 24 h OR anuria for 12 h
Loss of kidney function	Complete loss of kidney function >4 weeks	
End-stage kidney disease	Complete loss of kidney function >3 months	

Abbreviations: GFR: glomerular filtration rate, eGFR: estimated glomerular filtration rate. Please refer to text for references.

AKI Biomarkers

Neutrophil gelatinase-associated lipocalin (NGAL) is expressed in multiple cell types (e.g., renal, hepatic, cardiac, etc.) at relatively low, but constant levels [98]. NGAL generally functions as a bacteriostatic agent [99]. Urinary NGAL is the most widely studied biomarker of AKI [94]. Renal NGAL mRNA and protein are strongly upregulated after ischemic or toxic kidney injury in both human and animal models [100–103]. In the kidneys, NGAL is produced in the thick ascending limb of the loop of Henle and intercalated cells of the collecting duct [104]. In addition, circulating NGAL from extrarenal sources is filtered by the glomeruli and reabsorbed in the proximal tubules [105]. The increased urinary NGAL concentrations in the context of AKI are likely caused by endogenous NGAL production in the kidneys and reductions in tubular NGAL reabsorption [94,104], a hypothesis supported by clinical evidence that urinary NGAL is not elevated in isolated prerenal AKI [33,106], although these findings are not unanimous [107]. Therefore, urinary NGAL appears to be a marker of general tubular injury, without a specific etiology [93,94,104] (Figure 1). Plasma NGAL may also have some utility as a biomarker of AKI [93]. However, increases in plasma NGAL likely more readily reflect reductions in GFR, as well as renal ischemia and/or glomerular dysfunction [93,95] (Figure 1).

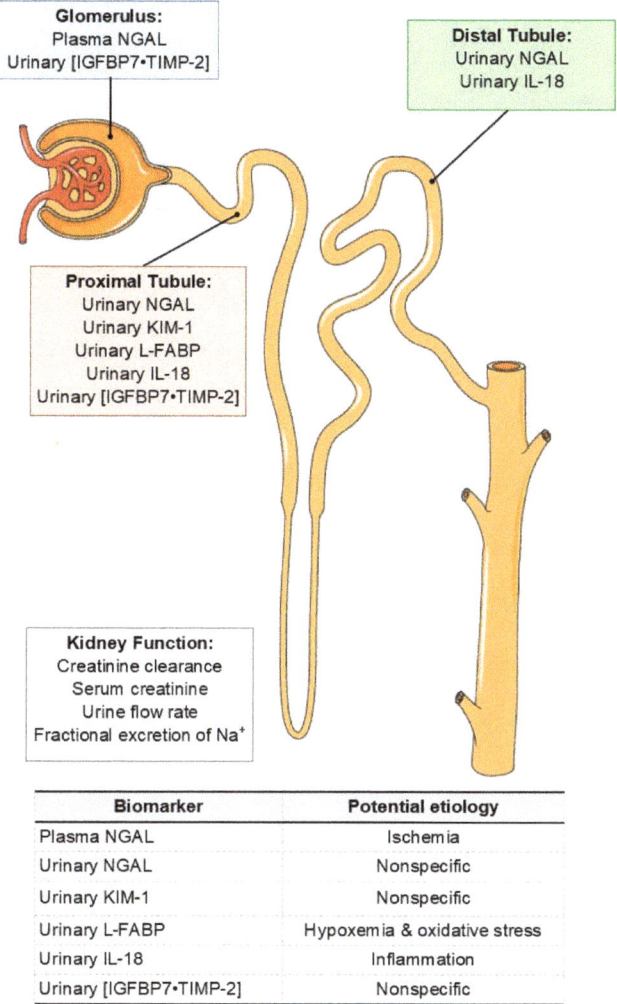

Figure 1. Top: Anatomical locations for biomarkers indicative of an increased risk of acute kidney injury (AKI) and common clinically relevant measures indicative of overall kidney function. Bottom: Potential etiology underlying increases in AKI biomarkers. Abbreviations—NGAL: Neutrophil gelatinase-associated lipocalin, [IGFBP7•TIMP-2]: the product of Insulin-like growth factor binding protein 7 (IGFBP7) and tissue inhibitor metalloproteinase 2 (TIMP-2), KIM-1: Kidney injury molecule-1, L-FABP: Liver-type fatty acid binding protein, IL-18: Interleukin-18. Please refer to text for references.

Kidney injury molecule-1 (KIM-1) is a transmembrane glycoprotein that is expressed at low levels in the normal kidney, but is further upregulated following ischemia-reperfusion and toxic kidney injury [108,109]. KIM-1 is mainly upregulated in proximal tubule cells during AKI [110,111]. Thus, increases in urinary KIM-1 likely indicate proximal tubule injury, although the etiology is nonspecific (Figure 1). Clinical studies investigating the utility of KIM-1 have shown variable results [94].

Liver-type fatty acid binding protein (L-FABP) is a cytoplasmic protein that protects against oxidative stress induced by peroxisomal metabolism [112], particularly in the presence of hypoxia given that the human L-FABP gene contains a hypoxia-inducible factor 1α response element [113]. L-FABP is excreted by proximal tubule epithelia into the tubular lumen together with bound peroxisomal products [113]. Urinary L-FABP can likely be used to identify patients at risk of developing AKI. This is supported by data indicating that patients with high L-FABP levels measured at the time of intensive care unit admission had a greater risk for developing AKI within 1 week, compared to a group of patients with lower L-FABP levels [114]. The genetic link with hypoxia-inducible factor 1α, together with findings indicating that urinary L-FABP levels are strongly correlated with the duration of ischemia in kidney transplant recipients [113], suggests that urinary L-FABP may provide an indication that the mechanism of this risk of AKI is related to proximal tubule hypoxemia and the development of oxidative stress (Figure 1).

Interleukin-18 (IL-18) is a proinflammatory cytokine that is produced in the intercalated cells of the collecting ducts of healthy kidneys [115], but is more broadly made in tubular epithelial cells as part of the inflammatory cascade induced by AKI [116]. Urinary IL-18 has been shown to be a promising biomarker of AKI in animal models [94]. Clinical studies also demonstrate that urinary IL-18 may have utility in predicting AKI [117]. However, its diagnostic value remains less clear [117]. Nevertheless, urinary IL-18 is likely a marker of general tubular injury and subsequent inflammatory-pathway activation (Figure 1).

Insulin-like growth factor binding protein 7 (IGFBP7) and *tissue inhibitor metalloproteinase 2* (TIMP-2) are proteins known to induce G1 cell cycle arrest [118]. In general, cell cycle arrest likely occurs to prevent potential DNA damage during cellular stress [119]. However, if cells stay in a phase too long or exit a phase too soon, the normal division and repair process can become maladaptive [120]. Cell cycle arrest occurs in renal epithelial cells in a variety of in vitro models of AKI [121] and is associated with the development of fibrosis following multiple types of AKI in rodents [122]. The arithmetic product of urinary IGFBP7 and urinary TIMP-2 ([IGFBP7•TIMP-2]) was identified as an AKI biomarker in a clinical study in which it outperformed ~338 other candidate biomarkers at predicting AKI based on standard clinical criteria (Table 1) [123]. In 2014, an [IGFBP7•TIMP-2] test system (better known by its proprietary name, NEPHROCHECK®) received FDA approval for marketing as a screening tool to estimate the risk of AKI development [124]. FDA approval carefully stipulated that increases in [IGFBP7•TIMP-2] should not necessarily be interpreted to indicate that AKI is ongoing. This indication is consistent with the fact that G1 cell cycle arrest occurs during the very early stages of cellular stress [125]. Notably, [IGFBP7•TIMP-2] is the only biomarker approved by the FDA for an AKI related indication [124]. Recent evidence indicates that increases in urinary [IGFBP7•TIMP-2] following diverse forms AKI is contributed to by a multitude of factors, which include decreases in glomerular permeability, proximal tubular cell leakage, and impaired reabsorption of IGFBP7 and TIMP-2 in the proximal tubule [126]. Thus, increases in [IGFBP7•TIMP-2] can be interpreted as evidence of the potential for renal injury of a nonspecific origin occurring in the glomeruli and proximal tubules (Figure 1).

3. Interpretation of AKI Biomarkers in Non-Clinical Settings

Recent advances in our understanding of AKI biomarkers have unexpectedly resulted in reports of the potential for AKI in situations traditionally considered to be clinically benign for the kidneys. This is highlighted by studies consistently demonstrating increases in AKI biomarkers following a single bout of prolonged endurance exercise [127–132]. Such findings have raised the question as to whether regularly engaging in endurance exercise may lead to poor renal health outcomes [133]. Arguments against this position are numerous and highlighted by the supposition that since the development of the 'jogging phenomenon' in the early 1960s [134] there has not been a profound increase in the incidence of AKI. Rather, the epidemic of AKI in the general population is largely attributed to patients hospitalized with acute illnesses and those undergoing major surgery, which may be partially contributed to by a greater recognition of AKI, and improved diagnostic and classification criteria [135]. Moreover, regularly engaging in vigorous physical activity (such as endurance exercise) reduces the risk of developing CKD [136], suggesting that the repeated exposures to exercise-induced elevations in AKI biomarkers does not lead to long-term sequelae. This has raised the question regarding how to interpret acute increases in AKI biomarkers in otherwise healthy individuals. This is an important consideration with regards to understanding the risk of AKI occurring subsequent to exercise in the heat.

The AKI biomarkers described herein were developed to identify AKI as would occur in clinical situations, in which large and sustained elevations were expected. In such instances, elevations in these AKI biomarkers would be indicative of intrinsic renal damage occurring at various locations along the nephron (Figure 1) [96,137]. Data obtained from otherwise healthy individuals engaging in endurance exercise demonstrate consistent increases in AKI biomarkers [127–132], but these elevations are often shorter in duration and not to the same extent as those observed in clinical situations [100–103,113,117,123]. These consistent elevations in AKI biomarkers are often interpreted as meaningful, but because the increases are small, they are usually not interpreted as being indicative of intrinsic renal injury. Rather, these small increases in AKI biomarkers likely reflect an increased potential to develop of AKI, although the possibility that increases in AKI biomarkers reflect some degree of intrinsic injury cannot be completely ruled out at this time. We believe this conclusion is indirectly supported by evidence that elevations in AKI biomarkers in the laboratory setting typically resolve ~24 h following exercise [127,130]. Thus, small, transient increases in AKI biomarkers are likely indicative of acute kidney stress [138]. This state likely represents a period in which there is an increased risk of developing AKI, with the magnitude of this risk occurring in proportion to the magnitude of elevations in AKI biomarkers. Notably, this definition is consistent with the FDA approved indication for urinary [IGFBP7•TIMP-2] as a biomarker of the magnitude of the risk associated with developing AKI.

Currently, there is no consensus regarding the best AKI biomarker to measure. Urinary NGAL may have the most robust evidence base [94], but only urinary [IGFBP7•TIMP-2] has an FDA approved indication for AKI [124]. That said, to our knowledge no study has measured urinary [IGFBP7•TIMP-2] under conditions of exercise, heat strain and/or exercise. In this context, there is likely value in employing a battery of assays for AKI biomarkers. This approach may provide important insights regarding: (i) the magnitude of the risk of AKI, (ii) the anatomical location where this risk originated, and (iii) the potential etiology of this risk (Figure 1). Such an understanding may provide important information towards determining countermeasures to reduce the risk of AKI in the context of exercise in the heat.

There is likely also value in combining the measurement of AKI biomarkers with traditional indices of kidney function (e.g., serum creatinine, urine flow rate, etc.) for interpreting the risk of AKI. This approach has been proposed in the clinical literature as a method to discern prerenal AKI (i.e., only a reduction in kidney function without increases in AKI biomarkers) from intrinsic AKI (i.e., a reduction in kidney function with increased AKI biomarkers) or subclinical AKI (i.e., increased biomarkers in the absence of a reduction in kidney function) [96,97,137,139]. In a similar manner, the risk of AKI can likely be assessed in the context of exercise in the heat (Figure 2). For instance, a decrease in kidney function without increases in AKI biomarkers may be indicative of a relatively mild risk for AKI because the change in function is unlikely to be pathological. This decline in kidney function may be the normal physiological response of the kidneys to a stressor (such as exercise) that is completely reversed once the stress has abated. That said, increases in AKI biomarkers without a change in kidney function may be interpreted as a slightly higher (i.e., moderate) risk of AKI, owing to the presence of potential pathological processes. Finally, the highest risk of AKI may occur when kidney function is reduced alongside increases in AKI biomarkers. Moreover, this risk could be further delineated based on the magnitude of the reductions in kidney function and/or increases in AKI biomarkers. For example, the condition invoking the greatest reductions in kidney function and largest increases in AKI biomarkers would be interpreted as having the highest risk of AKI. Notably, however, this AKI risk matrix is likely only useful in situations where comparisons between conditions might be considered the most important (i.e., it may only provide an index of relative AKI risk). The utility of this matrix for providing information regarding absolute AKI risk is currently unclear.

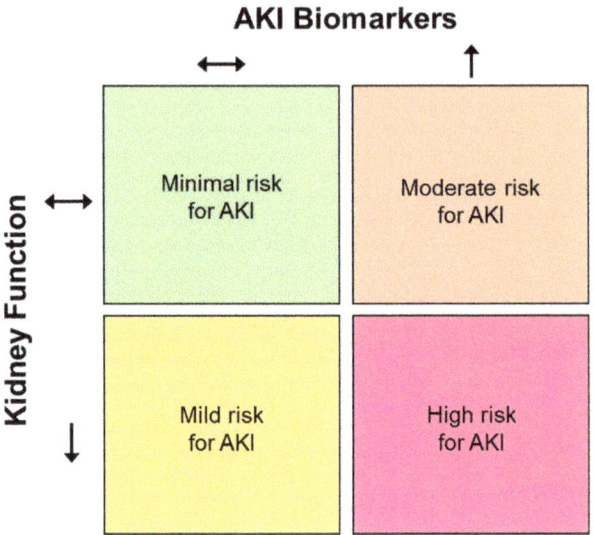

Figure 2. Proposed method for determining the relative risk of developing acute kidney injury (AKI) during exercise in the heat based on changes in kidney function and AKI biomarkers. A decrease in kidney function without increases in AKI biomarkers may be indicative of a relatively mild risk for AKI because the renal changes are unlikely to be pathological (bottom-left). Increases in AKI biomarkers without a change in kidney function may be interpreted as a slightly higher (i.e., moderate) risk of AKI, owing to the presence of potential pathological processes (top-right). The highest risk of AKI may occur when kidney function is reduced alongside increases in AKI biomarkers (bottom-right). AKI risk could be further delineated based on the magnitude of the reductions in kidney function and/or increases in AKI biomarkers.

Finally, an important methodological consideration is the normalization of urinary AKI biomarkers to urine concentration. It is common in clinical and research settings to correct urine-based AKI biomarkers by normalizing to urinary creatinine [140]. However, the application of urinary creatinine normalization in exercise models is likely flawed [36]. This is because urinary creatinine excretion becomes inconsistent both within and between subjects during and following exercise, owing to relatively large swings in GFR [141]. Thus, in controlled laboratory settings it is often suggested that the most accurate method to quantify renal biomarkers requires the collection of timed urine specimens to estimate the excretion rate of a given biomarker [140]. Therefore, concentrations of urinary AKI biomarkers in the context of exercise in the heat are often normalized to urine flow rate [30,36]. That said, normalization to other markers of urinary concentration (e.g., osmolality) may also be a valid approach [131,132].

4. AKI Susceptibility Evoked by Exercise in the Heat in Humans

Clinical AKI associated with exercise in the heat has occasionally been reported in the clinical literature. To our knowledge, the most complete clinical dataset was published in 1967, which reported the cases of eight previously healthy military recruits who had developed AKI during training exercises outdoors in the summer months [142]. The overall incidence of AKI is generally very low in this population of military recruits. However, it was later estimated that ~10% of the AKI cases treated at Walter Reed General (Military) Hospital from 1960 to 1966 were due to AKI occurring subsequent to exercise in the heat [143]. Thus, there is clinical evidence that exercise in the heat can bring about AKI, at least in a subset of individuals.

More recently, traditional measures of kidney function have been combined with AKI biomarkers to examine the risk of AKI during exercise in the heat. Generally, the findings from these studies suggest that exercise in the heat can increase the susceptibility to AKI. For instance, Junglee et al. demonstrated that mild heat strain (+1.3 °C increase in core temperature) and mild dehydration (~1% body weight loss) due to exercise in the heat resulted in elevations in serum creatinine, reductions in urine flow rate, and increases in plasma NGAL [36]. Our laboratory has furthered this work and found that elevations in serum creatinine and plasma NGAL were influenced by the magnitude of increases in core temperature and the extent of dehydration produced by exercise in the heat of two different durations [29] (Figure 3). Of the increases in serum creatinine, ~30% of the observations satisfied the criteria for stage 1 AKI according to the AKIN criteria (Table 1) [73] (Figure 3). We also showed that elevations in serum creatinine and plasma NGAL returned to baseline levels the following day [29] (Figure 3), which is supportive of the idea that this period of an increased risk of AKI is transient. Similarly, McDermott et al. found that 4–6 h of exercise in the heat, which evoked moderate dehydration (~1.6% body weight loss), elevated both serum creatinine and serum NGAL [70]. Collectively, the findings to date support that exercise in the heat can increase the risk of AKI in humans and that this increased risk occurs in proportion to the magnitude of heat strain and dehydration. To our knowledge, however, no study in the context of exercise in the heat has systematically examined markers of kidney function simultaneous with a panel of AKI biomarkers. This is a significant limitation with regards to the strength of the evidence base. Thus, future studies are necessary to conclusively determine the risk of AKI caused by exercise in the heat.

Importantly, many of the potential modulators of the magnitude of AKI risk evoked by exercise in the heat remain largely unexplored. This is important because resolving these unknowns will have important ramifications regarding the development of countermeasures to alleviate the risk of AKI during exercise in the heat. For instance, the relative importance of heat strain versus dehydration on the magnitude of the risk of AKI evoked by exercise in the heat is unknown. Although a formal body of evidence is lacking, there is evidence that hydration status may be a comparatively more important modulator of AKI risk compared to heat strain alone. For instance, allowing rodents full access to water during 4 weeks of repeated heat exposure prevented the renal injury and nephropathy that occurred in the rodents that were exposed to the same heat load, but were restricted from drinking during the heat exposures [47]. Thus, it can be speculated that hydration status is the most important modulator of AKI risk during exercise in the heat. That said, a limitation of this conclusion is that core temperature is often elevated to a greater extent in a dehydrated state during exercise and/or heat exposure [144]. In the aforementioned study, core temperature in the rats was not measured [47]. Therefore, the comparative importance of heat strain versus dehydration on the risk of AKI during exercise in the heat remains largely uncertain. Another important knowledge gap is the effect of substances that have nephrotoxic side effects on the risk of AKI during exercise in the heat. The best example is likely NSAIDs, which are commonly used in occupational settings [18,19]. Notably, a 1.2 g dose of the NSAID ibuprofen results in greater reductions in GFR during exercise in the heat compared to a placebo condition [145]. However, recent evidence indicates that this deleterious effect on kidney function does not translate to a greater risk of AKI, such that a 0.6 g dose of ibuprofen did not lead to greater increases in serum NGAL following 4–6 h of exercise in the heat [70]. However, these findings may be explained by the lower NSAID dose (0.6 vs. 1.2 g). Thus, future studies are required to elucidate the modulatory role of nephrotoxic substances (particularly NSAIDs) on the risk of AKI during exercise in the heat.

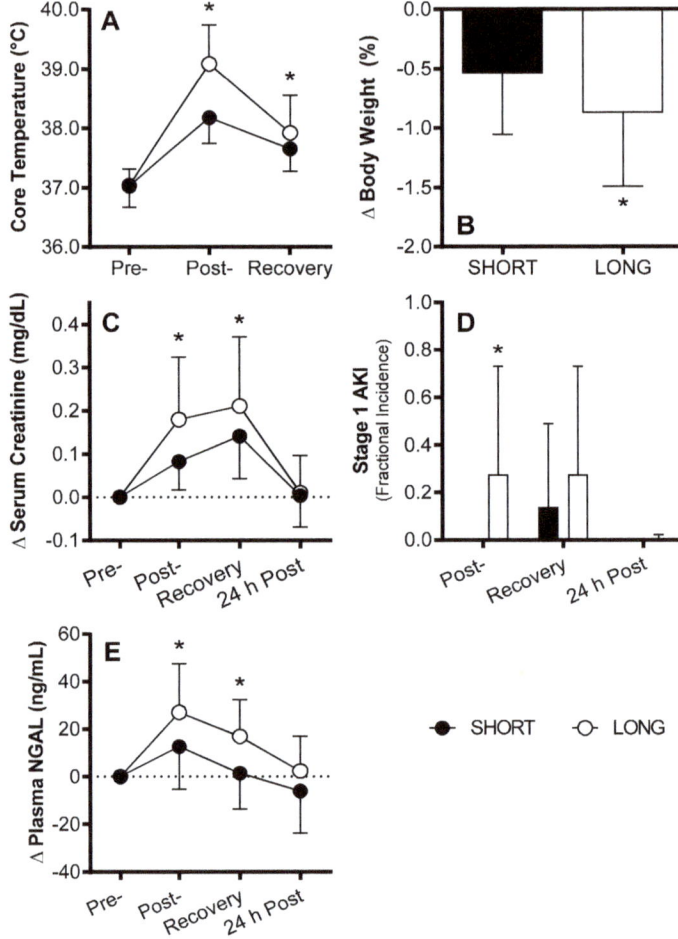

Figure 3. During the longer of two bouts of exercise in the heat (LONG vs. SHORT), greater heat strain (**A**) and dehydration (**B**) resulted in greater changes (Δ) in serum creatinine (**C**), which were sufficient to satisfy the criteria for Stage 1 acute kidney injury (AKI) in ~30% of the subjects (**D**), and greater increases in plasma neutrophil gelatinase-associated lipocalin (NGAL) (**E**). * different from SHORT ($p < 0.05$), Mean ± SD, n = 29. From Schlader et al. [29] with permission.

Mechanisms of AKI Susceptibility Evoked by Exercise in the Heat

In general, the mechanisms by which exercise in the heat may increase the risk of AKI in humans remain largely unexplored. That said, data from animal models, together with some fundamental physiological data in humans, suggest that the potential increased risk of AKI provoked by exercise in the heat is multifactorial.

Heat strain [145,146], dehydration [81,82] and exercise [147–149] independently reduce renal blood flow in humans, and even more profound reductions in perfusion are observed when these conditions are combined [150]. These reductions in renal perfusion are largely due to increases in renal sympathetic nerve activity [151] and circulating vasopressin levels [152], but may also be contributed to by activation of the renin–angiotensin–aldosterone system. For instance, angiotensin II has vasoconstrictor actions in the kidneys [153] and may modulate kidney function during exercise in the heat in humans [154]. Notably, these declines in renal perfusion typically resolve with recovery [36,145,146,150] and are generally considered to be clinically inconsequential [16]. That said, data from dehydrated rats indicate that reductions in overall renal perfusion can invoke a heterogenous distribution of blood flow within the kidneys [84]. Strikingly, in this same study a sub-analysis of data from one rat using a different experimental technique indicated that dehydration can produce localized ischemia, particularly in cortical regions [84]. These data are seemingly corroborated by data in dogs whereby heat strain-induced reductions in renal perfusion were solely caused by reductions in cortical blood flow, without a change in medullary blood flow [155]. This relatively low blood flow state can compromise oxygen delivery to the renal cortex, which could provoke ischemia and a localized reduction in ATP [84]. Importantly, a low ATP environment can theoretically increase the risk of AKI secondary to increased oxidative stress and inflammation [156].

Against this background, it is clearly important to understand how exercise in the heat may affect renal vascular control in humans, particularly as it relates to intrarenal blood flow distribution and oxygenation. To our knowledge, such studies have never been carried out. This knowledge gap may be important for understanding the mechanisms by which exercise in the heat may increase the risk of AKI. For instance, the renal cortex, which demonstrates reductions in blood flow during dehydration (in rats) [84] and heat strain (in dogs) [155], anatomically houses the majority of the proximal tubules [157], where upwards to 65% of sodium is reabsorbed [158]. Sodium reabsorption in the kidneys can be directly stimulated by aldosterone [159], angiotensin II [160] and/or increases in renal sympathetic nerve activity [161], all of which are increased with heat strain, dehydration and/or exercise in an effort to maintain fluid homeostasis [162–164]. Sodium reabsorption is energetically expensive, owing to the reliance on the Na^+/K^+ pump [165]. Thus, an increased demand for sodium reabsorption may increase the susceptibility of the kidneys to injury particularly in the presence of additional stressors that can compromise ATP production (e.g., low blood flow). This is supported by data demonstrating that blocking the actions of aldosterone via the administration of a mineralocorticoid receptor antagonist attenuates the severity of injury in a rat model of mild ischemia-induced AKI [166], and prevents the subsequent development of CKD in a similar rodent model of ischemic AKI [167]. Aldosterone exerts its sodium reabsorption actions via the Na^+/K^+ pump [159]. Thus, these data support the idea that increased energy demands associated with activation of the Na^+/K^+ pump can contribute to the incidence and severity of AKI. Whether this holds true in the context of exercise in the heat remains unknown. Notably, sodium reabsorption is greater during exercise in the heat compared to passive heat exposure to the same extent of dehydration and heat strain [164], suggesting that exercise in the heat evokes a relatively large renal ATP demand. Moreover, sodium reabsorption is greater during exercise in the heat in the presence of dehydration [168]. This increased ATP demand is further challenged by the relatively low renal cortical oxygen delivery that is likely occurring subsequent to heat strain, dehydration and exercise. Oxygen delivery is required to sustain ATP production. Moreover, any mismatch between oxygen delivery and oxygen demand increases the susceptibility of the kidneys to injury [169], which likely occurs subsequent to increased oxidative stress and inflammation [156]. Thus, it is possible that a redistribution of blood flow within the kidneys, together with an increased oxygen demand, contributes to the increased risk of AKI during exercise in the heat. However, direct evidence is warranted.

There is certainly reason to believe that reductions in renal blood flow contribute to the increased risk of AKI during exercise in the heat in humans. However, there are two arguments against this contention. First, heat acclimation (or acclimatization) invoked by repeated heat exposures stimulates greater reductions in renal blood flow during heat exposure in rats [170], which contributes to improvements in heat tolerance [171]. Recent evidence, however, indicates that heat acclimation over a 23 day period attenuated the rise in serum creatinine during exercise in the heat in humans [172]. This was interpreted as evidence that heat acclimation likely has a protective effect in the kidneys, such that the incidence of serum creatinine defined AKI was attenuated with heat acclimation [172]. Despite the limitations associated with using serum creatinine to define AKI risk, such findings suggest that the presumed greater reductions in renal blood flow during exercise in the heat following heat acclimation may not translate to a greater risk of AKI. That said, it is important to note that workers experiencing CKDu are likely heat acclimated. Thus, the presumed protective effect of heat acclimation on kidney health remains uncertain. Second, older adults have attenuated reductions in renal blood flow during exercise in the heat [173] and passive heat exposure [174]. However, the incidence of AKI during heat waves is disproportionately higher in older adults compared to younger adults [175–178]. Thus, the theoretical benefit conferred by the relative maintenance of renal blood flow during heat exposure may not be protective against the risk of AKI in older adults. That said, these findings may be confounded by other age-related changes in kidney function, such as overactivation of the polyol-fructokinase pathway [179] and augmented vasopressin responses [180,181], both of which are discussed below. Nonetheless, there is a clear need to discern the role of reductions in renal blood flow to the increased risk of AKI during exercise in the heat in humans.

Rodent models also convincingly demonstrate that nephropathy due to recurrent AKI elicited by repeated heat exposures is contributed to by activation of the intrarenal polyol-fructokinase pathway and the endogenous production of fructose [47–49,182,183]. The polyol pathway is stimulated by an increased plasma osmolality that upregulates the enzyme aldose reductase [184]. Aldose reductase catalyzes the conversion of glucose into sorbitol, which has a protective effect against a hyperosmolar renal environment [184]. However, this benefit is not sustainable. Recent evidence has uncovered the potential deleterious effect of the subsequent activation of the fructokinase pathway, particularly with recurrent heat exposure and/or dehydration [185]. Under such conditions, sorbitol can be metabolized to fructose by sorbitol dehydrogenase and this fructose is then broken down by the enzyme fructokinase [185]. The metabolic breakdown of fructose occurs rapidly and is energetically costly [186]. Thus, activation of the fructokinase pathway can further reduce ATP availability [187]. It should be noted that the anatomical location of the polyol-fructokinase pathway is the proximal tubules [185,186], a location that likely has experienced a selective reduction in blood flow [84,155] and already has a heightened ATP demand [165] due to sodium reabsorption [164,168] and the activation of the Na^+/K^+ pump [159]. Collectively, this reduced ability to generate ATP can promote oxidative stress and inflammation [156] and can stimulate uric acid production [186]. Notably, hyperuricemia can further reduce renal perfusion [188] and independently can incite the polyol-fructokinase pathway [49,189], thereby exacerbating the oxidative stress and inflammation [67] that ultimately causes AKI [156]. Importantly, the fructokinase pathway is at least partially mediated by actions associated with vasopressin release [48,183,190], the production of which is stimulated by increases in plasma osmolality and/or hypovolemia [191].

The importance of the polyol-fructokinase pathway in AKI associated with heat exposure is highlighted by data indicating that when rats consume a high fructose beverage, which exogenously increases substrate for the fructokinase pathway, the resulting AKI and kidney damage from recurrent heat exposure is exacerbated [182,183]. Moreover, when the ability to generate fructokinase is genetically knocked out, mice exposed to recurrent heat exposure do not demonstrate AKI or kidney damage [47]. We have recently provided similar evidence in humans such that drinking a soft drink with a high fructose content during and following 4 h of exercise in the heat exacerbates increases in serum creatinine, reductions in urine flow rate, and elevations urinary NGAL, compared to when drinking an equivalent amount of water [30] (Figure 4). Interestingly, this observation occurred alongside greater increases in copeptin (a stable surrogate for vasopressin) and serum uric acid (Figure 4). These latter findings support the animal data [48,182,183] and the mechanisms by which the activation of the polyol-fructokinase pathway may increase the risk of AKI [185]. This recent work suggests that polyol-fructokinase pathway activity may modulate kidney function and the risk of AKI following a single bout of exercise in the heat in humans. It is important to note, however, that to our knowledge there is no evidence regarding whether the polyol-fructokinase pathway directly modulates the risk of AKI during exercise in humans. This is likely due to a lack of established biomarkers for determining the activation of these pathways in humans. Further work is required to establish such biomarkers and to apply this knowledge to exercise in the heat.

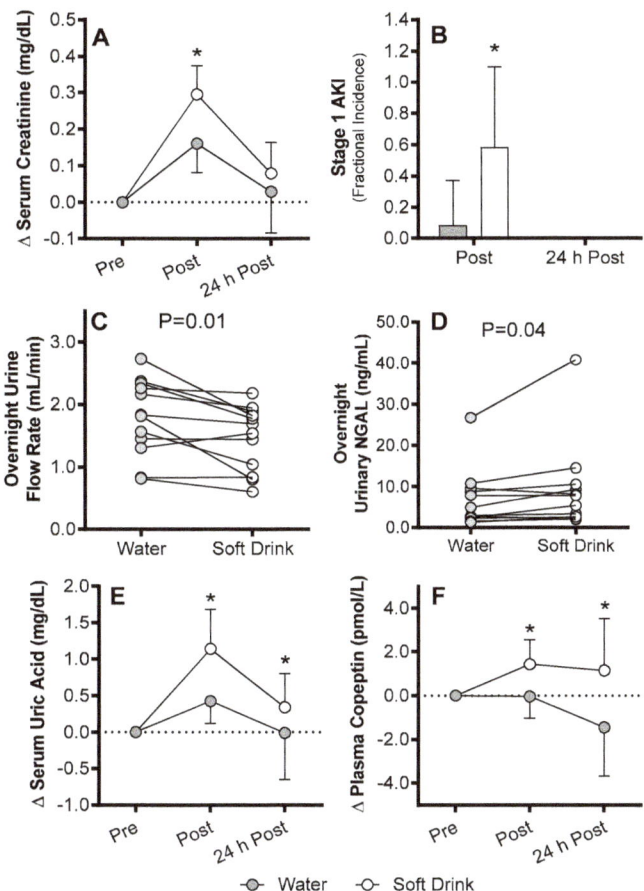

Figure 4. Despite no differences in core temperature or changes in body weight (data not shown), drinking a high fructose soft drink compared to water during and following 4 h of exercise in the heat resulted in greater changes (Δ) in serum creatinine (**A**), meeting the criteria for Stage 1 acute kidney injury (AKI) at Post exercise in ~60% of the subjects (**B**). During the overnight period (defined as the time from leaving the laboratory immediately after post-exercise data collection until returning to the laboratory 24 h following pre-exercise (~18 h following post-exercise)), drinking a soft drink reduced urine flow rate (despite drinking ~347 mL more fluid during the overnight period) (**C**) and elevated urinary neutrophil gelatinase-associated lipocalin (NGAL) (**D**). These changes in indices in kidney function and biomarkers of AKI in the soft drink trial were paralleled by greater elevations in serum uric acid (**E**) and plasma copeptin (**F**), a stable surrogate for vasopressin. * different from Water ($p < 0.05$), Mean ± SD or individual values, n = 12. From Chapman et al. [30] with permission.

5. Summary

The purpose of this narrative review was to present evidence that exercise in the heat increases the risk of developing AKI in humans. A growing body of evidence demonstrates that passive heat exposure in rodents causes kidney injury, and when this injury is chronically repeated it is capable of eliciting CKD. Experimental evidence in humans is more limited, with many gaps in the literature (Table 2). That said, studies consistently demonstrate that a single bout of exercise in the heat increases biomarkers of AKI and that the magnitude of these elevations in AKI biomarkers is dependent on the extent of heat strain and dehydration. In this context, elevations in AKI biomarkers are not necessarily indicative of intrinsic renal damage. Rather, a better interpretation is that they reflect an increased risk of AKI. Data largely derived from animal models indicate that the mechanism(s) underlying elevations in AKI biomarkers is multifactorial (Figure 5). For instance, heat-related reductions in renal blood flow may provoke a heterogenous blood flow distribution within the kidneys. In theory, this can promote localized ischemia, hypoxemia and ATP depletion, which may be exacerbated by an increased demand for sodium reabsorption—an energetically expensive process. Moreover, heightened polyol-fructokinase pathway activity likely exacerbates tissue hypoxemia and ATP depletion, occurring secondary to the intrarenal production of fructose and hyperuricemia. Collectively, these responses likely promote inflammation and oxidative stress, which can elevate biomarkers of AKI in otherwise healthy humans. Unfortunately, there is currently very little direct mechanistic evidence to support how exercise in the heat may increase the risk of AKI in humans (Table 2). This is an important knowledge gap that has ramifications regarding the development of countermeasures to safeguard the renal health of people who regularly engage in physical work in hot environments.

Table 2. Selected identified knowledge gaps regarding the link between exercise in the heat, acute kidney injury and the development of chronic kidney disease in humans.

• Acute Kidney Injury and the Development of Chronic kidney Disease:
• Can exercise in the heat induce intrinsic renal damage?
• How do we interpret increases in AKI biomarkers associated with exercise in the heat?
• Can repeated exposures to AKI caused by exercise in the heat lead to CKDu? How does the frequency and severity of this AKI relate to the development and severity of CKDu?
• Does heat acclimation alleviate the risk of AKI (and CKDu) associated with exercise in the heat?
Mechanisms by Which Exercise in the Heat May Increase the Risk Of Acute Kidney Injury:
• What is the relative importance of heat strain versus dehydration on the magnitude of the risk of AKI evoked by exercise in the heat?
• Do NSAIDs (or other common substances with nephrotoxic side effects) modulate the risk of AKI evoked by exercise in the heat?
• To what extent does exercise in the heat invoke a heterogenous distribution of blood flow in the kidneys? What are the contributions of heat strain and/or dehydration?
• Do reductions in renal blood flow during exercise in the heat cause localized ischemia, reductions in oxygenation, and/or decreases in ATP availability? Where do these changes occur within the kidneys?
• Does exercise in the heat promote inflammation and oxidative stress within the kidneys? What are the contributions of heat strain and/or dehydration?
• What is the extent by which activation of the Na^+/K^+ pump contributes to the risk of AKI during exercise in the heat?
• Does the polyol-fructokinase pathway directly contribute to the risk of AKI during exercise in the heat?
• What are the roles of vasopressin and hyperuricemia in the risk of AKI during exercise in the heat?

Abbreviations: AKI: acute kidney injury, CKDu: chronic kidney disease of unknown origins, NSAIDs: nonsteroidal anti-inflammatory drugs.

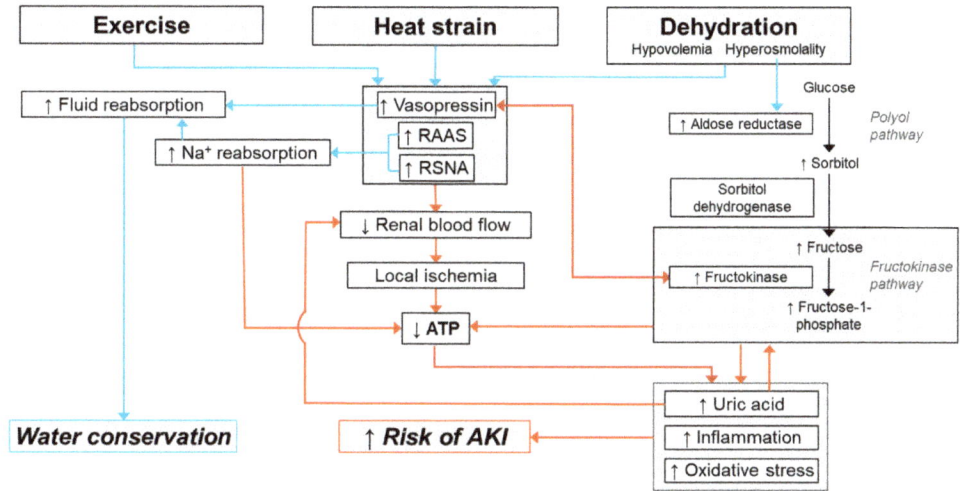

Figure 5. Potential mechanisms by which exercise in the heat and the subsequent development of heat strain (i.e., increases in core body temperature) and dehydration (a hypovolemic, hyperosmotic state) may increase the risk of acute kidney injury (AKI) while simultaneously promoting fluid conservation. Red arrows indicate potential pathophysiological pathways. Blue arrows indicate known beneficial physiological responses. Abbreviations—RAAS: Renin–angiotensin–aldosterone system, RSNA: Renal sympathetic nerve activity, ATP: adenosine triphosphate. Please refer to text for references.

Author Contributions: Z.J.S., D.H., M.D.P., R.R.P., J.W.L., B.D.J. and C.L.C. conceptualized the manuscript; Z.J.S. drafted the manuscript; Z.J.S. prepared figures; Z.J.S., D.H., M.D.P., R.R.P., J.W.L., B.D.J. and C.L.C. edited and revised the manuscript; Z.J.S., D.H., M.D.P., R.R.P., J.W.L., B.D.J. and C.L.C. approved the final version of the manuscript.

Funding: The writing of this manuscript and the work from our laboratory presented herein were not externally funded.

Acknowledgments: We thank the people who participated in the studies described herein.

Conflicts of Interest: The authors have no related conflicts of interest to report.

References

1. Chatterjee, R. Occupational hazard. *Science* **2016**, *352*, 24–27. [CrossRef] [PubMed]
2. Johnson, R.J.; Wesseling, C.; Newman, L.S. Chronic kidney disease of unknown cause in agricultural communities. *New Engl. J. Med.* **2019**, *380*, 1843–1852. [CrossRef] [PubMed]
3. Trabanino, R.G.; Aguilar, R.; Silva, C.R.; Mercado, M.O.; Merino, R.L. Nefropatía terminal en pacientes de un hospital de referencia en El Salvador. *Revista Panamericana de Salud Pública* **2002**, *12*, 202–206. [CrossRef] [PubMed]
4. Torres, C.; Aragón, A.; González, M.; Jakobsson, K.; Elinder, C.-G.; Lundberg, I.; Wesseling, C. Decreased kidney function of unknown cause in Nicaragua: A community-based survey. *Am. J. Kidney Dis.* **2010**, *55*, 485–496. [CrossRef] [PubMed]
5. O'Donnell, J.K.; Tobey, M.; Weiner, D.E.; Stevens, L.A.; Johnson, S.; Stringham, P.; Cohen, B.; Brooks, D.R. Prevalence of and risk factors for chronic kidney disease in rural Nicaragua. *Nephrol. Dial. Transplant.* **2011**, *26*, 2798–2805. [CrossRef] [PubMed]
6. Peraza, S.; Wesseling, C.; Aragon, A.; Leiva, R.; García-Trabanino, R.A.; Torres, C.; Jakobsson, K.; Elinder, C.G.; Hogstedt, C. Decreased kidney function among agricultural workers in El Salvador. *Am. J. Kidney Dis.* **2012**, *59*, 531–540. [CrossRef]

7. Glaser, J.; Lemery, J.; Rajagopalan, B.; Diaz, H.F.; García-Trabanino, R.; Taduri, G.; Madero, M.; Amarasinghe, M.; Abraham, G.; Anutrakulchai, S. Climate Change and the Emergent Epidemic of CKD from Heat Stress in Rural Communities: The Case for Heat Stress Nephropathy. *Clin. J. Am. Soc. Nephrol.* **2016**, *11*, 1472–1483. [CrossRef]
8. Flores, S.; Rider, A.C.; Alter, H.J. Mesoamerican nephropathy: A novel case of kidney failure in a US ED. *Am. J. Emerg Med.* **2015**, *34*, 1323.e5–1323.e6. [CrossRef]
9. Organization, P.A.H. *Epidemic of Chronic Kidney Disease in Agricultural Communities in Central America Case Definitions, Methodological Basis and Approaches for Public Health Surveillance*; Pan American Health Organization: Washington, DC, USA, 2017.
10. Elledge, M.F.; Redmon, J.H.; Levine, K.E.; Wickremasinghe, R.J.; Wanigasariya, K.P.; Peiris-John, R.J. *Chronic Kidney Disease of Unknown Etiology in Sri Lanka: Quest for Understanding and Global Implications*; RTI Research Brief. Research; RTI Press: Triangle Park, NC, USA, 2014.
11. Flouris, A.D.; Dinas, P.C.; Ioannou, L.G.; Nybo, L.; Havenith, G.; Kenny, G.P.; Kjellstrom, T. Workers' health and productivity under occupational heat strain: A systematic review and meta-analysis. *Lancet Planet. Health* **2018**, *2*, e521–e531. [CrossRef]
12. Pearce, N.; Caplin, B. *Let's Take the Heat OUT of the CKDu Debate: More Evidence Is Needed*; BMJ Publishing Group Ltd.: London, UK, 2019.
13. Wijkström, J.; Leiva, R.; Elinder, C.-G.; Leiva, S.; Trujillo, Z.; Trujillo, L.; Söderberg, M.; Hultenby, K.; Wernerson, A. Clinical and pathological characterization of Mesoamerican nephropathy: A new kidney disease in Central America. *Am. J. Kidney Dis.* **2013**, *62*, 908–918. [CrossRef]
14. Correa-Rotter, R.; Wesseling, C.; Johnson, R.J. CKD of unknown origin in Central America: The case for a Mesoamerican nephropathy. *Am. J. Kidney Dis.* **2014**, *63*, 506–520. [CrossRef] [PubMed]
15. Roncal-Jimenez, C.; Lanaspa, M.; Jensen, T.; Sanchez-Lozada, L.; Johnson, R. Mechanisms by which dehydration may lead to chronic kidney disease. *Ann. Nutr. Metab.* **2015**, *66*, 10–13. [CrossRef] [PubMed]
16. Roncal-Jimenez, C.A.; García-Trabanino, R.; Wesseling, C.; Johnson, R.J. Mesoamerican Nephropathy or Global Warming Nephropathy? *Blood Purif.* **2016**, *41*, 135–138. [CrossRef] [PubMed]
17. Orantes, C.M.; Herrera, R.; Almaguer, M.; Brizuela, E.G.; Hernández, C.E.; Bayarre, H.; Amaya, J.C.; Calero, D.J.; Orellana, P.; Colindres, R.M. Chronic kidney disease and associated risk factors in the Bajo Lempa region of El Salvador: Nefrolempa study, 2009. *Med. Rev.* **2011**, *13*, 14–22.
18. Herrera, R.; Orantes, C.M.; Almaguer, M.; Alfonso, P.; Bayarre, H.D.; Leiva, I.M.; Smith, M.J.; Cubias, R.A.; Almendárez, W.O.; Cubias, F.R. Clinical characteristics of chronic kidney disease of nontraditional causes in Salvadoran farming communities. *Med. Rev.* **2014**, *16*, 39–48.
19. Butler-Dawson, J.; Krisher, L.; Asensio, C.; Cruz, A.; Tenney, L.; Weitzenkamp, D.; Dally, M.; Asturias, E.J.; Newman, L.S. Risk factors for declines in kidney function in sugarcane workers in Guatemala. *J. Occup. Environ. Med.* **2018**, *60*, 548. [CrossRef] [PubMed]
20. González-Quiroz, M.; Pearce, N.; Caplin, B.; Nitsch, D. What do epidemiological studies tell us about chronic kidney disease of undetermined cause in Meso-America? A systematic review and meta-analysis. *Clin. Kidney J.* **2017**, *11*, 496–506. [CrossRef]
21. McClean, M.; Amador, J.J.; Laws, R.; Kaufman, J.S.; Weiner, D.E.; Sanchez-Rodriguez, J.; Brooks, D. *Biological Sampling Report: Investigating Biomarkers of Kidney Injury and Chronic Kidney Disease among Workers in Western Nicaragua*; University School of Public Health; Compliance Advisor Ombudsman: Boston, MA, USA, 2012.
22. Gifford, F.J.; Gifford, R.M.; Eddleston, M.; Dhaun, N. Endemic Nephropathy Across the World. *Kidney Int.* **2016**, *2*, 282–292. [CrossRef]
23. Johnson, R.J.; Glaser, J.; Sánchez-Lozada, L.G. Chronic kidney disease of unknown etiology: A disease related to global warming? *Med. Rev.* **2014**, *16*, 79.
24. Chapman, E.; Haby, M.M.; Illanes, E.; Sanchez-Viamonte, J.; Elias, V.; Reveiz, L. Risk factors for chronic kidney disease of non-traditional causes: A systematic review. *Pan Am. J. Pub. Health* **2019**, *43*, e35. [CrossRef]
25. Valcke, M.; Levasseur, M.-E.; da Silva, A.S.; Wesseling, C. Pesticide exposures and chronic kidney disease of unknown etiology: An epidemiologic review. *Environ. Health* **2017**, *16*, 49. [CrossRef] [PubMed]
26. Sorensen, C.J.; Butler-Dawson, J.; Dally, M.; Krisher, L.; Griffin, B.R.; Johnson, R.J.; Lemery, J.; Asensio, C.; Tenney, L.; Newman, L.S. Risk Factors and Mechanisms Underlying Cross-Shift Decline in Kidney Function in Guatemalan Sugarcane Workers. *J. Occup. Environ. Med.* **2019**, *61*, 239. [CrossRef] [PubMed]

27. Roncal-Jimenez, C.; García-Trabanino, R.; Barregard, L.; Lanaspa, M.A.; Wesseling, C.; Harra, T.; Aragón, A.; Grases, F.; Jarquin, E.R.; González, M.A. Heat stress nephropathy from exercise-induced uric acid crystalluria: A perspective on Mesoamerican nephropathy. *Am. J. Kidney Dis.* **2016**, *67*, 20–30. [CrossRef] [PubMed]
28. Madero, M.; García-Arroyo, F.E.; Sánchez-Lozada, L.-G. Pathophysiologic insight into MesoAmerican nephropathy. *Curr. Opin. Nephrol. Hypertens.* **2017**, *26*, 296–302. [CrossRef] [PubMed]
29. Schlader, Z.J.; Chapman, C.L.; Sarkar, S.; Russo, L.; Rideout, T.C.; Parker, M.D.; Johnson, B.D.; Hostler, D. Firefighter work duration influences the extent of acute kidney injury. *Med. Sci. Sport Exerc.* **2017**, *49*, 1745–1753. [CrossRef] [PubMed]
30. Chapman, C.L.; Johnson, B.D.; Sackett, J.R.; Parker, M.D.; Schlader, Z.J. Soft drink consumption during and following exercise in the heat elevates biomarkers of acute kidney injury. *Am. J. Physiol. Regul. Integr. Comp. Physiol.* **2019**, *316*, R189–R198. [CrossRef]
31. Laws, R.L.; Brooks, D.R.; Amador, J.J.; Weiner, D.E.; Kaufman, J.S.; Ramírez-Rubio, O.; Riefkohl, A.; Scammell, M.K.; López-Pilarte, D.; Sánchez, J.M. Biomarkers of kidney injury among Nicaraguan sugarcane workers. *Am. J. Kidney Dis.* **2016**, *67*, 209–217. [CrossRef]
32. Butler-Dawson, J.; Krisher, L.; Yoder, H.; Dally, M.; Sorensen, C.; Johnson, R.J.; Asensio, C.; Cruz, A.; Johnson, E.C.; Carlton, E.J. Evaluation of heat stress and cumulative incidence of acute kidney injury in sugarcane workers in Guatemala. *Int. Arch. Occup. Environ. Health* **2019**, 1–14. [CrossRef]
33. Au, V.; Feit, J.; Barasch, J.; Sladen, R.N.; Wagener, G. Urinary neutrophil gelatinase–associated lipocalin (NGAL) distinguishes sustained from transient acute kidney injury after general surgery. *Kidney Int. Rep.* **2016**, *1*, 3–9. [CrossRef]
34. Rawson, E.S.; Clarkson, P.M.; Tarnopolsky, M.A. Perspectives on exertional rhabdomyolysis. *Sports Med.* **2017**, *47*, 33–49. [CrossRef]
35. Correa-Rotter, R.; García-Trabanino, R. Mesoamerican nephropathy. *Semin. Nephrol.* **2019**, *39*, 263–271. [CrossRef] [PubMed]
36. Junglee, N.A.; Di Felice, U.; Dolci, A.; Fortes, M.B.; Jibani, M.M.; Lemmey, A.B.; Walsh, N.P.; Macdonald, J.H. Exercising in a hot environment with muscle damage: Effects on acute kidney injury biomarkers and kidney function. *Am. J. Physiol. Ren. Physiol.* **2013**, *305*, F813–F820. [CrossRef] [PubMed]
37. Sánchez-Lozada, L.-G.; García-Arroyo, F.E.; Gonzaga, G.; Silverio, O.; Blas-Marron, M.G.; Muñoz-Jimenez, I.; Tapia, E.; Osorio-Alonso, H.; Madero, M.; Roncal-Jiménez, C.A. Kidney Injury from Recurrent Heat Stress and Rhabdomyolysis: Protective Role of Allopurinol and Sodium Bicarbonate. *Am. J. Nephrol.* **2018**, *48*, 339–348. [CrossRef] [PubMed]
38. Brown, S.J.; Child, R.B.; Day, S.H.; Donnelly, A.E. Exercise-induced skeletal muscle damage and adaptation following repeated bouts of eccentric muscle contractions. *J. Sports Sci.* **1997**, *15*, 215–222. [CrossRef] [PubMed]
39. Herath, C.; Jayasumana, C.; De Silva, P.M.C.; De Silva, P.C.; Siribaddana, S.; De Broe, M.E. Kidney diseases in agricultural communities: A case against heat-stress nephropathy. *Kidney Int. Rep.* **2018**, *3*, 271–280. [CrossRef] [PubMed]
40. Basile, D.P.; Bonventre, J.V.; Mehta, R.; Nangaku, M.; Unwin, R.; Rosner, M.H.; Kellum, J.A.; Ronco, C. Progression after AKI: Understanding maladaptive repair processes to predict and identify therapeutic treatments. *J. Am. Soc. Nephrol.* **2015**, *27*, 687–697. [CrossRef]
41. Basile, D.P.; Anderson, M.D.; Sutton, T.A. Pathophysiology of acute kidney injury. *Compr. Physiol.* **2011**, *2*, 1303–1353.
42. Basile, D.P.; Donohoe, D.; Roethe, K.; Osborn, J.L. Renal ischemic injury results in permanent damage to peritubular capillaries and influences long-term function. *Am. J. Physiol. Ren. Physiol.* **2001**, *281*, F887–F899. [CrossRef]
43. Tanaka, S.; Tanaka, T.; Nangaku, M. Hypoxia as a key player in the AKI-to-CKD transition. *Am. J. Physiol. Ren. Physiol.* **2014**, *307*, F1187–F1195. [CrossRef]
44. Ferenbach, D.A.; Bonventre, J.V. Acute kidney injury and chronic kidney disease: From the laboratory to the clinic. *Nephrol. Ther.* **2016**, *12*, S41–S48. [CrossRef]
45. Humphreys, B.D. Fibrotic Changes Mediating Acute Kidney Injury to Chronic Kidney Disease Transition. *Nephron* **2017**, *137*, 264–267.

46. Ko, G.J.; Grigoryev, D.N.; Linfert, D.; Jang, H.R.; Watkins, T.; Cheadle, C.; Racusen, L.; Rabb, H. Transcriptional analysis of kidneys during repair from AKI reveals possible roles for NGAL and KIM-1 as biomarkers of AKI-to-CKD transition. *Am. J. Physiol. Ren. Physiol.* **2010**, *298*, F1472–F1483. [CrossRef] [PubMed]
47. Roncal-Jimenez, C.A.; Ishimoto, T.; Lanaspa, M.A.; Rivard, C.J.; Nakagawa, T.; Ejaz, A.A.; Cicerchi, C.; Inaba, S.; Le, M.; Miyazaki, M. Fructokinase activity mediates dehydration-induced renal injury. *Kidney Int.* **2014**, *86*, 294–302. [CrossRef] [PubMed]
48. Roncal-Jimenez, C.A.; Milagres, T.; Andres-Hernando, A.; Kuwabara, M.; Jensen, T.; Song, Z.; Bjornstad, P.; Garcia, G.E.; Sato, Y.; Sanchez-Lozada, L.G. Effects of exogenous desmopressin on a model of heat stress nephropathy in mice. *Am. J. Physiol. Ren. Physiol.* **2017**, *312*, F418–F426. [CrossRef] [PubMed]
49. Roncal-Jimenez, C.A.; Sato, Y.; Milagres, T.; Andres-Hernando, A.; Garcia, G.E.; Bjornstad, P.; Butler-Dawson, J.; Sorensen, C.; Newman, L.; Krisher, L. Experimental Heat Stress Nephropathy and Liver Injury are Improved by Allopurinol. *Am. J. Physiol. Ren. Physiol.* **2018**, *315*, F726–F733. [CrossRef]
50. Moyce, S.; Joseph, J.; Tancredi, D.; Mitchell, D.; Schenker, M. Cumulative Incidence of Acute Kidney Injury in California's Agricultural Workers. *J. Occup. Environ. Med.* **2016**, *58*, 391–397. [CrossRef] [PubMed]
51. García-Trabanino, R.; Jarquín, E.; Wesseling, C.; Johnson, R.J.; González-Quiroz, M.; Weiss, I.; Glaser, J.; Vindell, J.J.; Stockfelt, L.; Roncal, C. Heat stress, dehydration, and kidney function in sugarcane cutters in El Salvador—A cross-shift study of workers at risk of Mesoamerican nephropathy. *Environ. Res.* **2015**, *142*, 746–755. [CrossRef]
52. Laws, R.L.; Brooks, D.R.; Amador, J.J.; Weiner, D.E.; Kaufman, J.S.; Ramírez-Rubio, O.; Riefkohl, A.; Scammell, M.K.; López-Pilarte, D.; Sánchez, J.M. Changes in kidney function among Nicaraguan sugarcane workers. *Int. J. Occup. Environ. Health* **2015**, *21*, 241–250. [CrossRef]
53. Santos, U.P.; Zanetta, D.M.T.; Terra-Filho, M.; Burdmann, E.A. Burnt sugarcane harvesting is associated with acute renal dysfunction. *Kidney Int.* **2015**, *87*, 792–799. [CrossRef]
54. Wesseling, C.; Aragón, A.; González, M.; Weiss, I.; Glaser, J.; Bobadilla, N.A.; Roncal-Jiménez, C.; Correa-Rotter, R.; Johnson, R.J.; Barregard, L. Kidney function in sugarcane cutters in Nicaragua—A longitudinal study of workers at risk of Mesoamerican nephropathy. *Environ. Res.* **2016**, *147*, 125–132. [CrossRef]
55. Moyce, S.; Mitchell, D.; Armitage, T.; Tancredi, D.; Joseph, J.; Schenker, M. Heat strain, volume depletion and kidney function in California agricultural workers. *Occup. Environ. Med.* **2017**, *74*, 402–409. [CrossRef] [PubMed]
56. Wesseling, C.; García-Trabanino, R.; Wegman, D.H. Mesoamerican Nephropathy: Do Novel Biomarkers of Kidney Damage Have a Role to Play? *Am. J. Kidney Dis.* **2016**, *67*, 173–175. [CrossRef] [PubMed]
57. Heung, M.; Steffick, D.E.; Zivin, K.; Gillespie, B.W.; Banerjee, T.; Hsu, C.-Y.; Powe, N.R.; Pavkov, M.E.; Williams, D.E.; Saran, R. Acute kidney injury recovery pattern and subsequent risk of CKD: An analysis of veterans health administration data. *Am. J. Kidney Dis.* **2016**, *67*, 742–752. [CrossRef]
58. Coca, S.G.; Singanamala, S.; Parikh, C.R. Chronic kidney disease after acute kidney injury: A systematic review and meta-analysis. *Kidney Int.* **2012**, *81*, 442–448. [CrossRef]
59. Arias-Cabrales, C.; Rodríguez, E.; Bermejo, S.; Sierra, A.; Burballa, C.; Barrios, C.; Soler, M.J.; Pascual, J. Short-and long-term outcomes after non-severe acute kidney injury. *Clin. Exp. Nephrol.* **2017**, 1–7. [CrossRef] [PubMed]
60. Ishani, A.; Xue, J.L.; Himmelfarb, J.; Eggers, P.W.; Kimmel, P.L.; Molitoris, B.A.; Collins, A.J. Acute kidney injury increases risk of ESRD among elderly. *J. Am. Soc. Nephrol.* **2009**, *20*, 223–228. [CrossRef]
61. Schiffl, H.; Fischer, R. Five-year outcomes of severe acute kidney injury requiring renal replacement therapy. *Nephrol. Dial. Transplant.* **2008**, *23*, 2235–2241. [CrossRef]
62. Uchino, S.; Bellomo, R.; Bagshaw, S.M.; Goldsmith, D. Transient azotaemia is associated with a high risk of death in hospitalized patients. *Nephrol. Dial. Transplant.* **2010**, *25*, 1833–1839. [CrossRef]
63. Chawla, L.S.; Eggers, P.W.; Star, R.A.; Kimmel, P.L. Acute kidney injury and chronic kidney disease as interconnected syndromes. *New Engl. J. Med.* **2014**, *371*, 58–66. [CrossRef]
64. Chawla, L.S.; Kimmel, P.L. Acute kidney injury and chronic kidney disease: An integrated clinical syndrome. *Kidney Int.* **2012**, *82*, 516–524. [CrossRef]
65. Belayev, L.Y.; Palevsky, P.M. The link between AKI and CKD. *Curr. Opin. Nephrol. Hypertens.* **2014**, *23*, 149. [CrossRef] [PubMed]

66. Roncal, C.A.; Mu, W.; Croker, B.; Reungjui, S.; Ouyang, X.; Tabah-Fisch, I.; Johnson, R.J.; Ejaz, A.A. Effect of elevated serum uric acid on cisplatin-induced acute renal failure. *Am. J. Physiol. Ren. Physiol.* **2007**, *292*, F116–F122. [CrossRef] [PubMed]
67. Ryu, E.-S.; Kim, M.J.; Shin, H.-S.; Jang, Y.-H.; Choi, H.S.; Jo, I.; Johnson, R.J.; Kang, D.-H. Uric acid-induced phenotypic transition of renal tubular cells as a novel mechanism of chronic kidney disease. *Am. J. Physiol. Ren. Physiol.* **2013**, *304*, F471–F480. [CrossRef] [PubMed]
68. Suga, S.-I.; Phillips, M.I.; Ray, P.E.; Raleigh, J.A.; Vio, C.P.; Kim, Y.-G.; Mazzali, M.; Gordon, K.L.; Hughes, J.; Johnson, R.J. Hypokalemia induces renal injury and alterations in vasoactive mediators that favor salt sensitivity. *Am. J. Physiol. Ren. Physiol.* **2001**, *281*, F620–F629. [CrossRef] [PubMed]
69. Perner, A.; Prowle, J.; Joannidis, M.; Young, P.; Hjortrup, P.B.; Pettilä, V. Fluid management in acute kidney injury. *Intensive Care Med.* **2017**, *43*, 807–815. [CrossRef] [PubMed]
70. McDermott, B.P.; Smith, C.R.; Butts, C.L.; Caldwell, A.R.; Lee, E.C.; Vingren, J.L.; Munoz, C.X.; Kunces, L.J.; Williamson, K.; Ganio, M.S. Renal stress and kidney injury biomarkers in response to endurance cycling in the heat with and without ibuprofen. *J. Sci. Med. Sport* **2018**, *21*, 1180–1184. [CrossRef] [PubMed]
71. Kellum, J.A.; Lameire, N.; Aspelin, P.; Barsoum, R.S.; Burdmann, E.A.; Goldstein, S.L.; Herzog, C.A.; Joannidis, M.; Kribben, A.; Levey, A.S. Kidney disease: Improving global outcomes (KDIGO) acute kidney injury work group. KDIGO clinical practice guideline for acute kidney injury. *Kidney Int. Suppl.* **2012**, *2*, 1–138.
72. Levey, A.S.; Eckardt, K.-U.; Tsukamoto, Y.; Levin, A.; Coresh, J.; Rossert, J.; Zeeuw, D.D.; Hostetter, T.H.; Lameire, N.; Eknoyan, G. Definition and classification of chronic kidney disease: A position statement from Kidney Disease: Improving Global Outcomes (KDIGO). *Kidney Int.* **2005**, *67*, 2089–2100. [CrossRef]
73. Mehta, R.L.; Kellum, J.A.; Shah, S.V.; Molitoris, B.A.; Ronco, C.; Warnock, D.G.; Levin, A. Acute Kidney Injury Network: Report of an initiative to improve outcomes in acute kidney injury. *Crit. Care* **2007**, *11*, R31. [CrossRef]
74. Bellomo, R.; Ronco, C.; Kellum, J.A.; Mehta, R.L.; Palevsky, P. Acute renal failure–definition, outcome measures, animal models, fluid therapy and information technology needs: The Second International Consensus Conference of the Acute Dialysis Quality Initiative (ADQI) Group. *Crit. Care* **2004**, *8*, R204. [CrossRef]
75. Kellum, J.A.; Lameire, N. Diagnosis, evaluation, and management of acute kidney injury: A KDIGO summary (Part 1). *Crit. Care* **2013**, *17*, 204. [CrossRef] [PubMed]
76. Beierwaltes, W.H.; Harrison-Bernard, L.M.; Sullivan, J.C.; Mattson, D.L. Assessment of renal function; clearance, the renal microcirculation, renal blood flow, and metabolic balance. *Compr. Physiol.* **2013**, *3*, 165–200. [PubMed]
77. Traynor, J.; Mactier, R.; Geddes, C.C.; Fox, J.G. How to measure renal function in clinical practice. *BMJ* **2006**, *333*, 733–737. [CrossRef] [PubMed]
78. Yong, Z.; Pei, X.; Zhu, B.; Yuan, H.; Zhao, W. Predictive value of serum cystatin C for acute kidney injury in adults: A meta-analysis of prospective cohort trials. *Sci. Rep.* **2017**, *7*, 41012. [CrossRef] [PubMed]
79. Odutayo, A.; Cherney, D. Cystatin C and acute changes in glomerular filtration rate. *Clin. Nephrol.* **2012**, *78*, 64–75. [CrossRef] [PubMed]
80. Parikh, C.R.; Coca, S.G. Acute kidney injury: Defining prerenal azotemia in clinical practice and research. *Nat. Rev. Nephrol.* **2010**, *6*, 641. [CrossRef]
81. McCance, R.; Widdowson, E. The secretion of urine in man during experimental salt deficiency. *J. Physiol.* **1937**, *91*, 222–231. [CrossRef]
82. Nadal, J.W.; Pedersen, S.; Maddock, W.G. A comparison between dehydration from salt loss and from water deprivation. *J. Clin. Invest.* **1941**, *20*, 691. [CrossRef]
83. Kirkebø, A.; Tyssebotn, I. Effect of dehydration on renal blood flow in dog. *Acta Physiol. Scand.* **1977**, *101*, 257–263. [CrossRef]
84. Hope, A.; Tyssebotn, I. The effect of water deprivation on local renal blood flow and filtration in the laboratory rat. *Circ. Shock* **1982**, *11*, 175–186.
85. Stocker, S.D.; Hunwick, K.J.; Toney, G.M. Hypothalamic paraventricular nucleus differentially supports lumbar and renal sympathetic outflow in water-deprived rats. *J. Physiol.* **2005**, *563*, 249–263. [CrossRef] [PubMed]

86. Bardgett, M.E.; Chen, Q.-H.; Guo, Q.; Calderon, A.S.; Andrade, M.A.; Toney, G.M. Coping with dehydration: Sympathetic activation and regulation of glutamatergic transmission in the hypothalamic PVN. *Am. J. Physiol. Regul. Integr. Comp. Physiol.* **2014**, *306*, R804–R813. [CrossRef] [PubMed]
87. Bie, P. Osmoreceptors, vasopressin, and control of renal water excretion. *Physiol. Rev.* **1980**, *60*, 961–1048. [CrossRef] [PubMed]
88. Di Nicolantonio, R.; Mendelsohn, F. Plasma renin and angiotensin in dehydrated and rehydrated rats. *Am. J. Physiol. Regul. Integr. Comp. Physiol.* **1986**, *250*, R898–R901. [CrossRef] [PubMed]
89. Mack, G.W.; Nadel, E.R. Body fluid balance during heat stress in humans. In *Comprehensive Physiology*; Supplement 14: Handbook of Physiology, Environmental Physiology; Wiley: Hoboken, NJ, USA, 2011; pp. 187–214.
90. Cheuvront, S.N.; Ely, B.R.; Kenefick, R.W.; Sawka, M.N. Biological variation and diagnostic accuracy of dehydration assessment markers. *Am. J. Clin. Nutr.* **2010**, *92*, 565–573. [CrossRef]
91. Griffin, B.R.; Gist, K.M.; Faubel, S. Current status of novel biomarkers for the diagnosis of acute kidney injury: A historical perspective. *J. Intensive Care Med.* **2019**, 0885066618824531. [CrossRef] [PubMed]
92. Malhotra, R.; Siew, E.D. Biomarkers for the early detection and prognosis of acute kidney injury. *Clin. J. Am. Soc. Nephrol.* **2017**, *12*, 149–173. [CrossRef]
93. Koyner, J.L.; Parikh, C.R. Clinical utility of biomarkers of AKI in cardiac surgery and critical illness. *Clin. J. Am. Soc. Nephrol.* **2013**, *8*, 1034–1042. [CrossRef]
94. Schrezenmeier, E.; Barasch, J.; Budde, K.; Westhoff, T.; Schmidt-Ott, K. Biomarkers in acute kidney injury–pathophysiological basis and clinical performance. *Acta Physiol.* **2017**, *219*, 556–574. [CrossRef]
95. Schaub, J.A.; Parikh, C.R. Biomarkers of acute kidney injury and associations with short-and long-term outcomes. *F1000Research* **2016**, *5*. [CrossRef]
96. Kashani, K.; Kellum, J.A. Novel biomarkers indicating repair or progression after acute kidney injury. *Curr. Opin. Nephrol. Hypertens.* **2015**, *24*, 21–27. [CrossRef] [PubMed]
97. Haase, M.; Kellum, J.A.; Ronco, C. Subclinical AKI—An emerging syndrome with important consequences. *Nat. Rev. Nephrol.* **2012**, *8*, 735. [CrossRef] [PubMed]
98. Chakraborty, S.; Kaur, S.; Guha, S.; Batra, S.K. The multifaceted roles of neutrophil gelatinase associated lipocalin (NGAL) in inflammation and cancer. *Biochim. Biophys. Acta Rev. Cancer* **2012**, *1826*, 129–169. [CrossRef] [PubMed]
99. Goetz, D.H.; Holmes, M.A.; Borregaard, N.; Bluhm, M.E.; Raymond, K.N.; Strong, R.K. The neutrophil lipocalin NGAL is a bacteriostatic agent that interferes with siderophore-mediated iron acquisition. *Mol. Cell* **2002**, *10*, 1033–1043. [CrossRef]
100. Mishra, J.; Mori, K.; Ma, Q.; Kelly, C.; Barasch, J.; Devarajan, P. Neutrophil gelatinase-associated lipocalin: A novel early urinary biomarker for cisplatin nephrotoxicity. *Am. J. Nephrol.* **2004**, *24*, 307–315. [CrossRef]
101. Mishra, J.; Dent, C.; Tarabishi, R.; Mitsnefes, M.M.; Ma, Q.; Kelly, C.; Ruff, S.M.; Zahedi, K.; Shao, M.; Bean, J. Neutrophil gelatinase-associated lipocalin (NGAL) as a biomarker for acute renal injury after cardiac surgery. *Lancet* **2005**, *365*, 1231–1238. [CrossRef]
102. Mishra, J.; Ma, Q.; Prada, A.; Mitsnefes, M.; Zahedi, K.; Yang, J.; Barasch, J.; Devarajan, P. Identification of neutrophil gelatinase-associated lipocalin as a novel early urinary biomarker for ischemic renal injury. *J. Am. Soc. Nephrol.* **2003**, *14*, 2534–2543. [CrossRef]
103. Supavekin, S.; Zhang, W.; Kucherlapati, R.; Kaskel, F.J.; Moore, L.C.; Devarajan, P. Differential gene expression following early renal ischemia/reperfusion. *Kidney Int.* **2003**, *63*, 1714–1724. [CrossRef]
104. Schmidt-Ott, K.M.; Mori, K.; Li, J.Y.; Kalandadze, A.; Cohen, D.J.; Devarajan, P.; Barasch, J. Dual action of neutrophil gelatinase–associated lipocalin. *J. Am. Soc. Nephrol.* **2007**, *18*, 407–413. [CrossRef]
105. Hvidberg, V.; Jacobsen, C.; Strong, R.K.; Cowland, J.B.; Moestrup, S.K.; Borregaard, N. The endocytic receptor megalin binds the iron transporting neutrophil-gelatinase-associated lipocalin with high affinity and mediates its cellular uptake. *FEBS Lett.* **2005**, *579*, 773–777. [CrossRef]
106. Singer, E.; Elger, A.; Elitok, S.; Kettritz, R.; Nickolas, T.L.; Barasch, J.; Luft, F.C.; Schmidt-Ott, K.M. Urinary neutrophil gelatinase-associated lipocalin distinguishes pre-renal from intrinsic renal failure and predicts outcomes. *Kidney Int.* **2011**, *80*, 405–414. [CrossRef] [PubMed]
107. Nejat, M.; Pickering, J.W.; Devarajan, P.; Bonventre, J.V.; Edelstein, C.L.; Walker, R.J.; Endre, Z.H. Some biomarkers of acute kidney injury are increased in pre-renal acute injury. *Kidney Int.* **2012**, *81*, 1254–1262. [CrossRef] [PubMed]

108. Ichimura, T.; Bonventre, J.V.; Bailly, V.; Wei, H.; Hession, C.A.; Cate, R.L.; Sanicola, M. Kidney injury molecule-1 (KIM-1), a putative epithelial cell adhesion molecule containing a novel immunoglobulin domain, is up-regulated in renal cells after injury. *J. Biol. Chem.* **1998**, *273*, 4135–4142. [CrossRef] [PubMed]
109. Prozialeck, W.; Vaidya, V.; Liu, J.; Waalkes, M.; Edwards, J.; Lamar, P.; Bernard, A.; Dumont, X.; Bonventre, J. Kidney injury molecule-1 is an early biomarker of cadmium nephrotoxicity. *Kidney Int.* **2007**, *72*, 985–993. [CrossRef] [PubMed]
110. Ichimura, T.; Hung, C.C.; Yang, S.A.; Stevens, J.L.; Bonventre, J.V. Kidney injury molecule-1: A tissue and urinary biomarker for nephrotoxicant-induced renal injury. *Am. J. Physiol. Ren. Physiol.* **2004**, *286*, F552–F563. [CrossRef]
111. Han, W.K.; Bailly, V.; Abichandani, R.; Thadhani, R.; Bonventre, J.V. Kidney Injury Molecule-1 (KIM-1): A novel biomarker for human renal proximal tubule injury. *Kidney Int.* **2002**, *62*, 237–244. [CrossRef] [PubMed]
112. Wang, G.; Gong, Y.; Anderson, J.; Sun, D.; Minuk, G.; Roberts, M.S.; Burczynski, F.J. Antioxidative function of L-FABP in L-FABP stably transfected Chang liver cells. *Hepatology* **2005**, *42*, 871–879. [CrossRef]
113. Yamamoto, T.; Noiri, E.; Ono, Y.; Doi, K.; Negishi, K.; Kamijo, A.; Kimura, K.; Fujita, T.; Kinukawa, T.; Taniguchi, H. Renal L-type fatty acid–binding protein in acute ischemic injury. *J. Am. Soc. Nephrol.* **2007**, *18*, 2894–2902. [CrossRef]
114. Doi, K.; Negishi, K.; Ishizu, T.; Katagiri, D.; Fujita, T.; Matsubara, T.; Yahagi, N.; Sugaya, T.; Noiri, E. Evaluation of new acute kidney injury biomarkers in a mixed intensive care unit. *Crit. Care Med.* **2011**, *39*, 2464–2469. [CrossRef]
115. Gauer, S.; Sichler, O.; Obermüller, N.; Holzmann, Y.; Kiss, E.; Sobkowiak, E.; Pfeilschifter, J.; Geiger, H.; Mühl, H.; Hauser, I. IL-18 is expressed in the intercalated cell of human kidney. *Kidney Int.* **2007**, *72*, 1081–1087. [CrossRef]
116. Franke, E.I.; Vanderbrink, B.A.; Hile, K.L.; Zhang, H.; Cain, A.; Matsui, F.; Meldrum, K.K. Renal IL-18 production is macrophage independent during obstructive injury. *PLoS ONE* **2012**, *7*, e47417. [CrossRef] [PubMed]
117. Lin, X.; Yuan, J.; Zhao, Y.; Zha, Y. Urine interleukin-18 in prediction of acute kidney injury: A systemic review and meta-analysis. *J. Nephrol.* **2015**, *28*, 7–16. [CrossRef]
118. Kellum, J.A.; Chawla, L.S. Cell-cycle arrest and acute kidney injury: The light and the dark sides. *Nephrol. Dial. Transplant.* **2015**, *31*, 16–22. [CrossRef] [PubMed]
119. Rodier, F.; Campisi, J.; Bhaumik, D. Two faces of p53: Aging and tumor suppression. *Nucleic Acids Res.* **2007**, *35*, 7475–7484. [CrossRef] [PubMed]
120. Shankland, S.J. Cell cycle regulatory proteins in glomerular disease. *Kidney Int.* **1999**, *56*, 1208–1215. [CrossRef] [PubMed]
121. Witzgall, R.; Brown, D.; Schwarz, C.; Bonventre, J.V. Localization of proliferating cell nuclear antigen, vimentin, c-Fos, and clusterin in the postischemic kidney. Evidence for a heterogenous genetic response among nephron segments, and a large pool of mitotically active and dedifferentiated cells. *J. Clin. Investig.* **1994**, *93*, 2175–2188. [CrossRef] [PubMed]
122. Yang, L.; Besschetnova, T.Y.; Brooks, C.R.; Shah, J.V.; Bonventre, J.V. Epithelial cell cycle arrest in G2/M mediates kidney fibrosis after injury. *Nat. Med.* **2010**, *16*, 535. [CrossRef]
123. Kashani, K.; Al-Khafaji, A.; Ardiles, T.; Artigas, A.; Bagshaw, S.M.; Bell, M.; Bihorac, A.; Birkhahn, R.; Cely, C.M.; Chawla, L.S. Discovery and validation of cell cycle arrest biomarkers in human acute kidney injury. *Crit. Care* **2013**, *17*, R25. [CrossRef]
124. Endre, Z.H.; Pickering, J.W. Acute kidney injury: Cell cycle arrest biomarkers win race for AKI diagnosis. *Nat. Rev. Nephrol.* **2014**, *10*, 683. [CrossRef]
125. Price, P.M.; Safirstein, R.L.; Megyesi, J. The cell cycle and acute kidney injury. *Kidney Int.* **2009**, *76*, 604–613. [CrossRef]
126. Johnson, A.C.; Zager, R.A. Mechanisms Underlying Increased TIMP2 and IGFBP7 Urinary Excretion in Experimental AKI. *J. Am. Soc. Nephrol.* **2018**, *76*, 604–613. [CrossRef] [PubMed]
127. McCullough, P.A.; Chinnaiyan, K.M.; Gallagher, M.J.; Colar, J.M.; Geddes, T.; Gold, J.M.; Trivax, J.E. Changes in renal markers and acute kidney injury after marathon running. *Nephrology* **2011**, *16*, 194–199. [CrossRef] [PubMed]

128. Hoffman, M.D.; Stuempfle, K.J.; Fogard, K.; Hew-Butler, T.; Winger, J.; Weiss, R.H. Urine dipstick analysis for identification of runners susceptible to acute kidney injury following an ultramarathon. *J. Sport Sci.* **2013**, *31*, 20–31. [CrossRef] [PubMed]
129. Hou, S.-K.; Chiu, Y.-H.; Tsai, Y.-F.; Tai, L.-C.; Hou, P.C.; How, C.-K.; Yang, C.-C.; Kao, W.-F. Clinical impact of speed variability to identify ultramarathon runners at risk for acute kidney injury. *PLoS ONE* **2015**, *10*, e0133146. [CrossRef] [PubMed]
130. Mansour, S.G.; Verma, G.; Pata, R.W.; Martin, T.G.; Perazella, M.A.; Parikh, C.R. Kidney injury and repair biomarkers in marathon runners. *Am. J. Kidney Dis.* **2017**, *70*, 252–261. [CrossRef] [PubMed]
131. Bongers, C.C.; Alsady, M.; Nijenhuis, T.; Hartman, Y.A.; Eijsvogels, T.M.; Deen, P.M.; Hopman, M.T. Impact of acute versus repetitive moderate intensity endurance exercise on kidney injury markers. *Physiol. Rep.* **2017**, *5*, e13544. [CrossRef] [PubMed]
132. Bongers, C.C.; Alsady, M.; Nijenhuis, T.; Tulp, A.D.; Eijsvogels, T.M.; Deen, P.M.; Hopman, M.T. Impact of acute versus prolonged exercise and dehydration on kidney function and injury. *Physiol. Rep.* **2018**, *6*, e13734. [CrossRef] [PubMed]
133. Eichner, E.R. Is Heat Stress Nephropathy a Concern for Endurance Athletes? *Curr. Sport Med. Rep.* **2017**, *16*, 299–300. [CrossRef]
134. Latham, A. The history of a habit: Jogging as a palliative to sedentariness in 1960s America. *Cult. Geogr.* **2015**, *22*, 103–126. [CrossRef]
135. Rewa, O.; Bagshaw, S.M. Acute kidney injury—Epidemiology, outcomes and economics. *Nat. Rev. Nephrol.* **2014**, *10*, 193. [CrossRef]
136. Stump, C.S. Physical activity in the prevention of chronic kidney disease. *Cardiorenal Med.* **2011**, *1*, 164–173. [CrossRef] [PubMed]
137. Murray, P.T.; Mehta, R.L.; Shaw, A.; Ronco, C.; Endre, Z.; Kellum, J.A.; Chawla, L.S.; Cruz, D.; Ince, C.; Okusa, M.D. Potential use of biomarkers in acute kidney injury: Report and summary of recommendations from the 10th Acute Dialysis Quality Initiative consensus conference. *Kidney Int.* **2014**, *85*, 513–521. [CrossRef] [PubMed]
138. Katz, N.; Ronco, C. Acute kidney stress—A useful term based on evolution in the understanding of acute kidney injury. *Crit. Care* **2015**, *20*, 23. [CrossRef] [PubMed]
139. Kellum, J.A. Diagnostic criteria for acute kidney injury: Present and future. *Crit. Care Clin.* **2015**, *31*, 621–632. [CrossRef] [PubMed]
140. Waikar, S.S.; Sabbisetti, V.S.; Bonventre, J.V. Normalization of urinary biomarkers to creatinine during changes in glomerular filtration rate. *Kidney Int.* **2010**, *78*, 486–494. [CrossRef]
141. Junglee, N.A.; Lemmey, A.B.; Burton, M.; Searell, C.; Jones, D.; Lawley, J.S.; Jibani, M.M.; Macdonald, J.H. Does proteinuria-inducing physical activity increase biomarkers of acute kidney injury? *Kidney Blood Press. Res.* **2012**, *36*, 278–289. [CrossRef]
142. Schrier, R.W.; Henderson, H.S.; Tisher, C.C.; Tannen, R.L. Nephropathy associated with heat stress and exercise. *Ann. Intern. Med.* **1967**, *67*, 356–376. [CrossRef]
143. Schrier, R.W.; Hano, J.; Keller, H.I.; Finkel, R.M.; Gilliland, P.F.; Cirksena, W.J.; Teschan, P.E. Renal, metabolic, and circulatory responses to heat and exercise. Studies in military recruits during summer training, with implications for acute renal failure. *Ann. Intern. Med.* **1970**, *73*, 213–223. [CrossRef]
144. Montain, S.J.; Coyle, E.F. Influence of graded dehydration on hyperthermia and cardiovascular drift during exercise. *J. Appl. Physiol.* **1992**, *73*, 1340–1350. [CrossRef]
145. Farquhar, W.; Morgan, A.; Zambraski, E.; Kenney, W. Effects of acetaminophen and ibuprofen on renal function in the stressed kidney. *J. Appl. Physiol.* **1999**, *86*, 598–604. [CrossRef]
146. Radigan, L.R.; Robinson, S. Effects of environmental heat stress and exercise on renal blood flow and filtration rate. *J. Appl. Physiol.* **1949**, *2*, 185–191. [CrossRef] [PubMed]
147. Barclay, J.; Cooke, W.; Kenney, R.; Nutt, M.E. The effects of water diuresis and exercise on the volume and composition of the urine. *Am. J. Physiol.* **1947**, *148*, 327–337. [CrossRef] [PubMed]
148. Kenney, W.; Zappe, D. Effect of age on renal blood flow during exercise. *Aging Clin. Exp. Res.* **1994**, *6*, 293–302. [CrossRef]
149. Kawakami, S.; Yasuno, T.; Matsuda, T.; Fujimi, K.; Ito, A.; Yoshimura, S.; Uehara, Y.; Tanaka, H.; Saito, T.; Higaki, Y. Association between exercise intensity and renal blood flow evaluated using ultrasound echo. *Clin. Exp. Nephrol.* **2018**, *22*, 1061–1068. [CrossRef] [PubMed]

150. Smith, J.; Robinson, S.; Pearcy, M. Renal responses to exercise, heat and dehydration. *J. Appl. Physiol.* **1952**, *4*, 659–665. [CrossRef] [PubMed]
151. Wilson, T.E. Renal sympathetic nerve, blood flow, and epithelial transport responses to thermal stress. *Auton. Neurosci. Basic Clin.* **2017**, *204*, 25–34. [CrossRef] [PubMed]
152. Azzawi, S.; Shirley, D. The effect of vasopressin on renal blood flow and its distribution in the rat. *J. Physiol.* **1983**, *341*, 233–244. [CrossRef] [PubMed]
153. Freeman, R.H.; Davis, J.O.; Vitale, S.J.; Johnson, J.A. Intrarenal role of angiotensin II: Homeostatic regulation of renal blood flow in the dog. *Circ. Res.* **1973**, *32*, 692–698. [CrossRef] [PubMed]
154. Mittleman, K.D. Influence of angiotensin II blockade during exercise in the heat. *Eur. J. Appl. Physiol. Occup. Physiol.* **1996**, *72*, 542–547. [CrossRef]
155. Miyamoto, M. Renal cortical and medullary tissue blood flow during experimental hyperthermia in dogs. *Therm. Med* **1994**, *10*, 78–89. [CrossRef]
156. Devarajan, P. Update on mechanisms of ischemic acute kidney injury. *J. Am. Soc. Nephrol.* **2006**, *17*, 1503–1520. [CrossRef] [PubMed]
157. Zhuo, J.L.; Li, X.C. Proximal nephron. *Compr. Physiol.* **2013**, *3*, 1079–1123. [CrossRef] [PubMed]
158. Palmer, L.G.; Schnermann, J. Integrated control of Na transport along the nephron. *Clin. J. Am. Soc. Nephrol.* **2015**, *10*, 676–687. [CrossRef] [PubMed]
159. El Mernissi, G.; Doucet, A. Short-term effect of aldosterone on renal sodium transport and tubular Na−K-ATPase in the rat. *Pflügers Arch.* **1983**, *399*, 139–146. [CrossRef]
160. Johnson, M.D.; Malvin, R.L. Stimulation of renal sodium reabsorption by angiotensin II. *Am. J. Physiol. Ren. Physiol.* **1977**, *232*, F298–F306. [CrossRef]
161. Bell-Reuss, E.; Trevino, D.; Gottschalk, C. Effect of renal sympathetic nerve stimulation on proximal water and sodium reabsorption. *J. Clin. Investig.* **1976**, *57*, 1104–1107. [CrossRef]
162. Montain, S.J.; Laird, J.E.; Latzka, W.A.; Sawka, M.N. Aldosterone and vasopressin responses in the heat: Hydration level and exercise intensity effects. *Med. Sci. Sports Exerc.* **1997**, *29*, 661–668. [CrossRef]
163. Kenney, M.J.; Barney, C.C.; Hirai, T.; Gisolfi, C.V. Sympathetic nerve responses to hyperthermia in the anesthetized rat. *J. Appl. Physiol.* **1995**, *78*, 881–889. [CrossRef]
164. Melin, B.; Koulmann, N.; Jimenez, C.; Savourey, G.; Launay, J.-C.; Cottet-Emard, J.-M.; Pequignot, J.-M.; Allevard, A.-M.; Gharib, C. Comparison of passive heat or exercise-induced dehydration on renal water and electrolyte excretion: The hormonal involvement. *Eur. J. Appl. Physiol.* **2001**, *85*, 250–258. [CrossRef]
165. Doucet, A. Function and control of Na-K-ATPase in single nephron segments of the mammalian kidney. *Kidney Int.* **1988**, *34*, 749–760. [CrossRef]
166. Barrera-Chimal, J.; Pérez-Villalva, R.; Ortega, J.A.; Sánchez, A.; Rodríguez-Romo, R.; Durand, M.; Jaisser, F.; Bobadilla, N.A. Mild ischemic injury leads to long-term alterations in the kidney: Amelioration by spironolactone administration. *Int. J. Biol. Sci.* **2015**, *11*, 892. [CrossRef] [PubMed]
167. Lattenist, L.; Lechner, S.M.; Messaoudi, S.; Le Mercier, A.; El Moghrabi, S.; Prince, S.; Bobadilla, N.A.; Kolkhof, P.; Jaisser, F.; Barrera-Chimal, J. Nonsteroidal Mineralocorticoid Receptor Antagonist Finerenone Protects Against Acute Kidney Injury–Mediated Chronic Kidney Disease: Role of Oxidative Stress. *Hypertension* **2017**, *69*, 870–878. [CrossRef] [PubMed]
168. Otani, H.; Kaya, M.; Tsujita, J. Effect of the volume of fluid ingested on urine concentrating ability during prolonged heavy exercise in a hot environment. *J. Sports Sci. Med.* **2013**, *12*, 197. [PubMed]
169. Evans, R.G.; Ince, C.; Joles, J.A.; Smith, D.W.; May, C.N.; O'Connor, P.M.; Gardiner, B.S. Haemodynamic influences on kidney oxygenation: Clinical implications of integrative physiology. *Clin. Exp. Pharmacol. Physiol.* **2013**, *40*, 106–122. [CrossRef] [PubMed]
170. Chayoth, R.; Kleinman, D.; Kaplanski, J.; Sod Moriah, U. Renal clearance of urea, inulin, and p-aminohippurate in heat-acclimated rats. *J. Appl. Physiol.* **1984**, *57*, 731–732. [CrossRef] [PubMed]
171. Taylor, N.A. Human heat adaptation. *Compr. Physiol.* **2014**, *4*, 325–365. [PubMed]
172. Omassoli, J.; Hill, N.E.; Woods, D.R.; Delves, S.K.; Fallowfield, J.L.; Brett, S.J.; Wilson, D.; Corbett, R.W.; Allsopp, A.J.; Stacey, M.J. Variation in renal responses to exercise in the heat with progressive acclimatisation. *J. Sci. Med. Sport* **2019**, *22*, 1004–1009. [CrossRef] [PubMed]
173. Ho, C.W.; Beard, J.L.; Farrell, P.A.; Minson, C.T.; Kenney, W.L. Age, fitness, and regional blood flow during exercise in the heat. *J. Appl. Physiol.* **1997**, *82*, 1126–1135. [CrossRef]

174. Minson, C.T.; Wladkowski, S.L.; Cardell, A.F.; Pawelczyk, J.A.; Kenney, W.L. Age alters the cardiovascular response to direct passive heating. *J. Appl. Physiol.* **1998**, *84*, 1323–1332. [CrossRef]
175. Lim, Y.-H.; So, R.; Lee, C.; Hong, Y.-C.; Park, M.; Kim, L.; Yoon, H.-J. Ambient temperature and hospital admissions for acute kidney injury: A time-series analysis. *Sci. Total Environ.* **2018**, *616*, 1134–1138. [CrossRef]
176. McTavish, R.K.; Richard, L.; McArthur, E.; Shariff, S.Z.; Acedillo, R.; Parikh, C.R.; Wald, R.; Wilk, P.; Garg, A.X. Association between high environmental heat and risk of acute kidney injury among older adults in a northern climate: A matched case-control study. *Am. J. Kidney Dis.* **2018**, *71*, 200–208. [CrossRef] [PubMed]
177. Kim, E.; Kim, H.; Kim, Y.C.; Lee, J.P. Association between extreme temperature and kidney disease in South Korea, 2003–2013: Stratified by sex and age groups. *Sci. Total Environ.* **2018**, *642*, 800–808. [CrossRef] [PubMed]
178. Bobb, J.F.; Obermeyer, Z.; Wang, Y.; Dominici, F. Cause-specific risk of hospital admission related to extreme heat in older adults. *JAMA* **2014**, *312*, 2659–2667. [CrossRef] [PubMed]
179. Roncal-Jimenez, C.A.; Ishimoto, T.; Lanaspa, M.A.; Milagres, T.; Hernando, A.A.; Jensen, T.; Miyazaki, M.; Doke, T.; Hayasaki, T.; Nakagawa, T. Aging-associated renal disease in mice is fructokinase dependent. *Am. J. Physiol. Ren. Physiol.* **2016**, *311*, F722–F730. [CrossRef] [PubMed]
180. Stachenfeld, N.S.; Mack, G.W.; Takamata, A.; DiPietro, L.; Nadel, E.R. Thirst and fluid regulatory responses to hypertonicity in older adults. *Am. J. Physiol. Regul. Integr. Comp. Physiol.* **1996**, *271*, R757–R765. [CrossRef]
181. Phillips, P.A.; Rolls, B.J.; Ledingham, J.G.; Forsling, M.L.; Morton, J.J.; Crowe, M.J.; Wollner, L. Reduced thirst after water deprivation in healthy elderly men. *New Engl. J. Med.* **1984**, *311*, 753–759. [CrossRef]
182. Garcia-Arroyo, F.E.; Cristóbal, M.; Arellano-Buendía, A.S.; Osorio, H.; Tapia, E.; Soto, V.; Madero, M.; Lanaspa, M.A.; Roncal-Jimenez, C.A.; Bankir, L. Rehydration with Soft Drink-like Beverages Exacerbates Dehydration and Worsens Dehydration-associated Renal Injury. *Am. J. Physiol. Regul. Integr. Comp. Physiol.* **2016**, *111*, R57–R65. [CrossRef]
183. García-Arroyo, F.E.; Tapia, E.; Blas-Marron, M.G.; Gonzaga, G.; Silverio, O.; Cristóbal, M.; Osorio, H.; Arellano-Buendía, A.S.; Zazueta, C.; Aparicio-Trejo, O.E. Vasopressin Mediates the Renal Damage Induced by Limited Fructose Rehydration in Recurrently Dehydrated Rats. *Int. J. Biol. Sci.* **2017**, *13*, 961–975. [CrossRef]
184. Burg, M.B. Molecular basis of osmotic regulation. *Am. J. Physiol. Ren. Physiol.* **1995**, *268*, F983–F996. [CrossRef]
185. Johnson, R.J.; Rodriguez-Iturbe, B.; Roncal-Jimenez, C.; Lanaspa, M.A.; Ishimoto, T.; Nakagawa, T.; Correa-Rotter, R.; Wesseling, C.; Bankir, L.; Sanchez-Lozada, L.G. Hyperosmolarity drives hypertension and CKD–water and salt revisited. *Nat. Rev. Nephrol.* **2014**, *10*, 415–420. [CrossRef]
186. Cirillo, P.; Gersch, M.S.; Mu, W.; Scherer, P.M.; Kim, K.M.; Gesualdo, L.; Henderson, G.N.; Johnson, R.J.; Sautin, Y.Y. Ketohexokinase-dependent metabolism of fructose induces proinflammatory mediators in proximal tubular cells. *J. Am. Soc. Nephrol.* **2009**, *20*, 545–553. [CrossRef] [PubMed]
187. Lanaspa, M.A.; Ishimoto, T.; Cicerchi, C.; Tamura, Y.; Roncal-Jimenez, C.A.; Chen, W.; Tanabe, K.; Andres-Hernando, A.; Orlicky, D.J.; Finol, E. Endogenous fructose production and fructokinase activation mediate renal injury in diabetic nephropathy. *J. Am. Soc. Nephrol.* **2014**, *25*, 2526–2538. [CrossRef] [PubMed]
188. Sanchez-Lozada, L.G.; Tapia, E.; Santamaria, J.; Avila-Casado, C.; Soto, V.; Nepomuceno, T.; Rodriguez-Iturbe, B.; Johnson, R.J.; Herrera-Acosta, J. Mild hyperuricemia induces vasoconstriction and maintains glomerular hypertension in normal and remnant kidney rats. *Kidney Int.* **2005**, *67*, 237–247. [CrossRef] [PubMed]
189. Huang, Z.; Hong, Q.; Zhang, X.; Xiao, W.; Wang, L.; Cui, S.; Feng, Z.; Lv, Y.; Cai, G.; Chen, X. Aldose reductase mediates endothelial cell dysfunction induced by high uric acid concentrations. *Cell Commun. Signal.* **2017**, *15*, 3. [CrossRef] [PubMed]
190. Song, Z.; Roncal-Jimenez, C.A.; Lanaspa-Garcia, M.A.; Oppelt, S.A.; Kuwabara, M.; Jensen, T.; Milagres, T.; Andres-Hernando, A.; Ishimoto, T.; Garcia, G.E. Role of fructose and fructokinase in acute dehydration-induced vasopressin gene expression and secretion in mice. *J. Neurophysiol.* **2016**, *117*, 646–654. [CrossRef] [PubMed]
191. Schrier, R.; Berl, T.; Anderson, R. Osmotic and nonosmotic control of vasopressin release. *Am. J. Physiol. Ren. Physiol.* **1979**, *236*, F321–F332. [CrossRef] [PubMed]

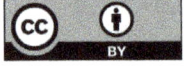

© 2019 by the authors. Licensee MDPI, Basel, Switzerland. This article is an open access article distributed under the terms and conditions of the Creative Commons Attribution (CC BY) license (http://creativecommons.org/licenses/by/4.0/).

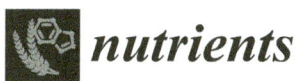

Review

Pediatric Thermoregulation: Considerations in the Face of Global Climate Change

Caroline J. Smith

Department of Health and Exercise Science, Appalachian State University, Boone, NC 28608, USA; smithcj7@appstate.edu

Received: 1 July 2019; Accepted: 16 August 2019; Published: 26 August 2019

Abstract: Predicted global climate change, including rising average temperatures, increasing airborne pollution, and ultraviolet radiation exposure, presents multiple environmental stressors contributing to increased morbidity and mortality. Extreme temperatures and more frequent and severe heat events will increase the risk of heat-related illness and associated complications in vulnerable populations, including infants and children. Historically, children have been viewed to possess inferior thermoregulatory capabilities, owing to lower sweat rates and higher core temperature responses compared to adults. Accumulating evidence counters this notion, with limited child–adult differences in thermoregulation evident during mild and moderate heat exposure, with increased risk of heat illness only at environmental extremes. In the context of predicted global climate change, extreme environmental temperatures will be encountered more frequently, placing children at increased risk. Thermoregulatory and overall physiological strain in high temperatures may be further exacerbated by exposure to/presence of physiological and environmental stressors including pollution, ultraviolet radiation, obesity, diabetes, associated comorbidities, and polypharmacy that are more commonly occurring at younger ages. The aim of this review is to revisit fundamental differences in child–adult thermoregulation in the face of these multifaceted climate challenges, address emerging concerns, and emphasize risk reduction strategies for the health and performance of children in the heat.

Keywords: thermoregulation; children; sweating; skin blood flow; heat stress; climate change; pollution; ultraviolet radiation; hydration; environmental stressors

---

1. Introduction

Globally, increased variability in environmental extremes and rising average global temperatures [1], coupled with increasing ultraviolet (UV) exposure [2] and pollution [3–6], are greatly impacting human health and performance [7–9]. The very limits of human thermoregulation may be tested, with multiple combined stressors of heat, dehydration, UV radiation, pollution, and noise and disease transmission all exacerbating physiological strain [10,11]. This review aims to address the topic of thermoregulation in the context of global climate challenges with emphasis placed on children, who are considered an 'at risk' population for increased morbidity and mortality during heat events and a range of environmental stressors.

Concepts in pediatric thermoregulation have been revisited and challenged over the past 20 years, countering the argument that children possess inferior thermoregulatory capabilities [12], particularly in mild and moderate environmental conditions. However, greater risk of adverse health events compared to healthy adults is widely recognized in more extreme environmental conditions and during physical exertion. Considering the rapidity and magnitude of predicted global climate change and adverse environmental conditions, it is prudent to understand the effects on physiological function resulting from high ambient temperatures, UV radiation [2,13,14], and pollution [4,15–18]. In addition, understanding the interplay between multiple environmental stressors and increasingly common childhood diseases and comorbidities, including obesity and the onset of preventable 'adult' diseases in children, is important in accurately predicting thermoregulatory responses and long-term health effects in a rapidly changing environmental landscape. This review is not a comprehensive and exhaustive review of thermoregulation in children, for which the reader is directed to other articles [19,20]. Rather, the focus of the present review will be adult–child differences in thermoregulation, with an emphasis on the adverse impact of projected environmental and climate change on thermoregulation, physiological function, overall health, and precautions for risk reduction.

2. Thermoregulation

Humans regulate internal body temperature at ~37 °C via complex autonomic control of skin blood flow (SkBF) and sweating, with further local modulation [21]. Afferent inputs from central and peripheral (skin) thermoreceptors are sent to the thermoregulatory control center in the preoptic anterior hypothalamus (POAH) [22–24]. Inputs are integrated in the POAH before efferent sympathetic signals elicit appropriate sudomotor and vasomotor adjustments to regulate core body temperature (T_c) [21]. Heat exchange and T_c responses are conceptually demonstrated via the human heat balance Equation (1), with additional adjustments for respiratory heat losses:

$$S = M - W \pm K \pm R \pm C - E. \tag{1}$$

Metabolic energy (M) is either converted into external work (W; negligible in most conditions) or thermal energy, which must be dissipated from the body to avoid an increase in heat storage (S). Heat exchange (both losses and gains) occurs via dry heat loss mechanisms; conduction (K), radiation (R), convection (C), in addition to evaporative heat loss (E), primarily from sweat on the skin surface but to a minor extent via the respiratory tract. Rates of heat gain and dissipation must be equivalent to maintain heat balance ($S = 0$) and a stable T_c [25]. Under normothermic conditions, cutaneous vasomotor adjustments facilitate convective heat loss (or gain) at the skin surface to counter minor fluctuations in body temperature. During exercise and/or exposure to high ambient temperatures, heat gains exceed heat losses ($S > 0$), and increased T_c and skin (T_{sk}) temperatures elicit more pronounced cutaneous vasodilation and initiation of sudomotor responses [26–28]. SkBF can increase from ~0.25–0.30 L/min during normothermic conditions to 6–7 L/min during extreme heat exposure. To facilitate increased SkBF (and muscle blood flow during exercise in the heat), in addition to providing blood plasma as a precursor for sweat production, cardiac output (Q) increases to meet demands. Notably, when ambient temperature (T_a) exceeds T_{sk}, a reversal of the temperature gradient prevents dry heat losses from the body, and heat is gained, increasing thermal load. Evaporation of sweat is the greatest avenue of heat loss from the body during exercise and heat exposure, varying with age, exercise intensity, and hydration status. Thermoregulatory function is influenced by many factors, including cardiovascular responses, sweating rate (SR), body surface area (BSA) to mass ratio, body composition, hydration status, and nonthermal inputs. During hyperthermia, increased T_c and T_{sk} elicit thermoregulatory responses to balance heat losses and gains and stabilize T_c (compensable conditions) [25]. If heat loss mechanisms are not sufficient, conditions are said to be uncompensable and T_c will continue to rise, with potential progression to heat-related illness and injury, including fatal heat stroke [29].

Adult–child differences in thermoregulatory responses to warm environments are evident, largely owing to immaturity of their physiological systems, morphological, and neuroendocrine differences. Children exhibit a lower Q [30], lower whole-body SRs [31–34], and greater increases in T_c during passive exercise in the heat [33,35]. Children consistently show higher SkBF responses in warm conditions compared to adults, directing a significantly greater proportion of their lower Q to the skin. Combined with significantly lower SRs, children are reported to rely more heavily on dry heat losses compared to adults [31,35]. Historically, these differences have led to the view that children possess inferior thermoregulatory responses and poorer tolerance to heat compared to adults, defined as an inability to maintain heat balance, resulting in an amplified T_c response that may progress to serious heat illness without intervention [36]. This notion has been challenged [37], with accumulating evidence of compromised thermoregulatory function only at environmental extremes. This warrants further investigation with rising average global temperatures and increased frequency of heat events.

The concept of children being classified as "at risk" of heat-related illness relates to increased vulnerability to the effects of heat stress, with increased morbidity or mortality versus a healthy adult reference population [38]. Epidemiological evidence is mixed but does indicate a distinct age-related variation in heat-related morbidity and mortality [38]. Age groups at greatest risk of health-related morbidity and mortality include older adults (≥75 years) and "young children" (0–4 years) [38,39]. Death rates are lowest among children aged 5–14 years at 0.1 per million, with considerably higher infant death rates at 4.2 per million, in part owing to infants and younger children being unable to operate locks or being restrained in vehicles, in which ambient temperature is exacerbated [38]. Between 17–74 years of age, a progressive, moderate increase in heat-related deaths occurs, with considerable increases with more advanced age (≥85 years, 12.8 deaths per million). Prediction models of weather-related deaths due to excessive natural heat exposure suggest an odds ratio of 4.4 in infants (<1 year), 1.9 in young children (1–4) versus an odds ratio of 1.0 in the young adult reference population (25–34 years) [38]. Overall, the World Health Organization (WHO) predicts child mortality related to heat exposure at >100,000 deaths per year by 2050, with greatest climate change related mortality occurring in South Asia [40].

3. Global Climate Change

Climate fluctuations are recognized to increase the risk and exacerbate the impact of a broad range of diseases, with extreme heat (and cold), pollution and UV exposure increasing human morbidity and mortality [41,42]. Compelling evidence from predictive models of climate change indicate with virtual certainty rising global temperatures and increasing heat wave frequency and severity, but the overall impact of climate change on human health is not fully understood [43].

Climate change will disproportionally affect certain global regions, with extreme temperatures occurring not only in traditionally warm countries, but also in regions not accustomed to high ambient temperatures. A direct temperature–mortality relationship exists and varies by geographical region and climate, with heat events causing significantly greater deaths in historically cooler areas. Predicted heat-related illness and injury could be reduced with heat acclimatization and physiological adaptation, improving the temperature–mortality relationship in cooler areas closer to that observed in warmer geographical regions [44]. In areas frequently exposed to heat, increasing frequency and severity of heat events will occur, with projected temperatures challenging the limits of human thermoregulation and acclimatization [44–46]. In Europe, estimates for predicted heat-related mortality in the 2080's ranges from 60,000–165,000 in the absence of acclimatization or acclimation [44]. Notably, not only is the increase in average global land and sea temperatures important, but close attention should be given to the frequency, duration, and overall impact of heat events, during which fatalities dramatically increase [44].

Global climate change has been evident for several decades, with anticipated increases in average global temperatures of approximately 1.5 °C (2.7 °F) by 2100, with predictions ranging from 0.3 to 4.8 °C (0.5–8.6 °F) depending on varying emission scenarios predicted utilizing climate models [47,48] (pp. 1037, 1065–1068). In the United States, predictive climate models indicate increases of 1.7–6.7 °C (3–12 °F) by 2100, varying by the emission scenario. There will be an increased frequency and intensity of heat waves and related events, with altered patterns and frequency of storms (both heat- and cold-related) and precipitation [47]. Regional variation in severity of climate change will occur, with amplified arctic warming at rates ~2.2–2.4 times greater than the global average [48] (pp. 1037, 1065–1068). Predicted heat events and extremes will continue to exceed prior records, causing hundreds of thousands of additional deaths, crop destruction, and subsequent food shortages, altered disease transmission, and significantly affected economic burden [41].

Despite wide-scale scientific evidence associating greenhouse emissions and global climate change, there is limited evidence of emission reductions. The accelerated rate of increase is unparalleled in human history. Populations who are heat-sensitive or possess underdeveloped or compromised thermoregulatory responses will be most at risk of heat-related morbidity and mortality. Particular attention should be focused on the elderly, infants and children, individuals with cardiovascular, renal, metabolic diseases and related comorbidities, and individuals using medications that alter or limit mechanisms of heat dissipation. The limits of human thermal tolerance and ability to adapt to increasing global temperatures, even in healthy populations, will be tested.

4. Adult–Child Differences in Thermoregulation during Heat Exposure

The American Academy of Pediatrics defines pediatrics as "the specialty of medical science concerned with the physical, mental, and social health of children from birth to young adulthood." [49]. Discrepancies in pediatric thermoregulation literature are therefore not surprising given the large age range and developmental stages encompassed by this field. For the purposes of this review, pediatric age categories follow US Food and Drug Agency (FDA) [50] and World Health Organization (WHO) [51] guidelines for clinical pharmacology, reflecting the underlying principle of a liner relationship between weight and growth. Based on these guidelines, pediatric subpopulations are defined as (a) neonates, 0–1 month, (b) infants, 1 month to 2 years, (c) children, 2–12 years, and (d) adolescents 12–16 years. If considering adolescent, further sub-classifications based on pubertal maturational stage should be considered. Physiological responses to exercise and heat exposure differ between infants, children, adolescents, and adults owing to differences in morphological, endocrine, cardiovascular, metabolic, and thermoregulatory responses, yet guidelines are often modified from adult data. Infants and children have traditionally been considered an 'at risk' group with greater susceptibility to adverse physiological responses and health events during environmental extremes owing to inferior thermoregulatory capabilities [12]. Over the past twenty five years, this notion has been challenged, with limited physiological or epidemiological evidence of compromised or insufficient thermoregulatory capabilities in a wide range of environmental conditions when compared to healthy adults [19,37,52]. Many identified risk factors for heat illness in children, including hydration status, clothing, training and recovery periods, are modifiable and thus largely preventable [52]. The importance of many of these factors in pediatric thermoregulation will be reviewed, with an emphasis on recent advances and future challenges associated with climate change.

4.1. Morphology

Understanding alterations in thermoregulation in the context of growth and development is complex and multifaceted. Not only do children grow and mature at differing rates, but the many physical and physiological changes that impact thermoregulation during this time also occur at varied rates and times, making the pediatric population challenging to assess. Understandably, as children and adolescents grow and develop towards full maturity, adult–child differences become less pronounced. During the 1990s, several investigators suggested that thermoregulation in children differed from adults for physiological reasons beyond morphology [53–55], but this remains a prominent physical difference with important consequences for thermoregulation. Children are smaller than adults, with associated smaller total body surface area (BSA), lower total muscle mass, and metabolic heat production during exercise [37,56]. Notably, children have a larger BSA to mass ratio, with more effective dry heat loss and evaporative efficiency versus adults. This is advantageous in cooler and moderate conditions when $T_a < T_{sk}$ [32,57] but also provides a greater surface area to take on heat in hot conditions. Several studies support the beneficial larger BSA:mass ratio in children during exercise in the heat [58], but this may increase the risk of heat illness as global temperatures continue to rise.

4.2. Body Composition

Obesity is widely recognized as a risk factor for heat-related illness and injury in both adults and children [59–61]. The most recent nationally representative estimates from the United States indicate that the prevalence of childhood obesity is continuing to increase: In 2015–2016, 35% of 2–19-year-olds in the National Health and Examination Survey (NHANES) were overweight (BMI ≥85th CDC percentile), and a further 24.5% obese (BMI ≥95th percentile) [62]. Globally, 50 (24–89) million girls and 70 (39–125) boys aged 5–19 years are estimated to be obese (2SD above the WHO median) [63]. In the context of the increasing incidence of overweight and obesity in children both in the USA and internationally, coupled with increasing average global temperatures, appropriate risk assessment and safety guidelines for exercise in the heat are critically important [64]. The majority of data regarding body composition and thermoregulation concerns adults, with considerable discrepancies in the literature. Several studies indicate similar responses during passive heating [65] or exercise in the heat [66], whilst others demonstrate blunted thermoregulatory (sweating) responses [67] and increased thermal strain (T_c) in obese versus normal weight individuals [67]. Notably, most studies appear confounded by the effects of body mass and/or heat production introducing a systematic bias owing to study design and not adiposity per se [68]. When metabolic heat production is fixed, some of the differences are mitigated [69]. Several studies in children similarly demonstrate the physiological disadvantage of higher adiposity during exercise in the heat [70–72]. Higher visceral and subcutaneous fat deposits, combined with a typically lower BSA to mass ratio, may contribute to hindered heat loss in obese versus lean children [73]. By contrast, a small number of studies indicate similar heat tolerance of obese or overweight compared to normal weight children during exercise in the heat [70,74]. This has been suggested by other authors to result in part from three exercise heat acclimation sessions conducted prior to testing, which were not discussed in the studies themselves [72]. Studies incorporating exercise/heat acclimation sessions prior to experimental testing may reduce differences in thermoregulatory responses between groups but in applied terms have important implications for reducing heat illness risk in obese children.

Importantly, total body mass is typically greater in obese compared to lean children, resulting in a greater heat production and therefore evaporative requirement during similar absolute workloads. In addition, obese children typically possess a lower maximal aerobic capacity, and therefore, when exercising at the same intensity, obese children are achieving a higher absolute workload and heat production [74]. Adipose tissue has a lower water content and lower specific heat compared to muscle (2.97 kJ·kg^{-1}·°C^{-1} versus 3.66 kJ·kg^{-1}·°C^{-1}), with less heat necessary to increase a specific mass of adipose tissue a given temperature. It is logical to assume that both children and adults with higher adiposity may therefore experience a greater T_c rise for a given heat production compared to lean individuals. Notably, the physiological impact of adiposity on thermoregulation and practical considerations for prescribing comparable workloads has recently been challenged [68]. In adults, Dervis and colleagues [68] eloquently demonstrated that during exercise in the heat, overweight or obese individuals experience a greater T_c increase versus those with lower body fat, independently of differences in mass and metabolic heat production [68]. They further suggest that body fat percentage has a relatively small influence on T_c, with independent influences on thermoregulatory function during exercise only with large differences (>20%) between groups or individuals (e.g., obesity). Dervis and colleagues calculated (based on another authors data [75]) that a 20% difference in body fat only elicits a ~3%–5% difference in whole-body mean specific heat, perhaps explaining the similarities between groups in some studies. Obese individuals pose a lower mean specific heat capacity compared to lean individuals, which, coupled with blunted sudomotor responses, may explain the greater T_c rise [68]. Prior studies have also suggested the insulative properties of adipose tissue may attenuate heat loss at the skin [76], but this was not observed by Dervis et al. [68] and may only be relevant in cool conditions when SkBF is minimal and subcutaneous fat is of greater importance. Many of these biophysical principles may hold true in children but warrant further research to explore the independent effects of adiposity on thermoregulation, with appropriate physiological adult–child comparisons requiring workload adjustment for body mass and BSA to avoid systematic bias.

Body composition is an important factor for consideration in outdoor physical activity guidelines for children, in addition to hydration, fitness level, acclimation status, disease, and medications, all of which can modulate thermoregulatory responses and ultimately risk of heat-related illness and injury. Although beyond the scope of this review, it is also pertinent to recognize that obesity is associated with a multitude of risk factors for the development of cardiovascular disease, including insulin resistance, dyslipidemia, and hypertension. Obesity is a proinflammatory condition that contributes to the pathogenesis of obesity-linked diseases, including metabolic dysfunction, cardiovascular diseases, and associated comorbidities [77]. In light of the growing incidence of childhood obesity [62,63], associated comorbidities [78], and increased polypharmacy at increasing younger ages [79,80], development of significant vascular dysfunction and cardiovascular disease in children and young adults is a sobering reality [78,81,82]. This has serious implications for long-term cardiometabolic risk profiles [82,83], in addition to thermoregulatory dysfunction contributing to increased heat illness risk [84–87], exacerbated by a warming global climate.

4.3. Metabolic Heat Production

Children have less efficient locomotion than adults, producing more heat per unit body mass during weight-bearing activities [88,89]. Metabolic heat production can be ~10%–15% higher in children for a given workload [88], although is less pronounced during nonweight bearing activities including cycling. Studies investigating the metabolic cost of locomotion in relation to individual biomechanical variables have typically observed poor relationships. Rather, economy appears related to results from the combined effects of a multitude of factors [90]. Frost and colleagues [91] investigated metabolic, kinematic, and electromyographic responses of varying ages of children (7–8 years, 10–12 years, and 15–16 years) to 4 minute bouts of treadmill walking and running at increasing speeds. The best predictor of both VO_2 and efficiency was age, but specific growth-related factors that may influence the metabolic cost of locomotion remain unclear [91]. Resting metabolic rate (per kg TBW) is higher in children than adults, decreasing during childhood [92,93]. Differences in total mechanical work, stride length [92], knee joint range of motion, gait efficiency [94], and higher respiratory frequency (and a higher cost of ventilation) may all contribute to a greater submaximal VO_2 in children versus adults [92,93].

For children with disabilities or disease that affects mobility, low locomotion efficiency results in large energy expenditure compared to healthy or typically developing children. For example, cerebral palsy, the most common childhood disability in the United States, causes a high metabolic demand on daily activates. Walking efficiency is three times higher in cerebral palsy children, affecting participation in daily activities and overall quality of life [94]. Specific metabolic demands of activities in children are important in the context of safe exercise practices and thermoregulation in extreme environments, with important consideration and modifications to activities for children with disabilities affecting movement.

4.4. Cardiovascular Responses

In comparison to adults, children produce a lower Q during similar absolute submaximal workloads [30,95,96]. Several studies have reported similar Q during exercise in children and adults, but an explanation for these discrepancies is not clear [97,98]. Lower Q in children results from a lower stroke volume (SV), attributed to their smaller body size and therefore smaller heart (left ventricle) compared to adults [95]. Partial compensation is provided by a higher heart rate, with more complete compensation resulting from a greater arterial–venous O_2 difference, ultimately providing similar adult–child VO_2 values despite a lower Q. Children therefore have an appropriate cardiovascular response for their size during exercise. This is demonstrated when SV is scaled to body size, virtually eliminating child–adult SV differences [95]. Similarly, Falk and Dotan calculated cardiovascular responses at fixed relative workloads corrected to provide a body mass specific Q (based on the data of Turley and Wilmore [95]), with values that were in fact ~10% higher in children than adults.

Despite the lower, albeit size-appropriate exercise Q in children, differences in cardiovascular responses associated with thermoregulatory challenges become apparent. Children possess a greater (~20%) BSA compared to adults, shunting a greater proportion of Q to the skin to maximize dry heat losses [31,33,35]. Higher SkBF responses are evident during exercise (50% VO_{2max}) in hot–dry conditions [55] and for similar rectal temperature (T_{re}) responses [31]. Notably, comparisons of cardiovascular responses to heat are typically standardized to metabolic load (relative intensity). If absolute workloads were utilized, group differences would be artificially exaggerated owing to factors including differing locomotion and therefore greater physiological strain in children, differences in body mass and size, and potentially greater SkBF responses for dissipation of additional heat [19]. The high SkBF response declines with increasing maturational development throughout adolescence. Falk and colleagues [55] observed progressively lower SkBF responses in pre-, mid-, and late pubertal boys (significant between all groups) during cycling at 50% VO_{2max} in a hot–dry environment (42 °C, 20% rh). Considering the proportionally higher SkBF responses in children, declines in performance are understandable. Venous return and thus Q are compromised, coupled with relatively lower muscle blood flow, presenting competing demands on the cardiovascular system during exercise in the heat [99]. If conditions (heat and exercise intensity) are sufficiently extreme and exposure continues, particularly without adequate rehydration, SkBF and sweating responses may decline, compromising thermoregulatory function with potential development of heat illness [100].

4.5. Thermoregulatory Sweating

Many authors have reported lower local and whole-body SRs in children compared to adults [31–34]. This is typically true regardless of normalization for BSA or per sweat gland, exercise intensity, environmental conditions, and T_{re} [55–57]. Further, the significantly lower SRs in children appear more pronounced in comparison to adults when exposed to greater environmental extremes, higher workloads [20] or during hypohydration [101]. This leads to the widespread view that children possess inferior thermoregulatory capabilities, a notion that was challenged by Falk and Dotan [37]. Despite lower whole-body SRs, T_c responses are often similar when workloads are adjusted or during passive heating, leading some to suggest that children may actually possess greater thermoregulatory efficiency during exercise and/or exposure to mild and moderate conditions [34,37]. This does not hold true in extreme ambient conditions, with children displaying greater physiological strain and increased heat illness risk.

The main focus on thermoregulatory sweating in children is typically whole-body sweating, with a paucity of data regarding RSR. Regional SRs are widely recognized in adults [102–106], with differences in children depending on maturational stage [34]. This was observed by Shibasaki and colleagues [34] following passive heating of prepubertal boys (7–11 years) and young men (21–25 years) via lower leg immersion in a 42 °C water bath for 60 min. RSRs varied, with some sites significantly higher than adults (forearm), some significantly lower (chest, thigh during latter 30 minutes only), and others showing no differences (back) between groups. The sweating threshold (T_b) was slightly higher in boys, albeit nonsignificant ($p < 0.10$), regardless of body region. Heat-activated sweat gland density (HASG) was higher in boys at all sites, but this is not surprising given their developmental stage and smaller body size and surface area. The authors suggest regional variation in sweating associated with maturational stage and argue a peripheral 'underdevelopment' at the level of the sweat gland versus central drive [34]. This highlights the necessity for measuring RSR at multiple sites and the need for more detailed regional sweating data in children and adolescents at varying maturational stages. Notably, ambient conditions were 25 °C, 45% rh, providing a favorable temperature gradient for dry heat losses on which children typically rely more heavily. The authors focus on sweating in relation to maturational age, but other heat loss mechanisms should be considered. Despite lower RSR, change in T_{re} did not differ between groups, indicating that prepubertal boys could adequately thermoregulate under mild to moderate passive heat stress in the specified conditions, relying on differing mechanisms and perhaps displaying greater efficiency.

Greater evaporative efficiency can also be attributed to the lower sweat electrolyte concentration in children [107] and serves to conserve body fluids. Children typically have higher T_{sk}, and thus higher sweat temperatures, resulting in higher water partial pressure. The result is increased water vapor pressure and higher sweat evaporation [37]. A greater evaporative efficiency and the ability to conserve water may actually serve as an argument for thermoregulatory superiority in children versus adults in mild and moderate conditions. Maximal SRs in children have never been established for ethical reasons, but it is reasonable to assume that in the context of global climate change and increasing heat waves, children may be unable to achieve sufficient sweating rates for heat balance (maximal evaporation < required evaporation) more frequently. Maximal SRs may be improved with heat acclimation, but in uncompensable conditions, children will be unable to thermoregulate adequately, with the potential for progression to developing heat illness if precautionary measures are not employed.

4.6. Heat Acclimation

Heat acclimation (HA) involves a series of beneficial physiological adaptations resulting from repeated exposure to heat stress that facilitate a greater ability to deal with subsequent heat exposure. Considering children are vulnerable to heat illness under extreme conditions, employing HA strategies provides a feasible risk reduction strategy in the face of climate change. Differing HA regimens may be utilized, with conditions closest to the anticipated exposure environment, typically lasting 7–14 days [108–111] and often incorporating exercise to elicit a maximally heat acclimated phenotype [112,113]. Physiological adaptations to HA have been extensively documented in adults [104,114–120], including reduced cardiovascular strain (heart rate (HR) and Q) at a given workload, a lower T_c threshold for sweating, increased thermosensitivity resulting in a higher SR for a given T_c, and greater maximal SRs [111,116,119,121–125]. Children acclimate similarly to adults yet do so more slowly, requiring several more days of exposure for complete HA [72]. The reduced sweating onset threshold and HA-associated increases in SR are highly beneficial during subsequent exposure to high ambient temperatures in a population that has significantly lower sweating responses compared to adults. Children display lower sweat NaCl concentrations compared to adults [107], with reductions in sweat Na$^+$ and Cl$^-$ concentrations in both groups following HA [126,127]. Further acclimation increases the responsiveness of the duct to aldosterone in adults [128], but this mechanism has not been investigated in children.

A pertinent consideration with increasing prevalence of childhood obesity (Section 2.4. Body Composition) is that obese children appear to possess a lower level of acclimation versus lean boys, likely resulting from the partial acclimation acquired through training. Obese boys show higher resting and exercise T_c, elevated HR responses, and lower SRs, indicating higher physiological strain [72]. Sedentary, obese children may therefore benefit most from carefully monitored HA regimens prior to summer months. In the instance of athletes, similarly to adults, exercise intensity should be progressively increased to emulate competition. A gradual increase in the number of training sessions per day and progressive introduction of protective clothing that may hinder heat loss should be adopted [129]. Considering the tendency for children to voluntarily dehydrate, special attention should be given to rehydration strategies during HA to limit hypohydration and maximize cardiovascular adaptations [130].

Ultimately, HA reduces cardiovascular strain, improves performance, and increases survivability to extreme environmental conditions, making this a critical component in reducing heat-related illness and injury in the pediatric population [72,111,116,119,121–125,129]. Most of the evidence available indicates similar HA responses between children and adults, but further work is warranted if HA regimens become widely adopted as ambient temperatures continue to increase, with additional consideration for body composition, disease conditions, and medication use.

4.7. Sweat Composition and Fluid Intake

Fluid intake is of considerable importance in relation to thermoregulatory function, with hypohydration considered a major risk factor in the development of heat illness [100,131–135]. In adults, even mild hypohydration (<2% body weight) impacts cardiovascular and sudomotor responses, reducing SkBF [136,137], delaying both the vasodilatory and sweating onset thresholds, and reducing sweating rates for a given T_c (reduced gain) [137,138], attenuating thermoregulatory function and heat tolerance [137]. For extensive reviews regarding the physiology of water balance, hydration assessment, strategies, and pathology, please refer to other reviews within this Special Issue. In the context of this review, hypohydration in children with consideration for rising global temperatures and concerns over predicted water shortages accompanying climate change are addressed.

In the pediatric population, voluntary dehydration is common, largely owing to children feeling a limited need to replenish fluids even when intake is insufficient [139]. This increases susceptibility to hypohydration and subsequent physiological and psychological impairments. Fluid intake and euhydration are essential for physiological function and health, in addition to cognitive function and mood in both children [140,141] and adults [142]. Hypohydration attenuates SRs in both populations, with notable thermoregulatory impact on children due to their already lower sweating responses for a given workload. Children experience a greater rise in T_c for a given level of hypohydration versus their adult counterparts, increasing physiological strain and thus reducing tolerance to the heat. Hypoydration is recognized as a major risk factor for heat-related illness and injury, including progression to life threating heat stroke [52,101].

Both adults [143] and children [139] often hydrate inadequately, but the effects of chronic low fluid intake and dehydration on health are not well understood. As global climate change progresses, knowledge of the complex and multifaceted interplay of factors influencing thermoregulatory function is important. Although speculative, consideration needs to be given to pediatric fluid intake as it pertains to chronic health, with the mindset of encouraging "preventative" habits for long-term health and risk reduction. In adults, fluid intake (typically self-reported) provides conflicting results regarding cardiometabolic disease risk, in part due to failure of investigators to report plain water consumption versus intake of other fluids, including sweetened beverages [144]. Evidence does indicate low fluid intake is independently associated with developing hyperglycemia [145], type 2 diabetes mellitus [146], and renal dysfunction including chronic kidney disease (CKD) [144], with inconsistent evidence of cardiovascular disease risk. The putative link between hydration and long-term health in adults remains controversial but certainly warrants consideration in children. This is particularly concerning in light of climate change potentially exacerbating dehydration risk, coupled with the high incidence of overweight and obese children in the western world, already at increased risk of cardiometabolic disease. Limited research has assessed the relationship between fluid intake and childhood obesity, but there is some indication that obese children are less hydrated compared to those of normal weight. Maffeis and colleagues [144] determined significantly lower hydration in obese versus normal weight children (7–11 years), based on average free water reserve over 48 h. In adults, Guelinckx and colleagues [144] raise the concept of increased plain water intake as a mechanism to reduce renal and metabolic dysfunction. Risk reduction for CKD and vascular dysfunction in adults has also been observed with high water intake (>2.6 L/day) but not sweetened beverages [147–149]. In children, albeit speculative, perhaps this approach serves to not only improve hydration and thermoregulatory function but reduce or limit the risk of renal and metabolic dysfunction.

Appropriate replacement of both electrolytes and water should be achieved during exercise and/or in warm conditions, yet limited data concerning sweat composition in children and adolescents are available, with subsequent hydration guidelines for children derived from adult data. Maintaining appropriate water balance is important, but beverage flavor and composition are of particular significance when SRs are high. During exercise in the heat, children consume significantly more fluid when beverages are flavored compared to plain water [150]. Bar Or and colleagues [150] observed that voluntary dehydration was significantly reduced when chilled water (8–10 °C) was grape-flavored versus plain during 3 h of intermittent exercise in the heat (35 °C, 40–45% rh). Further increases in fluid consumption were observed when the beverage was not only flavored but also contained carbohydrates (6%) and NaCl (18 mmol/L), resulting in mild overhydration (0.47% increase body weight). Physiological and perceptual variables, including T_{re}, T_{sk}, HR, thirst, and stomach fullness did not differ between conditions, which may be explained by the relatively minimal dehydration of only −0.65%, −0.32%, and +0.47% of body weight for plain water, flavored water, and flavored carbohydrate/NaCl water, respectively. Current guidelines by The American Association of Pediatricians [52] recommend consumption of cooled, flavored beverages to mitigate dehydration in the heat, with the addition of 15–20 mmol/L NaCl increasing ad libitum drinking by up to 90% versus plain water. Sweat composition and optimal composition of fluid-replacement beverages has been extensively studied in adults [150–154], but limited data are available in children, with an emphasis on pathophysiology, specifically cystic fibrosis.

There are many individual factors that can influence sweat electrolyte losses and therefore replacement, including age, physical fitness [155,156], and acclimation status [126,157]. Sweat electrolyte concentrations are a function of SR [158], with higher sweat Na^+ and Cl^- concentrations evident at higher SRs resulting from reduced reabsorption in the sweat duct [157,159]. Wide variation in sweat lactate concentrations has been reported, with data indicating an inverse correlation with SR [160,161], positive correlation [162], or no correlation [163]. Several studies have demonstrated significantly lower sweat lactate concentrations with maturational age (pre- versus late-pubescent boys) [164] and in children versus adults [160] during the initial stages of moderate exercise in the heat, but not during subsequent bouts. Despite varying data concerning the relationship between sweat lactate and SR, it has been proposed that sweat lactate is higher in children owing to their lower SR compared to adults. However, sweat lactate tends to decrease with increasing exercise duration in the heat [160], and the similarity in child and adult sweat lactate during latter stages of exercise cannot be explained by SR. One proposed mechanism is the reliance on anaerobic metabolism in a sweat gland during the initial stages of sweating, and an increasing reliance on oxidative phosphorylation as exercise progresses [160]. Regardless of the mechanism, identifying sweat electrolyte losses and adapting hydration strategies is vital.

Similarly to lactate, sweat NH_3 is significantly higher during initial stages of exercise than adults, which is thought to prevent further decreases in sweat pH through protonation of NH_3 to NH_4^+. This is also reflected in the lower sweat pH observed in children during the initial stages of moderate exercise in the heat (≤20 min) [160]. Further, an inverse correlation has been observed between sweat H^+ and Na^+, thought to relate to acidification of sweat via tubular antiporters reabsorbing HCO^- and/or secreting H^+ in exchange for Na^+ reabsorption, potentially explaining the greater Na^+ reabsorption in children [160].

Understanding optimal fluid composition and replacement strategies should be a priority in children, not only for performance but also overall health and safety. Hydration guidelines in children are often based on adult data, yet adult–child differences in sweat electrolyte concentrations, variation with intensity and duration, and marked differences in SR are evident. Coupled with greater voluntary dehydration in children [101], beverage composition and hydration guidelines need tailoring specifically to children and the intensity and environment in which they are exercising. Drink palatability, including flavor and temperature, are also important when considering fluid replacement in children. In the face of predicted rising average global temperatures, increased severity and frequency of heatwaves, and predicted water shortages, tailored hydration strategies will be increasingly important not only for those exercising in the heat, but for daily activates and prolonged periods outside in the heat (i.e., summer camps).

5. Emerging Environmental Challenges: Effects on Thermoregulation and Health

The World Health Organization (WHO) first published an atlas outlining global environmental challenges to children's health in 2004, which has since been expanded and updated to highlight emerging environmental stressors and strategies for exposure reduction [165]. Rising global temperatures and heat waves are only one component of environmental hazards facing children, with exposure to multiple physiological and psychological stressors influencing growth, development, and long-term health. In the context of thermoregulation, stressors including pollution, UV exposure, and water shortages may not only directly affect physiological function, but a complex interplay of multiple stressors may plausibly modulate thermoregulatory function in children (e.g., via impacts on the cardiovascular system), potentially increasing risk associated with heat-related illness and associated complications. Currently, little is known about the effects of multiple stressors on thermoregulatory function in children.

5.1. Pollution

Acute exposure to pollutants and toxic substances can impair thermoregulatory responses [166], with chronic exposure resulting in a multitude of long-term health complications. Children are reported to spend significantly greater periods of time outdoors compared to adults, potentially increasing their likelihood for exposure to toxicants. It is widely recognized that high ambient temperatures increase the uptake of many pollutants and play a critical role in increasing toxicity [167], which may be further compounded by exercise in the heat [167]. Pollutants and toxins that alter metabolism, SkBF, and/or sweating responses may have a profound effect upon thermoregulation responses of both children and adults [168]. In rodents, an acute, protective hypothermia followed by a rebound, sustained hyperthermia is observed following dosing with many toxic substances, including insecticides. Humans do not typically experience the magnitude of hypothermia observed in rodents following toxicant exposure, although marked hypothermia has been observed in specific instances [169]. More common is a hyperthermic or fever response that may persist for several days after exposure to a toxic agent [167]. Importantly, T_b affects both uptake and toxicity of substances, which in turn impacts T_b regulation. Based on increasing levels of pollution from vehicles, insecticide use, and byproducts from industry, an understanding of routes of absorption, toxicity, modulation of physiological responses, including temperature regulation, and long-term health effects is necessary. Increasing interest in the complex interplay among pollutants, mortality, and heat stress in older individuals is evident [17,170], which should be extended to other vulnerable populations.

The WHO estimates the global cost resulting from pollution at 1.7 million children deaths per year [171]. High ambient temperatures and airborne pollutants independently increase morbidity and mortality, but few studies have investigated the interplay between both stressors [172,173]. A limited number of studies have attempted to do so, yielding mixed results. Several studies indicate an interaction effect, with pollution effects being greater on days with higher ambient temperature [17], whilst others found limited or no interaction [172]. Toxicity of air pollutants can be modified by atmospheric transformations, with greater primary pollutants forming toxic secondary products under conditions of higher temperature, greater sunlight exposure, and in the presence of copollutants [174]. Considering predicted elevations of both stressors in the future, and limited current knowledge of how their interactions affect thermoregulation and overall health, further research is urgently needed. The physiological strain associated with exposure to high ambient temperatures may alter the physiological response to pollutants and other chemicals, increasing susceptibility to the negative health effects [172,173]. A further plausible consideration is the deleterious cardiovascular and respiratory effects of airborne pollution that may lead to compromised thermoregulatory function both in children and later in life, raising health risks in an already vulnerable population during extreme heat exposure.

An increasing number of studies have elucidated an association between residential proximity to high traffic roads and, thus, airborne vehicle pollution and a multitude of adverse health events and conditions. Impacts on the respiratory system have been widely studied [175], and increasing literature is indicating a concerning impact on the cardiovascular system.

Air pollution has been implicated as proatherogenic, increasing likelihood of cardiovascular events [176]. Vehicle emissions are a major contributor to outdoor pollution, accounting for up to 90% of pollutants, including carbon dioxide (CO_2), carbon monoxide (CO), oxides of nitrogen (NO_x), particulate matter (PM), ozone (O_3), volatile organic compounds (VOCs) including benzene and formaldehyde, and other byproducts. Many of these pollutants are linked to numerous adverse health conditions and events, particularly relating to respiratory function [177] and cancer risk [178]. Specifically, PM from vehicle exhaust emissions has been linked to adverse cardiovascular events [179,180]. Of concern to climate change, higher ambient temperatures are linked to greater respiratory uptake of pollutants such as O_3 and greater toxicity [167].

In adults, literature is varied, with some evidence that long-term exposure to urban pollution may increase arterial stiffness and carotid intima–media thickness, regardless of pre-existing Cardiovascular disease (CVD) [181]. Potential mechanisms include signaling cascades stimulating pro-inflammatory cytokine release, ROS production, endothelial dysfunction, and vascular smooth muscle remodeling, ultimately attenuating vascular function and promoting atherogenesis [182,183]. Children are at greater risk of negative health effects associated with pollution, owing to a complex interplay of factors, including immature immune responses, small lung volumes, higher respiratory rates, tendency for mouth breathing, and longer time periods spent outside [184]. Children exposed to urban air pollution show increased markers of oxidative stress, inflammation, and endothelial dysfunction [16,185]. Notably, this an understudied area of toxicology and physiology, with only one study indicating that long-term urban residency of children living in close proximity to a major road (30–300 m) was linked to increased carotid arterial stiffness versus those living further away.

Armijos and colleagues [186] observed that long-term residency in close proximity to a high traffic road (<100 m), and thus airborne pollution, stimulates arterial remodeling (carotid intima–media thickness) in children aged 7–12 years versus those living further away (>200 m), with control for covariates and risk factors for atherosclerosis [186]. Many factors can influence inflammation and CVD risk, but there is a need for long-term, longitudinal, epidemiological studies to determine the cumulative effects of pollution on cardiovascular health, with putative implications for thermoregulatory function and exercise capacity. Exposure to proatherogenic environmental factors may cause early progression to clinical disease, rendering current knowledge of vascular responses in children inaccurate with the potential for overestimating heat loss potential in certain conditions. Whilst currently speculative, elucidating if pollution has functional consequences for thermoregulation in children is vital in the face of multifaceted physiological stressors, including climate change and increasing prevalence of noncommunicable diseases.

5.2. Ultraviolet Exposure

Exposure to UV radiation can have beneficial or detrimental effects depending on a complex interplay of factors, including the wavelength of UV radiation, extent of exposure, skin pigmentation, and other individual factors [2]. Depletion of protective stratospheric ozone has led to increased UVB (315–400 nm) levels reaching the earth's surface [187] and is therefore of concern to human health. The epidermis absorbs the majority of UV that irradiates the skin, with only longer wavelengths transmitted deeper into the dermis. UVB has therefore been the predominant focus of research, but interest is growing in the effects of the UVA waveband (315–400 nm). Environmental change coupled with lifestyle choices in recent decades, including increased leisure time, popularity of beach/sunshine vacations, poor sunscreen habits, use of tanning beds, and fewer clothes worn outdoors, places individuals at risk of irradiation. This has pertinence to both adults and children; however, some evidence indicates that UV radiation exposure during childhood may be of greater importance for both beneficial and detrimental effects compared to exposure later in life [188].

Despite the largely negative literature surrounding UV exposure, it is important in many physiological processes, with skeletal disease and vitamin D insufficiency associated with inadequate exposure. Some evidence indicates a regulatory role in blood pressure via calcium homeostasis and vitamin D_3, with artificial UVB exposure lowering blood pressure in mild, unmedicated hypertensives [189]. Photoimmunology, an emerging field of study regarding how UV radiation impacts immune function, is a reminder of how limited current knowledge is on topics such as UV and effects on many physiological processes. UV radiation is typically immunosuppressive, yet increasing evidence suggests a protective role of UV radiation in autoimmune diseases, including Type 1 diabetes, rheumatoid arthritis, and multiple sclerosis [14]. This occurs via multiple signaling mechanisms, including local and systemic immunosuppression, the immunomodulatory effects of vitamin D (1,25-dihydroxycholecalciferol), and suppression of melatonin secretion and subsequent T cell responses [190–193]. Overall, it appears that UV radiation exerts immunomodulatory effects, primarily via suppression of helper T cell type-1 mediated responses thorough multiple mechanisms. This may be beneficial in specific circumstances, including autoimmune diseases, but requires further investigation in humans.

Excessive exposure to UV radiation is associated with many negative health effects, including increased skin cancer risk [13,194,195], eye damage, and suppressed immune function [196], with further deleterious health effects becoming more apparent. In instances of sunburn, skin injury results from penetration of UVB into the dermal and epidermal layers, causing damage to cutaneous blood vessels and eccrine sweat glands [197]. Mild artificial sunburn appears to attenuate SRs and sensitivity for at least 24 h, with potential for impaired thermoregulatory function if this occurs over a large body surface area [197]. Greater time spent outdoors by children compared to adults, poor sunscreen habits, and increasing UVB levels increase the likelihood of sunburn in a pediatric population, with potential for thermoregulatory dysfunction. Specific dermal conditions have been shown to impair thermoregulation and reduce heat tolerance [198]. Evidence is currently limited with regard to sunburn and thermal tolerance, but further studies examining the acute and chronic effects on eccrine sweat gland function and vascular responses are necessary in light of changing environmental conditions. Evidence of UVB-induced alterations in cutaneous vasodilation have recently been reported in adults but, as an important component of the thermoregulatory response, may have relevance for thermoregulation in both children and adults. Children rely more heavily on cutaneous vasodilation and 'dry' heat losses for thermoregulation compared to adults, making decrements in this response potentially more problematic. Nitric oxide (NO) is a potent vasodilator, produced from the substrate L-arginine via nitric oxide synthase (NOS) isoforms, and is necessary for full expression of the cutaneous vascular response to both local [199–201] and whole-body heating [202]. Recent work by Wolf et al. [203,204] indicates deleterious effects of acute UV radiation exposure on cutaneous microvascular function. Specifically, an acute dose of UVB radiation (300 mJ.cm^2, 75 s) was shown to attenuate NO-dependent vasodilation on the ventral forearm, likely via its putative degradation of 5-methyltetrahydrofolate (5-MTHF) and subsequent reactive oxygen species (ROS) signaling [203]. A further study by this group [204] indicated attenuated NO-dependent skin blood flow responses to a local heating protocol (42 °C) following acute broad spectrum UV radiation exposure (450 mJ.cm^{-2}, 75 s) versus control (non-exposure). UV radiation-mediated reductions in NO-dependent vasodilation were prevented with application of SPF 50 sunscreen or 'simulated sweat'. Notably, this was conducted under very acute conditions (60–75 s) in a young, healthy adult population, but consideration must be given to implications in children and adolescents. Children often spend greater time outdoors than adults, and rely more heavily on dry heat losses, shunting a greater proportion of Q to the skin during passive and exercise heat exposure. Whether long-term effects of chronic, repeated UV exposure on cutaneous vascular reactivity translate to meaningful physiological outcomes and compromised thermoregulatory function is currently unknown. As average global temperatures rise and broad spectrum UV radiation exposure increases, in part due to decreasing atmospheric ozone [187], understanding if these factors modulate cutaneous vascular responses, and thus thermoregulation, is certainly warranted.

6. Child Health, Safety, and Risk Reduction

Based on global climate predictions, awareness of the factors increasing risk of heat-illness in children is important in prevention, with particular emphasis on dehydration, current or recent illness, chronic conditions, and specific medications [52]. In particular, illness involving gastrointestinal distress (particularly vomiting and diarrhea), and conditions and medications that affect thermoregulation, exercise tolerance, and water–electrolyte balance should be addressed. Common examples include type 2 diabetes [205–207], obesity [72,208], cystic fibrosis [209], diabetes insipidus, anticholinergic medications, diuretics, dopamine [210], and serotonin uptake inhibitors.

A second important step in the prevention of heat-related illness and injury is understanding and implementing HA. Children acclimate to heat more slowly than adults [72] but will beneficially increase sweat capacity, reduce the onset threshold for sweating, and reduce overall physiological strain [72,208]. Obese children possess lower levels of acclimation and therefore should be acclimated more progressively during summer months [72]. When exercising in the heat, children should follow appropriate hydration and exposure guidelines for the ambient conditions, with special consideration and awareness of their propensity for greater voluntary dehydration [101]. Hypohydration compromises thermoregulatory function to a greater extent in children compared to adults, making it an import factor to mitigate health risks during exposure. The American Academy of Pediatrics position stand addressing "Climatic Heat Stress and Exercising Children and Adolescents" [52] recommends multiple risk reduction strategies, including but not limited to:

1. Increasing rest periods. Activities lasting >15 min should be reduced in conditions of high solar radiation, high humidity, and ambient temperatures above critical limits.
2. When beginning a strenuous exercise program or travelling to a warmer climate, HA over 10–14 days should be planned with reduced exercise intensity, duration, and protective clothing.
3. Ensure adequate hydration prior to extended exercise in the heat. Intermittent drinking periods should be enforced, regardless of thirst (100–250 mL every 20 min). Weighing a child pre/post-exercise can assist with verifying hydration.
4. Lightweight, light-colored, single-layer clothing should be worn that is absorbent. Sweat-soaked garments should be replaced.
5. Child education on heat illness and hydration practices should be adopted to help raise awareness of prevention, and recognition of the signs and symptoms of heat-related illness and injury. Trained staff should be present, and an emergency plan should be in place.

Considering the increasing incidence of a multitude of childhood diseases, awareness of diseases that alter thermoregulatory responses, recent illness, specific medications, and mental retardation (for example, a compromised ability to recognize dangers of heat, not rehydrating) are also important. Education surrounding behavioral thermoregulation is vital, including seeking shade, requesting help when needed, and using cool water and damp towels to help to reduce body temperature during hyperthermia. Sunscreen should be applied to reduce acute effects of UV radiation on cutaneous vascular responses in the heat and avoid sunburn. Clothing insulation and requirements in children in varying environmental conditions are beyond the scope of this review but are an important consideration. Readers are directed to other excellent reviews [211]. Emerging evidence highlights the complex interplay between multiple stressors, modulating physiological responses, and, therefore, morbidity and mortality risk. Exposure to increasing global temperatures necessitates consideration of heat stress in cumulative risk assessment [43], due to potential temperature-related modulation of toxicity of air pollution and other abundant chemicals, for example, pesticides [174], exacerbating health effects. Children are exposed to many physical and chemical stressors, including heat, UV radiation, sunlight, noise, infection, psychosocial stressors, and pollution. Long-term exposure may facilitate earlier progression to clinical disease, altered physiological responses versus those observed in healthy children, and ultimately premature mortality. The long-term impact of multiple environmental–physiological factors on physiological function are currently not fully understood. Combined efforts between thermal physiologists, epidemiologists, climate physiologists, and regulatory bodies/policymakers are necessary to produce more comprehensive heat protection policies, incorporating technology, clothing, and behavioral adaptations as global climate change advances and limits of human tolerance are reached [45].

7. Summary

Understanding physiological responses to heat exposure is of increasing importance in the face of extraordinary environmental and climate change facing humans. In particular, emphasis should be placed on 'at risk populations', including children and infants, the elderly, and individuals with obesity and chronic pathologies, including cardiovascular, renal, and metabolic diseases. Many physiological differences exist between adults and children of varying developmental stages in their responses to exercise and exposure to environmental extremes, including morphological, endocrine, cardiovascular, metabolic, and thermoregulatory responses. The classic notion that children possess inferior thermoregulatory capabilities and reduced thermal tolerance has been vigorously challenged over the past 25 years and may only hold true in extreme conditions. Of course, this is particularly relevant in light of global climate change where 'extremes' are more likely to be encountered, evidenced by patterns of increasing average global ambient temperatures, increased frequency and severity of heat waves, and increased pollution and UV exposure. The complex interplay between increasing environmental stressors should be carefully considered when coupled with concerning health statistics that negatively affect thermoregulation in children, including prevalence of inactivity, childhood obesity, and the earlier onset of preventable 'adult' diseases, including type 2 diabetes and dyslipidemia. The long-term impact of multiple environmental–physiological stressors, including heat, UV exposure, and pollution on physiological function in children, is not fully understood and warrants further investigation as a significant future global health challenge.

Funding: This research received no external funding.

Conflicts of Interest: The authors declare no conflict of interest.

References

1. Sherbakov, T.; Malig, B.; Guirguis, K.; Gershunov, A.; Basu, R. Ambient temperature and added heat wave effects on hospitalizations in California from 1999 to 2009. *Environ. Res.* **2018**, *160*, 83–90. [CrossRef] [PubMed]
2. Lucas, R.M.; Ponsonby, A.-L. Ultraviolet radiation and health: Friend and foe. *Med. J. Aust.* **2002**, *177*, 594–598. [PubMed]
3. Pope, C.A., 3rd; Muhlestein, J.B.; May, H.T.; Renlund, D.G.; Anderson, J.L.; Horne, B.D. Ischemic heart disease events triggered by short-term exposure to fine particulate air pollution. *Circulation* **2006**, *114*, 2443–2448. [CrossRef] [PubMed]
4. Ibald-Mulli, A.; Stieber, J.; Wichmann, H.E.; Koenig, W.; Peters, A. Effects of air pollution on blood pressure: A population-based approach. *Am. J. Public Health* **2001**, *91*, 571–577. [PubMed]
5. Urch, B.; Silverman, F.; Corey, P.; Brook, J.R.; Lukic, K.Z.; Rajagopalan, S.; Brook, R.D. Acute Blood Pressure Responses in Healthy Adults During Controlled Air Pollution Exposures. *Environ. Health Perspect.* **2005**, *113*, 1052–1055. [CrossRef] [PubMed]
6. Brook, R.D.; Urch, B.; Dvonch, J.T.; Bard, R.L.; Speck, M.; Keeler, G.; Morishita, M.; Marsik, F.J.; Kamal, A.S.; Kaciroti, N.; et al. Insights into the Mechanisms and Mediators of the Effects of Air Pollution Exposure on Blood Pressure and Vascular Function in Healthy Humans. *Hypertens* **2009**, *54*, 659–667. [CrossRef] [PubMed]
7. Van Loenhout, J.A.F.; Delbiso, T.D.; Kiriliouk, A.; Rodriguez-Llanes, J.M.; Segers, J.; Guha-Sapir, D. Heat and emergency room admissions in the Netherlands. *BMC Public Health* **2018**, *18*, 108. [CrossRef] [PubMed]
8. Wang, X.; Lavigne, E.; Ouellette-Kuntz, H.; Chen, B.E. Acute impacts of extreme temperature exposure on emergency room admissions related to mental and behavior disorders in Toronto, Canada. *J. Affect. Disord.* **2014**, *155*, 154–161. [CrossRef]
9. Sheffield, P.E.; Landrigan, P.J. Global climate change and children's health: Threats and strategies for prevention. *Environ. Health Perspect.* **2011**, *119*, 291–298. [CrossRef]
10. Xu, Z.; Sheffield, P.E.; Hu, W.; Su, H.; Yu, W.; Qi, X.; Tong, S. Climate Change and Children's Health—A Call for Research on What Works to Protect Children. *Int. J. Environ. Res. Public Health* **2012**, *9*, 3298–3316. [CrossRef]

11. UNICEF. *Climate Change and Children: A Human Security Challenge*; Hellenic Foundation for European and Foreign Policy; UNICEF and UNICEF Innocenti Research Centre: New York, NY, USA, 2008.
12. Inbar, O.; Bar-Or, O.; Dotan, R.; Gutin, B. Conditioning versus exercise in heat as methods for acclimatizing 8- to 10-yr-old boys to dry heat. *J. Appl. Physiol.* **1981**, *50*, 406–411. [CrossRef]
13. Anna, B.; Blazej, Z.; Jacqueline, G.; Andrew, C.J.; Jeffrey, R.; Andrzej, S. Mechanism of UV-related carcinogenesis and its contribution to nevi/melanoma. *Expert Rev. Dermatol.* **2007**, *2*, 451–469.
14. Hart, P.H.; Norval, M.; Byrne, S.N.; Rhodes, L.E. Exposure to Ultraviolet Radiation in the Modulation of Human Diseases. *Annu. Rev. Pathol. Mech. Dis.* **2019**, *14*, 55–81. [CrossRef]
15. Franchini, M.; Mannucci, P.M. Air pollution and cardiovascular disease. *Thromb. Res.* **2012**, *129*, 230–234. [CrossRef]
16. Iannuzzi, A.; Verga, M.C.; Renis, M.; Schiavo, A.; Salvatore, V.; Santoriello, C.; Pazzano, D.; Licenziati, M.R.; Polverino, M. Air pollution and carotid arterial stiffness in children. *Cardiol. Young* **2010**, *20*, 186–190. [CrossRef]
17. Katsouyanni, K.; Pantazopoulou, A.; Touloumi, G.; Tselepidaki, I.; Moustris, K.P.; Asimakopoulos, D.; Poulopoulou, G.; Trichopoulos, D. Evidence for Interaction between Air Pollution and High Temperature in the Causation of Excess Mortality. *Arch. Environ. Health Int. J.* **1993**, *48*, 235–242. [CrossRef]
18. Bowatte, G.; Lodge, C.; Lowe, A.J.; Erbas, B.; Perret, J.; Abramson, M.J.; Matheson, M.; Dharmage, S.C. The influence of childhood traffic-related air pollution exposure on asthma, allergy and sensitization: A systematic review and a meta-analysis of birth cohort studies. *Allergy* **2015**, *70*, 245–256. [CrossRef]
19. Falk, B. Effects of Thermal Stress during Rest and Exercise in the Paediatric Population. *Sports Med.* **1998**, *25*, 221–240. [CrossRef]
20. Inoue, Y.; Kuwahara, T.; Araki, T. Maturation- and Aging-related Changes in Heat Loss Effector Function. *J. Physiol. Anthr. Appl. Hum. Sci.* **2004**, *23*, 289–294. [CrossRef]
21. Smith, C.J.; Johnson, J.M. Responses to hyperthermia. Optimizing heat dissipation by convection and evaporation: Neural control of skin blood flow and sweating in humans. *Auton. Neurosci.* **2016**, *196*, 25–36. [CrossRef]
22. Moorhouse, V.H.K. Effect of Increased Temperature of the Carotid Blood. *Am. J. Physiol. Content* **1911**, *28*, 223–234. [CrossRef]
23. Ott, I. The Heat-Center in the Brain. *J. Nerv. Ment. Dis.* **1887**, *14*, 152–162. [CrossRef]
24. Benzinger, T.H. On physical heat regulation and the sense of temperature in man. *Proc. Natl. Acad. Sci. USA* **1959**, *45*, 645–659. [CrossRef]
25. Cramer, M.N.; Jay, O. Biophysical aspects of human thermoregulation during heat stress. *Auton. Neurosci.* **2016**, *196*, 3–13. [CrossRef]
26. Kellogg, D.L.; John, M.J. Thermoregulatory and thermal control in the human cutaneous circulation. *Front. Biosci.* **2010**, *2*, 825–853. [CrossRef]
27. Johnson, J.M.; Minson, C.T.; Kellogg, D.L. Cutaneous Vasodilator and Vasoconstrictor Mechanisms in Temperature Regulation. *Compr. Physiol.* **2014**, *4*, 33–89.
28. Kenney, W.L.; Johnson, J.M. Control of skin blood flow during exercise. *Med. Sci. Sports Exerc.* **1992**, *24*, 303. [CrossRef]
29. Bouchama, A.; Knochel, J.P. Heat stroke. *N. Engl. J. Med.* **2002**, *346*, 1978–1988. [CrossRef]
30. Bar-Or, O.; Shephard, R.J.; Allen, C.L. Cardiac output of 10- to 13-year-old boys and girls during submaximal exercise. *J. Appl. Physiol.* **1971**, *30*, 219–223. [CrossRef]
31. Shibasaki, M.; Inoue, Y.; Kondo, N.; Iwata, A. Thermoregulatory responses of prepubertal boys and young men during moderate exercise. *Graefe Arch. Clin. Exp. Ophthalmol.* **1997**, *75*, 212–218. [CrossRef]
32. Davies, C.T.M. Thermal responses to exercise in children. *Ergonomics* **1981**, *24*, 55–61. [CrossRef]
33. Wagner, J.A.; Robinson, S.; Tzankoff, S.P.; Marino, R.P. Heat tolerance and acclimatization to work in the heat in relation to age. *J. Appl. Physiol.* **1972**, *33*, 616–622. [CrossRef]
34. Shibasaki, M.; Inoue, Y.; Kondo, N. Mechanisms of underdeveloped sweating responses in prepubertal boys. *Graefe's Arch. Clin. Exp. Ophthalmol.* **1997**, *76*, 340–345. [CrossRef]
35. Drinkwater, B.L.; Kupprat, I.C.; Denton, J.E.; Crist, J.L.; Horvath, S.M. Response of prepubertal girls and college women to work in the heat. *J. Appl. Physiol.* **1977**, *43*, 1046–1053. [CrossRef]
36. Hosokawa, Y.; Stearns, R.L.; Casa, D.J. Is Heat Intolerance State or Trait? *Sports Med.* **2019**, *49*, 365–370. [CrossRef]

37. Falk, B.; Dotan, R. Children's thermoregulation during exercise in the heat—A revisit. *Appl. Physiol. Nutr. Metab.* **2008**, *33*, 420–427. [CrossRef]
38. Berko, J.; Ingram, D.D.; Saha, S.; Parker, J.D. *Deaths Attributed to Heat, Cold, and Other Weather Events in the United States, 2006–2010*; National Health Statistics Reports; no 76; National Center for Health Statistics: Hyattsville, MD, USA, 2014; pp. 1–15.
39. Semenza, J.C.; Rubin, C.H.; Falter, K.H.; Selanikio, J.D.; Wilhelm, J.L.; Flanders, W.D.; Howe, H.L. Heat-Related Deaths during the July 1995 Heat Wave in Chicago. *N. Engl. J. Med.* **1996**, *335*, 84–90. [CrossRef]
40. WHO. *Quantitative Risk Assessment of the Effects of Climate Change on Selected Causes of Death, 2030s and 2050s*; WHO Press: Geneva, Switzerland, 2014.
41. Patz, J.A.; Campbell-Lendrum, D.; Holloway, T.; Foley, J.A. Impact of regional climate change on human health. *Nature* **2005**, *438*, 310–317. [CrossRef]
42. Guo, Y.; Gasparrini, A.; Armstrong, B.G.; Tawatsupa, B.; Tobias, A.; Lavigne, E.; Coelho, M.; Pan, X.; Kim, H.; Hashizume, M.; et al. Heat Wave and Mortality: A Multicountry, Multicommunity Study. *Environ. Health Perspect.* **2017**, *125*, 087006. [CrossRef]
43. Peng, R.D.; Bobb, J.F.; Tebaldi, C.; McDaniel, L.; Bell, M.L.; Dominici, F. Toward a quantitative estimate of future heat wave mortality under global climate change. *Environ. Health Perspect.* **2011**, *119*, 701–706. [CrossRef]
44. Ciscar, J.C.; Iglesias, A.; Feyen, L.; Szabó, L.; Van Regemorter, D.; Amelung, B.; Nicholls, R.; Watkiss, P.; Christensen, O.B.; Dankers, R.; et al. Physical and economic consequences of climate change in Europe. *Proc. Natl. Acad. Sci. USA* **2011**, *108*, 2678–2683. [CrossRef]
45. Hanna, E.G.; Tait, P.W. Limitations to Thermoregulation and Acclimatization Challenge Human Adaptation to Global Warming. *Int. J. Environ. Res. Public Health* **2015**, *12*, 8034–8074. [CrossRef]
46. Basu, R.; Samet, J.M. Relation between Elevated Ambient Temperature and Mortality: A Review of the Epidemiologic Evidence. *Epidemiologic Rev.* **2002**, *24*, 190–202. [CrossRef]
47. Walsh, J.; Wuebbles, D.; Hayhoe, K.; Kossin, J.; Kunkel, K.; Stephens, G.; Thorne, P.; Vose, R.; Wehner, M.; Willis, J.; et al. Chapter 2: Our Changing Climate. In *Climate Change Impacts in the United States: The Third National Climate Assessment*; Melillo, J.M., Richmond, T., Yohe, G.W., Eds.; U.S. Global Change Research Program: Washington, DC, USA, 2014.
48. Collins, M.; Knutti, R.; Arblaster, J.; Dufresne, J.L.; Fichefet, T.; Friedlingstein, P.; Gao, X.J.; Gutowski, W.J.; Johns, T.; Krinner, G.; et al. Long-term Climate Change: Projections, Commitments and Irreversibility. In *Climate Change 2013: The Physical Science Basis. Contribution of Working Group I to the Fifth Assessment Report of the Intergovernmental Panel on Climate Change*; Stocker, T.F., Qin, D., Plattner, G.-K., Tignor, M., Allen, S.K., Boschung, J., Nauels, A., Xia, Y., Bex, V., Midgley, P.M., Eds.; Cambridge University Press: Cambridge, UK; New York, NY, USA, 2014; pp. 1037, 1065–1068.
49. Rimsza, M.E.; Hotaling, A.J.; Keown, M.E.; Marcin, J.P.; Moskowitz, W.B.; Sigrest, T.D.; Simon, H.K.; Harris, C.E.; McGuinness, G.A.; Mulvey, H.J.; et al. Definition of a Pediatrician. *Pediatrics* **2015**, *135*, 780–781.
50. US Food and Drug Administration. General Clinical Pharmacology Considerations for Pediatric Studies for Drugs and Biological Products: Guidance for Industry. FDA Website. Available online: www.fda.gov/downloads/drugs/guidancecomplianceregulatoryinformation/guidances/ucm425885.pdf (accessed on 26 December 2014).
51. WHO. *Paediatric Age Categories to be Used in Differentiating Between Listing on a Model Essential Medicines List for Children*; Position Paper; WHO: Geneva, Switzerland, 2007.
52. Med, C.S.; Hlth, F.C.S. Policy Statement-Climatic Heat Stress and Exercising Children and Adolescents. *Pediatrics* **2011**, *128*, E741–E747.
53. Falk, B.; Bar-Or, O.; Calvert, R.; MacDougall, J.D. Sweat gland response to exercise in the heat among pre-, mid-, and late-pubertal boys. *Med. Sci. Sports Exerc.* **1992**, *24*, 313–319. [CrossRef]
54. Falk, B.; Bar-OR, O.; MacDougall, J.D.; Goldsmith, C.H.; McGillis, L. Longitudinal analysis of the sweating response of pre-, mid-, and late-pubertal boys during exercise in the heat. *Am. J. Hum. Boil.* **1992**, *4*, 527–535. [CrossRef]
55. Falk, B.; Bar-Or, O.; MacDougall, J.D. Thermoregulatory responses of pre-, mid-, and late-pubertal boys to exercise in dry heat. *Med. Sci. Sports Exerc.* **1992**, *24*, 688–694. [CrossRef]
56. Bar-Or, O. Climate and the Exercising Child—A Review. *Int. J. Sports Med.* **1980**, *01*, 53–65. [CrossRef]

57. Inbar, O.; Morris, N.; Epstein, Y.; Gass, G. Comparison of thermoregulatory responses to exercise in dry heat among prepubertal boys, young adults and older males. *Exp. Physiol.* **2004**, *89*, 691–700. [CrossRef]
58. Epstein, Y.; Shapiro, Y.; Brill, S. Role of surface area-to-mass ratio and work efficiency in heat intolerance. *J. Appl. Physiol.* **1983**, *54*, 831–836. [CrossRef]
59. Chung, N.K.; Pin, C.H. Obesity and the Occurrence of Heat Disorders. *Mil. Med.* **1996**, *161*, 739–742. [CrossRef]
60. Bedno, S.A.; Urban, N.; Boivin, M.R.; Cowan, D.N. Fitness, obesity and risk of heat illness among army trainees. *Occup. Med.* **2014**, *64*, 461–467. [CrossRef]
61. Bedno, S.A.; Li, Y.; Han, W.; Cowan, D.N.; Scott, C.T.; Cavicchia, M.A.; Niebuhr, D.W. Exertional heat illness among overweight U.S. Army recruits in basic training. *Aviat. Space Environ. Med.* **2010**, *81*, 107–111. [CrossRef]
62. Skinner, A.C.; Ravanbakht, S.N.; Skelton, J.A.; Perrin, E.M.; Armstrong, S.C. Prevalence of Obesity and Severe Obesity in US Children, 1999–2016. *Pediatrics* **2018**, *141*, e20173459. [CrossRef]
63. Abarca-Gómez, L.; Abdeen, Z.A.; Hamid, Z.A.; Abu-Rmeileh, N.M.; Acosta-Cazares, B.; Acuin, C.; Adams, R.J.; Aekplakorn, W.; Afsana, K.; Aguilai-Salinas, C.A.; et al. Worldwide trends in body-mass index, underweight, overweight, and obesity from 1975 to 2016: A pooled analysis of 2416 population-based measurement studies in 128·9 million children, adolescents, and adults. *Lancet* **2017**, *390*, 2627–2642. [CrossRef]
64. American College of Sports Medicine; Armstrong, L.E.; Casa, D.J.; Millard-Stafford, M.; Moran, D.S.; Pyne, S.W.; Roberts, W.O. American College of Sports Medicine position stand. Exertional heat illness during training and competition. *Med. Sci. Sports Exerc.* **2007**, *39*, 556–572. [CrossRef]
65. Miller, A.T.; Blyth, C.S. Lack of Insulating Effect of Body Fat during Exposure to Internal and External Heat Loads. *J. Appl. Physiol.* **1958**, *12*, 17–19. [CrossRef]
66. Limbaugh, J.D.; Wimer, G.S.; Long, L.H.; Baird, W.H. Body fatness, body core temperature, and heat loss during moderate-intensity exercise. *Aviat. Space Environ. Med.* **2013**, *84*, 1153–1158. [CrossRef]
67. Moyen, N.E.; Burchfield, J.M.; Butts, C.L.; Glenn, J.M.; Tucker, M.A.; Treece, K.; Smith, A.J.; McDermott, B.P.; Ganio, M.S. Effects of obesity and mild hypohydration on local sweating and cutaneous vascular responses during passive heat stress in females. *Appl. Physiol. Nutr. Metab.* **2016**, *41*, 879–887. [CrossRef]
68. Dervis, S.; Coombs, G.B.; Chaseling, G.K.; Filingeri, D.; Smoljanic, J.; Jay, O. A comparison of thermoregulatory responses to exercise between mass-matched groups with large differences in body fat. *J. Appl. Physiol.* **2016**, *120*, 615–623. [CrossRef]
69. Adams, J.D.; Ganio, M.S.; Burchfield, J.M.; Matthews, A.C.; Werner, R.N.; Chokbengboun, A.J.; Dougherty, E.K.; LaChance, A.A. Effects of obesity on body temperature in otherwise-healthy females when controlling hydration and heat production during exercise in the heat. *Eur. J. Appl. Physiol.* **2015**, *115*, 167–176. [CrossRef]
70. Haymes, E.M.; McCormick, R.J.; Buskirk, E.R. Heat tolerance of exercising lean and obese prepubertal boys. *J. Appl. Physiol.* **1975**, *39*, 457–461. [CrossRef]
71. Bar-Or, O.; Lundegren, H.M.; Buskirk, E.R. Heat tolerance of exercising obese and lean women. *J. Appl. Physiol.* **1969**, *26*, 403–409. [CrossRef]
72. Dougherty, K.A.; Chow, M.; Kenney, W.L. Responses of lean and obese boys to repeated summer exercise in the heat bouts. *Med. Sci. Sport Exerc.* **2009**, *41*, 279–289. [CrossRef]
73. Robinson, S. The effect of body size upon energy exchange in work. *Am. J. Physiol. Content* **1942**, *136*, 363–368. [CrossRef]
74. Haymes, E.M.; Buskirk, E.R.; Hodgson, J.L.; Lundegren, H.M.; Nicholas, W.C. Heat tolerance of exercising lean and heavy prepubertal girls. *J. Appl. Physiol.* **1974**, *36*, 566–571. [CrossRef]
75. Geddes, L.A.; Baker, L.E. The specific resistance of biological material—A compendium of data for the biomedical engineer and physiologist. *Med. Boil. Eng.* **1967**, *5*, 271–293. [CrossRef]
76. Koppe, C.; Kovats, S.; Menne, B.; Jendritzky, G.; Baumuller, J.; Bitan, A.; Jimenez, J.D.; Ebi, K.L.; Havenith, G.; World Health Oragnization; et al. *Heat Waves: Risks and Responses*; WHO Regional Office for Europe: Copenhagen, Denmark, 2004.
77. Shibata, R.; Ouchi, N.; Ohashi, K.; Murohara, T. The role of adipokines in cardiovascular disease. *J. Cardiol.* **2017**, *70*, 329–334. [CrossRef]
78. Perrin, J.M.; Anderson, L.E.; Van Cleave, J. The Rise in Chronic Conditions Among Infants, Children, And Youth Can Be Met with Continued Health System Innovations. *Health Aff.* **2014**, *33*, 2099–2105. [CrossRef]

79. Horace, A.E.; Ahmed, F. Polypharmacy in pediatric patients and opportunities for pharmacists' involvement. *Integr. Pharm. Res. Pr.* **2015**, *4*, 113–126. [CrossRef]
80. Cox, E.R.; Halloran, D.R.; Homan, S.M.; Welliver, S.; Mager, D.E. Trends in the Prevalence of Chronic Medication Use in Children: 2002–2005. *Pediatrics* **2008**, *122*, 1053–1061. [CrossRef]
81. Wirix, A.J.G.; Kaspers, P.J.; Nauta, J.; Chinapaw, M.J.M.; Kist-van Holthe, J.E. Pathophysiology of hypertension in obese children: A systematic review. *Obes. Rev.* **2015**, *16*, 831–842. [CrossRef]
82. Din-Dzietham, R.; Liu, Y.; Bielo, M.V.; Shamsa, F. High blood pressure trends in children and adolescents in national surveys, 1963 to 2002. *Circulation* **2007**, *116*, 1488–1496. [CrossRef]
83. Magge, S.N.; Goodman, E.; Armstrong, S.C. The Metabolic Syndrome in Children and Adolescents: Shifting the Focus to Cardiometabolic Risk Factor Clustering. *Pediatrics* **2017**, *140*, 20171603. [CrossRef]
84. Balmain, B.N.; Sabapathy, S.; Jay, O.; Adsett, J.; Stewart, G.M.; Jayasinghe, R.; Morris, N.R. Heart Failure and Thermoregulatory Control: Can Patients with Heart Failure Handle the Heat? *J. Card. Fail.* **2017**, *23*, 621–627. [CrossRef]
85. Kenney, W.L.; Morgan, A.L.; Farquhar, W.B.; Brooks, E.M.; Pierzga, J.M.; Derr, J.A. Decreased active vasodilator sensitivity in aged skin. *Am. J. Physiol. Circ. Physiol.* **1997**, *272*, 1609. [CrossRef]
86. Balmain, B.N.; Jay, O.; Morris, N.R.; Shiino, K.; Stewart, G.M.; Jayasinghe, R.; Chan, J.; Sabapathy, S. Thermoeffector Responses at a Fixed Rate of Heat Production in Heart Failure Patients. *Med. Sci. Sports Exerc.* **2018**, *50*, 417–426. [CrossRef]
87. Balmain, B.N.; Jay, O.; Sabapathy, S.; Royston, D.; Stewart, G.M.; Jayasinghe, R.; Morris, N.R. Altered thermoregulatory responses in heart failure patients exercising in the heat. *Physiol. Rep.* **2016**, *4*, e13022. [CrossRef]
88. Åstrand, P.O. Experimental Studies of Physical Working Capacity in Relation to Sex and Age. Ph.D. Thesis, Munksgaard Forlag, Copenhagen, Denmark, 1952.
89. MacDougall, J.D.; Roche, P.D.; Bar-Or, O.; Moroz, J.R. Maximal Aerobic Capacity of Canadian Schoolchildren: Prediction Based on Age-Related Oxygen Cost of Running. *Int. J. Sports Med.* **1983**, *4*, 194–198. [CrossRef]
90. Frost, G.; Dowling, J.; Bar-Or, O.; Dyson, K. Ability of mechanical power estimations to explain differences in metabolic cost of walking and running among children. *Gait Posture* **1997**, *5*, 120–127. [CrossRef]
91. Frost, G.; Bar-Or, O.; Dowling, J.; Dyson, K. Explaining differences in the metabolic cost and efficiency of treadmill locomotion in children. *J. Sports Sci.* **2002**, *20*, 451–461. [CrossRef]
92. Unnithan, V.B.; Eston, R.G. Stride Frequency and Submaximal Treadmill Running Economy in Adults and Children. *Pediatr. Exerc. Sci.* **1990**, *2*, 149–155. [CrossRef]
93. Ebbeling, C.J.; Hamill, J.; Freedson, P.S.; Rowland, T.W. An Examination of Efficiency during Walking in Children and Adults. *Pediatr. Exerc. Sci.* **1992**, *4*, 36–49. [CrossRef]
94. Ries, A.J.; Schwartz, M.H. Low gait efficiency is the primary reason for the increased metabolic demand during gait in children with cerebral palsy. *Hum. Mov. Sci.* **2018**, *57*, 426–433. [CrossRef]
95. Turley, K.R.; Wilmore, J.H. Cardiovascular responses to treadmill and cycle ergometer exercise in children and adults. *J. Appl. Physiol.* **1997**, *83*, 948–957. [CrossRef]
96. Katsuura, T. Influences of age and sex on cardiac output during submaximal exercise. *Ann. Physiol. Anthr.* **1986**, *5*, 39–57. [CrossRef]
97. Gadhoke, S.; Jones, N.L. The responses to exercise in boys aged 9–15 years. *Clin. Sci.* **1969**, *37*, 789–801.
98. Godfrey, S.; Davies, C.T.M.; Woźniak, E.; Barnes, C.A. Cardio-Respiratory Response to Exercise in Normal Children. *Clin. Sci.* **1971**, *40*, 419–431. [CrossRef]
99. Kenney, W.L.; Stanhewicz, A.E.; Bruning, R.S.; Alexander, L.M. Blood pressure regulation III: What happens when one system must serve two masters: Temperature and pressure regulation? *Eur. J. Appl. Physiol.* **2014**, *114*, 467–479. [CrossRef]
100. Kenefick, R.W.; Cheuvront, S.N. Physiological adjustments to hypohydration: Impact on thermoregulation. *Auton. Neurosci.* **2016**, *196*, 47–51. [CrossRef]
101. Bar-Or, O.; Dotan, R.; Inbar, O.; Rotshtein, A.; Zonder, H. Voluntary hypohydration in 10- to 12-year-old boys. *J. Appl. Physiol.* **1980**, *48*, 104–108. [CrossRef]
102. Havenith, G.; Fogarty, A.; Bartlett, R.; Smith, C.J.; Ventenat, V. Male and female upper body sweat distribution during running measured with technical absorbents. *Eur. J. Appl. Physiol.* **2008**, *104*, 245–255. [CrossRef]
103. Smith, C.J.; Havenith, G. Body mapping of sweating patterns in athletes: A sex comparison. *Med. Sci. Sports Exerc.* **2012**, *44*, 2350–2361. [CrossRef]

104. Smith, C.J.; Havenith, G. Upper body sweat mapping provides evidence of relative sweat redistribution towards the periphery following hot-dry heat acclimation. *Temperature* **2019**, *6*, 50–65. [CrossRef]
105. Taylor, N.A.S.; Machado-Moreira, C.A. Regional variations in transepidermal water loss, eccrine sweat gland density, sweat secretion rates and electrolyte composition in resting and exercising humans. *Extrem. Physiol. Med.* **2013**, *2*, 4. [CrossRef]
106. Machado-Moreira, C.A.; Smith, F.M.; van den Heuvel, A.M.; Mekjavic, I.B.; Taylor, N.A. Sweat secretion from the torso during passively-induced and exercise-related hyperthermia. *Eur. J. Appl. Physiol.* **2008**, *104*, 265–270. [CrossRef]
107. Meyer, F.; Bar-Or, O.; MacDougall, D.; Heigenhauser, G.J. Sweat electrolyte loss during exercise in the heat: Effects of gender and maturation. *Med. Sci. Sports Exerc.* **1992**, *24*, 776–781. [CrossRef]
108. Poirier, M.P.; Gagnon, D.; Kenny, G.P. Local versus whole-body sweating adaptations following 14 days of traditional heat acclimation. *Appl. Physiol. Nutr. Metab.* **2016**, *41*, 816–824. [CrossRef]
109. Havenith, G.; Van Middendorp, H. *Determination of the Individual State of Acclimatization*; IZF Report 1986-27; TNO Institute for Perception: Soesterberg, The Netherlands, 1986; p. 24.
110. Patterson, M.J.; Stocks, J.M.; Taylor, N.A. Humid heat acclimation does not elicit a preferential sweat redistribution toward the limbs. *Am. J. Physiol. Integr. Comp. Physiol.* **2004**, *286*, 512–518. [CrossRef]
111. Sawka, M.N.; Young, A.J.; Cadarette, B.S.; Levine, L.; Pandolf, K.B. Influence of heat stress and acclimation on maximal aerobic power. *Graefe's Arch. Clin. Exp. Ophthalmol.* **1985**, *53*, 294–298. [CrossRef]
112. Kodesh, E.; Nesher, N.; Simaan, A.; Hochner, B.; Beeri, R.; Gilon, D.; Stern, M.D.; Gerstenblith, G.; Horowitz, M. Heat acclimation and exercise training interact when combined in an overriding and trade-off manner: Physiologic-genomic linkage. *Am. J. Physiol. Integr. Comp. Physiol.* **2011**, *301*, R1786–R1797. [CrossRef]
113. Pandolf, K.B. Effects of physical training and cardiorespiratory physical fitness on exercise-heat tolerance: Recent observations. *Med. Sci. Sports* **1979**, *11*, 60–65.
114. Taylor, N.A. Eccrine sweat glands. Adaptations to physical training and heat acclimation. *Sports Med.* **1986**, *3*, 387–397. [CrossRef]
115. Taylor, N.A.S. Principles and practices of heat adaptation. *J. Hum.-Environ. Syst.* **2000**, *4*, 11–22. [CrossRef]
116. Inoue, Y.; Havenith, G.; Kenney, W.L.; Loomis, J.L.; Buskirk, E.R. Exercise- and methylcholine-induced sweating responses in older and younger men: Effect of heat acclimation and aerobic fitness. *Int. J. Biometeorol.* **1999**, *42*, 210–216. [CrossRef]
117. Périard, J.D.; Travers, G.J.S.; Racinais, S.; Sawka, M.N. Cardiovascular adaptations supporting human exercise-heat acclimation. *Auton. Neurosci.* **2016**, *196*, 52–62. [CrossRef]
118. Pandolf, K.B.; Burse, R.L.; Goldman, R.F. Role of Physical Fitness in Heat Acclimatisation, Decay and Reinduction. *Ergonomics* **1977**, *20*, 399–408. [CrossRef]
119. Lorenzo, S.; Halliwill, J.R.; Sawka, M.N.; Minson, C.T. Heat acclimation improves exercise performance. *J. Appl. Physiol.* **2010**, *109*, 1140–1147. [CrossRef]
120. Jay, O.; Imbeault, P.; Ravanelli, N. The Sweating and Core Temperature Response to Compensable and Uncompensable Heat Stress Following Heat Acclimation. *FASEB J.* **2018**, *32*, 590–16124.
121. Havenith, G. Individualized model of human thermoregulation for the simulation of heat stress response. *J. Appl. Physiol.* **2001**, *90*, 1943–1954. [CrossRef]
122. Wyndham, C.H.; Rogers, G.G.; Senay, L.C.; Mitchell, D. Acclimization in a hot, humid environment: Cardiovascular adjustments. *J. Appl. Physiol.* **1976**, *40*, 779–785. [CrossRef]
123. Nielsen, B.; Hales, J.R.; Strange, S.; Christensen, N.J.; Warberg, J.; Saltin, B. Human circulatory and thermoregulatory adaptations with heat acclimation and exercise in a hot, dry environment. *J. Physiol.* **1993**, *460*, 467–485. [CrossRef]
124. Sato, F.; Owen, M.; Matthes, R.; Sato, K.; Gisolfi, C.V. Functional and morphological changes in the eccrine sweat gland with heat acclimation. *J. Appl. Physiol.* **1990**, *69*, 232–236. [CrossRef]
125. Candas, V.; Libert, J.P.; Vogt, J.J. Sweating and sweat decline of resting men in hot humid environments. *Graefe's Arch. Clin. Exp. Ophthalmol.* **1983**, *50*, 223–234. [CrossRef]
126. Buono, M.J.; Ball, K.D.; Kolkhorst, F.W. Sodium ion concentration vs. sweat rate relationship in humans. *J. Appl. Physiol.* **2007**, *103*, 990–994. [CrossRef]
127. Ogawa, T.; Asayama, M.; Miyagawa, T. Effects of sweat gland training by repeated local heating. *Jpn. J. Physiol.* **1982**, *32*, 971–981. [CrossRef]

128. Kirby, C.R.; Convertino, V.A. Plasma aldosterone and sweat sodium concentrations after exercise and heat acclimation. *J. Appl. Physiol.* **1986**, *61*, 967–970. [CrossRef]
129. Bytomski, J.R.; Squire, D.L. Heat illness in children. *Curr. Sports Med. Rep.* **2003**, *2*, 320–324. [CrossRef]
130. Zappe, D.H.; Bell, G.W.; Swartzentruber, H.; Wideman, R.F.; Kenney, W.L. Age and regulation of fluid and electrolyte balance during repeated exercise sessions. *Am. J. Physiol. Integr. Comp. Physiol.* **1996**, *270*, 71. [CrossRef]
131. Kenny, G.P.; Wilson, T.E.; Flouris, A.D.; Fujii, N. Heat exhaustion. *Handb. Clin. Neurol.* **2018**, *157*, 505–529.
132. Claremont, A.D.; Costill, D.L.; Fink, W.; Van Handel, P. Heat tolerance following diuretic induced dehydration. *Med. Sci. Sports Exerc.* **1976**, *8*, 239. [CrossRef]
133. Sawka, M.N.; Montain, S.J.; Latzka, W.A. Hydration effects on thermoregulation and performance in the heat. Comp. *Biochem. Physiol. Part A Mol. Integr. Physiol.* **2001**, *128*, 679–690. [CrossRef]
134. Cheuvront, S.N.; Carter, R.I.; Sawka, M.N. Fluid Balance and Endurance Exercise Performance. *Curr. Sports Med. Rep.* **2003**, *2*, 202–208. [CrossRef]
135. Sawka, M.N.; Burke, L.M.; Eichner, E.R.; Maughan, R.J.; Montain, S.J.; Stachenfeld, N.S. American College of Sports Medicine position stand. Exercise and fluid replacement. *Med. Sci. Sports Exerc.* **2007**, *39*, 377–390.
136. Kenney, W.L.; Tankersley, C.G.; Newswanger, D.L.; Hyde, D.E.; Puhl, S.M.; Turner, N.L. Age and hypohydration independently influence the peripheral vascular response to heat stress. *J. Appl. Physiol.* **1990**, *68*, 1902–1908. [CrossRef]
137. Fortney, S.M.; Wenger, C.B.; Bove, J.R.; Nadel, E.R. Effect of hyperosmolality on control of blood flow and sweating. *J. Appl. Physiol.* **1984**, *57*, 1688–1695. [CrossRef]
138. Sawka, M.N.; Young, A.J.; Francesconi, R.P.; Muza, S.R.; Pandolf, K.B. Thermoregulatory and blood responses during exercise at graded hypohydration levels. *J. Appl. Physiol.* **1985**, *59*, 1394–1401. [CrossRef]
139. Bar-David, Y.; Urkin, J.; Kozminsky, E. The effect of voluntary dehydration on cognitive functions of elementary school children. *Acta Paediatr.* **2005**, *94*, 1667–1673. [CrossRef]
140. Benton, D.; Burgess, N. The effect of the consumption of water on the memory and attention of children. *Appetite* **2009**, *53*, 143–146. [CrossRef]
141. Perry, C.S., 3rd; Rapinett, G.; Glaser, N.S.; Ghetti, S. Hydration status moderates the effects of drinking water on children's cognitive performance. *Appetite* **2015**, *95*, 520–527. [CrossRef]
142. Masento, N.A.; Golightly, M.; Field, D.T.; Butler, L.T.; van Reekum, C.M. Effects of hydration status on cognitive performance and mood. *Br. J. Nutr.* **2014**, *111*, 1841–1852. [CrossRef]
143. Braun, H.; von Andrian-Werburg, J.; Malisova, O.; Athanasatou, A.; Kapsokefalou, M.; Ortega, J.F.; Mora-Rodriguez, R.; Thevis, M. Differing Water Intake and Hydration Status in Three European Countries—A Day-to-Day Analysis. *Nutrients* **2019**, *11*, 773. [CrossRef]
144. Guelinckx, I.; Vecchio, M.; Perrier, E.T.; Lemetais, G. Fluid Intake and Vasopressin: Connecting the Dots. *Ann. Nutr. Metab.* **2016**, *68*, 6–11. [CrossRef]
145. Roussel, R.; Fezeu, L.; Bouby, N.; Balkau, B.; Lantieri, O.; Alhenc-Gelas, F.; Marre, M.; Bankir, L. Low Water Intake and Risk for New-Onset Hyperglycemia. *Diabetes Care* **2011**, *34*, 2551–2554. [CrossRef]
146. Enhoörning, S.; Wang, T.J.; Nilsson, P.M.; Almgren, P.; Hedblad, B.; Berglund, G.; Struck, J.; Morgenthaler, N.G.; Bergmann, A.; Lindholm, E.; et al. Plasma copeptin and the risk of diabetes mellitus. *Circulation* **2010**, *121*, 2102–2108. [CrossRef]
147. Sontrop, J.M.; Dixon, S.N.; Garg, A.X.; Buendia-Jimenez, I.; Dohein, O.; Huang, S.H.; Clark, W.F. Association between Water Intake, Chronic Kidney Disease, and Cardiovascular Disease: A Cross-Sectional Analysis of NHANES Data. *Am. J. Nephrol.* **2013**, *37*, 434–442. [CrossRef]
148. Shoham, D.A.; Durazo-Arvizu, R.; Kramer, H.; Luke, A.; Vupputuri, S.; Kshirsagar, A.; Cooper, R.S. Sugary Soda Consumption and Albuminuria: Results from the National Health and Nutrition Examination Survey, 1999–2004. *PLoS ONE* **2008**, *3*, e3431. [CrossRef]
149. Fung, T.T.; Malik, V.; Rexrode, K.M.; Manson, J.E.; Willett, W.C.; Hu, F.B. Sweetened beverage consumption and risk of coronary heart disease in women1234. *Am. J. Clin. Nutr.* **2009**, *89*, 1037–1042. [CrossRef]
150. Wilk, B.; Bar-Or, O. Effect of drink flavor and NaCL on voluntary drinking and hydration in boys exercising in the heat. *J. Appl. Physiol.* **1996**, *80*, 1112–1117. [CrossRef]
151. Barnes, K.A.; Anderson, M.L.; Stofan, J.R.; Dalrymple, K.J.; Reimel, A.J.; Roberts, T.J.; Randell, R.K.; Ungaro, C.T.; Baker, L.B. Normative data for sweating rate, sweat sodium concentration, and sweat sodium loss in athletes: An update and analysis by sport. *J. Sports Sci.* **2019**. [CrossRef]

152. Baker, L.B.; De Chavez, P.J.D.; Ungaro, C.T.; Sopena, B.C.; Nuccio, R.P.; Reimel, A.J.; Barnes, K.A. Exercise intensity effects on total sweat electrolyte losses and regional vs. whole-body sweat [Na(+)], [Cl(-)], and [K(+)]. *Eur. J. Appl. Physiol.* **2019**, *119*, 361–375. [CrossRef]
153. Baker, L.B.; Ungaro, C.T.; Sopeña, B.C.; Nuccio, R.P.; Reimel, A.J.; Carter, J.M.; Stofan, J.R.; Barnes, K.A. Body map of regional vs. whole body sweating rate and sweat electrolyte concentrations in men and women during moderate exercise-heat stress. *J. Appl. Physiol.* **2018**, *124*, 1304–1318. [CrossRef]
154. Baker, L.B.; Jeukendrup, A.E. Optimal Composition of Fluid-Replacement Beverages. *Compr. Physiol.* **2014**, *4*, 575–620.
155. Amano, T.; Hirose, M.; Konishi, K.; Gerrett, N.; Ueda, H.; Kondo, N.; Inoue, Y. Maximum rate of sweat ions reabsorption during exercise with regional differences, sex, and exercise training. *Eur. J. Appl. Physiol. Occup. Physiol.* **2017**, *30*, 708–1327. [CrossRef]
156. Henkin, S.D.; Sehl, P.L.; Meyer, F. Sweat rate and electrolyte concentration in swimmers, runners, and nonathletes. *Int. J. Sports Physiol. Perform.* **2010**, *5*, 359–366. [CrossRef]
157. Buono, M.J.; Kolding, M.; Leslie, E.; Moreno, D.; Norwood, S.; Ordille, A.; Weller, R. Heat acclimation causes a linear decrease in sweat sodium ion concentration. *J. Therm. Boil.* **2018**, *71*, 237–240. [CrossRef]
158. Pilardeau, P.A.; Lavie, F.; Vaysse, J.; Garnier, M.; Harichaux, P.; Margo, J.N.; Chalumeau, M.T. Effect of different work-loads on sweat production and composition in man. *J. Sports Med. Phys. Fit.* **1988**, *28*, 247–252.
159. Gerrett, N.; Amano, T.; Inoue, Y.; Havenith, G.; Kondo, N. The effects of exercise and passive heating on the sweat glands ion reabsorption rates. *Physiol. Rep.* **2018**, *6*, e13619. [CrossRef]
160. Meyer, F.; Laitano, O.; Bar-Or, O.; McDougall, D.; Heigenhauser, G.J. Effect of age and gender on sweat lactate and ammonia concentrations during exercise in the heat. *Braz. J. Med Boil. Res.* **2007**, *40*, 135–143. [CrossRef]
161. Lamont, L.S. Sweat lactate secretion during exercise in relation to women's aerobic capacity. *J. Appl. Physiol.* **1987**, *62*, 194–198. [CrossRef]
162. Bijman, J.; Quinton, P.M. Lactate and Bicarbonate Uptake in the Sweat Duct of Cystic Fibrosis and Normal Subjects. *Pediatr. Res.* **1987**, *21*, 79–82. [CrossRef]
163. Kaiser, D.; Songo-Williams, R.; Drack, E. Hydrogen ion and electrolyte excretion of the single human sweat gland. *Pflügers Arch. Eur. J. Physiol.* **1974**, *349*, 63–72. [CrossRef]
164. Falk, B.; Bar-Or, O.; MacDougall, J.D.; McGillis, L.; Calvert, R.; Meyer, F. Sweat lactate in exercising children and adolescents of varying physical maturity. *J. Appl. Physiol.* **1991**, *71*, 1735–1740. [CrossRef]
165. WHO. *Inheriting a Sustainable World? Atlas on Children's Health and the Environment*; World Health Organization: Geneva, Switzerland, 2017.
166. Lomax, P.; Schönbaum, E. Chapter 12 the Effects of Drugs on Thermoregulation during Exposure to Hot Environments. In *Progress in Brain Research*; Elsevier: Amsterdam, The Netherlands, 1998; Volume 115, pp. 193–204.
167. Gordon, C.J.; Johnstone, A.F.; Aydin, C. Thermal stress and toxicity. *Compr. Physiol.* **2014**, *4*, 995–1016.
168. Gordon, C.J. Response of the Thermoregulatory System to Toxic Chemicals. In *Theory and Applications of Heat Transfer in Humans*; Wiley: Hoboken, NJ, USA, 2018; Volume 1, pp. 529–552.
169. Moffatt, A.; Mohammed, F.; Eddleston, M.; Azher, S.; Eyer, P.; Buckley, N.A. Hypothermia and Fever After Organophosphorus Poisoning in Humans—A Prospective Case Series. *J. Med Toxicol.* **2010**, *6*, 379–385. [CrossRef]
170. Michelozzi, P.; Forastiere, F.; Fusco, D.; Perucci, C.A.; Ostro, B.; Ancona, C.; Pallotti, G. Air pollution and daily mortality in Rome, Italy. *Occup. Environ. Med.* **1998**, *55*, 605–610. [CrossRef]
171. WHO. The Cost of a Polluted Environment: 1.7 Million Child Deaths a Year, Says WHO. Available online: https://www.who.int/en/news-room/detail/06-03-2017-the-cost-of-a-polluted-environment-1-7-million-child-deaths-a-year-says-who (accessed on 29 June 2019).
172. Cheng, Y.; Kan, H. Effect of the Interaction between Outdoor Air Pollution and Extreme Temperature on Daily Mortality in Shanghai, China. *J. Epidemiol.* **2012**, *22*, 28–36. [CrossRef]
173. Li, G.; Zhou, M.; Cai, Y.; Zhang, Y.; Pan, X. Does temperature enhance acute mortality effects of ambient particle pollution in Tianjin City, China. *Sci. Total. Environ.* **2011**, *409*, 1811–1817. [CrossRef]
174. Rider, C.V.; Boekelheide, K.; Catlin, N.; Gordon, C.J.; Morata, T.; Selgrade, M.K.; Sexton, K.; Simmons, J.E. Cumulative risk: Toxicity and interactions of physical and chemical stressors. *Toxicol. Sci.* **2014**, *137*, 3–11. [CrossRef]

175. Heinzerling, A.; Hsu, J.; Yip, F. Respiratory Health Effects of Ultrafine Particles in Children: A Literature Review. *Water Air Soil Pollut.* **2016**, *227*, 32. [CrossRef]
176. Franchini, M.; Mannucci, P.M. Short-term effects of air pollution on cardiovascular diseases: Outcomes and mechanisms. *J. Thromb. Haemost.* **2007**, *5*, 2169–2174. [CrossRef]
177. Tager, I.B.; Balmes, J.; Lurmann, F.; Ngo, L.; Alcorn, S.; Künzli, N. Chronic Exposure to Ambient Ozone and Lung Function in Young Adults. *Epidemiology* **2005**, *16*, 751–759. [CrossRef]
178. Hemminki, K.; Pershagen, G. Cancer risk of air pollution: Epidemiological evidence. *Environ. Health Perspect.* **1994**, *102*, 187–192.
179. He, F.; Shaffer, M.L.; Rodriguez-Colon, S.; Yanosky, J.D.; Bixler, E.; Cascio, W.E.; Liao, D. Acute Effects of Fine Particulate Air Pollution on Cardiac Arrhythmia: The APACR Study. *Environ. Health Perspect.* **2011**, *119*, 927–932. [CrossRef]
180. Liao, D.; Shaffer, M.L.; He, F.; Rodriguez-Colon, S.; Wu, R.; Whitsel, E.A.; Bixler, E.O.; Cascio, W.E. Fine Particulate air Pollution is Associated with Higher Vulnerability to Atrial Fibrillation—The APACR Study. *J. Toxicol. Environ. Health Part A* **2011**, *74*, 693–705. [CrossRef]
181. Su, T.C.; Hwang, J.J.; Shen, Y.C.; Chan, C.C. Carotid Intima-Media Thickness and Long-Term Exposure to Traffic-Related Air Pollution in Middle-Aged Residents of Taiwan: A Cross-Sectional Study. *Environ. Health Perspect.* **2015**, *123*, 773–778. [CrossRef]
182. Rao, X.; Zhong, J.; Brook, R.D.; Rajagopalan, S. Effect of Particulate Matter Air Pollution on Cardiovascular Oxidative Stress Pathways. *Antioxid. Redox Signal* **2018**, *28*, 797–818. [CrossRef]
183. Lawal, A.O. Air particulate matter induced oxidative stress and inflammation in cardiovascular disease and atherosclerosis: The role of Nrf2 and AhR-mediated pathways. *Toxicol. Lett.* **2017**, *270*, 88–95. [CrossRef]
184. Schwartz, J. Air pollution and children's health. *Pediatrics* **2004**, *113*, 1037–1043.
185. Calderón-Garcidueñas, L.; Villarreal-Calderon, R.; Valencia-Salazar, G.; Henríquez-Roldán, C.; Gutiérrez-Castrellón, P.; Torres-Jardón, R.; Osnaya-Brizuela, N.; Romero, L.; Torres-Jardón, R.; Solt, A.; et al. Systemic Inflammation, Endothelial Dysfunction, and Activation in Clinically Healthy Children Exposed to Air Pollutants. *Inhal. Toxicol.* **2008**, *20*, 499–506. [CrossRef]
186. Armijos, R.X.; Weigel, M.M.; Myers, O.B.; Li, W.W.; Racines, M.; Berwick, M. Residential Exposure to Urban Traffic Is Associated with Increased Carotid Intima-Media Thickness in Children. *J. Environ. Public Health* **2015**, *2015*, 1–11. [CrossRef]
187. Bais, A.F.; McKenzie, R.L.; Bernhard, G.; Aucamp, P.J.; Ilyas, M.; Madronich, S.; Tourpali, K. Ozone depletion and climate change: Impacts on UV radiation. *Photochem. Photobiol. Sci.* **2015**, *14*, 19–52. [CrossRef]
188. Armstrong, B.K.; Kricker, A. The epidemiology of UV induced skin cancer. *J. Photochem. Photobiol. B: Boil.* **2001**, *63*, 8–18. [CrossRef]
189. Krause, R.; Bühring, M.; Hopfenmüller, W.; Holick, M.F.; Sharma, A.M. Ultraviolet B and blood pressure. *Lancet* **1998**, *352*, 709–710. [CrossRef]
190. Liebmann, P.M.; Wölfler, A.; Felsner, P.; Hofer, D.; Schauenstein, K. Melatonin and the Immune System. *Int. Arch. Allergy Immunol.* **1997**, *112*, 203–211. [CrossRef]
191. Maestroni, G.J.M. The immunotherapeutic potential of melatonin. *Expert Opin. Investig. Drugs* **2001**, *10*, 467–476. [CrossRef]
192. Constantinescu, C.S.; Hilliard, B.; Ventura, E.; Rostami, A. Luzindole, a Melatonin Receptor Antagonist, Suppresses Experimental Autoimmune Encephalomyelitis. *Pathobiology* **1997**, *65*, 190–194. [CrossRef]
193. Ren, W.; Liu, G.; Chen, S.; Yin, J.; Wang, J.; Tan, B.; Wu, G.; Bazer, F.W.; Peng, Y.; Li, T.; et al. Melatonin signaling in T cells: Functions and applications. *J. Pineal Res.* **2017**, *62*, e12394. [CrossRef]
194. De Gruijl, F.R. Skin cancer and solar UV radiation. *Eur. J. Cancer* **1999**, *35*, 2003–2009. [CrossRef]
195. Rass, K.; Reichrath, J. UV damage and DNA repair in malignant melanoma and nonmelanoma skin cancer. *Adv. Exp. Med. Biol.* **2008**, *624*, 162–178.
196. Ponsonby, A.L.; McMichael, A.; van der Mei, I. Ultraviolet radiation and autoimmune disease: Insights from epidemiological research. *Toxicology* **2002**, *181*, 71–78. [CrossRef]
197. Pandolf, K.B.; Gange, R.W.; Latzka, W.A.; Blank, I.H.; Kraning, K.K., 2nd; Gonzalez, R.R. Human thermoregulatory responses during heat exposure after artificially induced sunburn. *Am. J. Physiol.* **1992**, *262*, R610–R616. [CrossRef]
198. Pandolf, K.B.; Griffin, T.B.; Munro, E.H.; Goldman, R.F. Persistence of impaired heat tolerance from artificially induced miliaria rubra. *Am. J. Physiol. Integr. Comp. Physiol.* **1980**, *239*, R226–R232. [CrossRef]

199. Bruning, R.S.; Santhanam, L.; Stanhewicz, A.E.; Smith, C.J.; Berkowitz, D.E.; Kenney, W.L.; Holowatz, L.A. Endothelial nitric oxide synthase mediates cutaneous vasodilation during local heating and is attenuated in middle-aged human skin. *J. Appl. Physiol.* **2012**, *112*, 2019–2026. [CrossRef]
200. Kellogg, D.L., Jr.; Liu, Y.; Kosiba, I.F.; O'Donnell, D. Role of nitric oxide in the vascular effects of local warming of the skin in humans. *J. Appl. Physiol.* **1999**, *86*, 1185–1190. [CrossRef]
201. Minson, C.T.; Berry, L.T.; Joyner, M.J. Nitric oxide and neurally mediated regulation of skin blood flow during local heating. *J. Appl. Physiol.* **2001**, *91*, 1619–1626. [CrossRef]
202. Kellogg, D.L., Jr.; Crandall, C.G.; Liu, Y.; Charkoudian, N.; Johnson, J.M. Nitric oxide and cutaneous active vasodilation during heat stress in humans. *J. Appl. Physiol.* **1998**, *85*, 824–829. [CrossRef]
203. Wolf, S.T.; Stanhewicz, A.E.; Jablonski, N.G.; Kenney, W.L. Acute ultraviolet radiation exposure attenuates nitric oxide-mediated vasodilation in the cutaneous microvasculature of healthy humans. *J. Appl. Physiol.* **2018**. [CrossRef]
204. Wolf, S.T.; Berry, C.W.; Stanhewicz, A.E.; Kenney, L.E.; Ferguson, S.B.; Kenney, W.L. Sunscreen or simulated sweat minimizes the impact of acute ultraviolet radiation on cutaneous microvascular function in healthy humans. *Exp. Physiol.* **2019**. [CrossRef]
205. Wick, D.E.; Roberts, S.K.; Basu, A.; Sandroni, P.; Fealey, R.D.; Sletten, D.; Charkoudian, N. Delayed threshold for active cutaneous vasodilation in patients with Type 2 diabetes mellitus. *J. Appl. Physiol.* **2006**, *100*, 637–641. [CrossRef]
206. Petrofsky, J.S.; Lee, S.; Patterson, C.; Cole, M.; Stewart, B. Sweat production during global heating and during isometric exercise in people with diabetes. *Med Sci. Monit.* **2005**, *11*, 515–521.
207. Fealey, R.D.; Low, P.A.; Thomas, J.E. Thermoregulatory Sweating Abnormalities in Diabetes Mellitus. *Mayo Clin. Proc.* **1989**, *64*, 617–628. [CrossRef]
208. Dougherty, K.A.; Chow, M.; Kenney, W.L. Critical environmental limits for exercising heat-acclimated lean and obese boys. *Eur. J. Appl. Physiol.* **2010**, *108*, 779–789. [CrossRef]
209. Bar-Or, O.; Blimkie, C.; Hay, J.A.; MacDougall, J.D.; Ward, D.S.; Wilson, W.M. Voluntary dehydration and heat intolerance in cystic fibrosis. *Lancet* **1992**, *339*, 696–699. [CrossRef]
210. Roelands, B.; Hasegawa, H.; Watson, P.; Piacentini, M.F.; Buyse, L.; De Schutter, G.; Meeusen, R.R. The Effects of Acute Dopamine Reuptake Inhibition on Performance. *Med. Sci. Sports Exerc.* **2008**, *40*, 879–885. [CrossRef]
211. Havenith, G. Metabolic rate and clothing insulation data of children and adolescents during various school activities. *Ergonomics* **2007**, *50*, 1689–1701. [CrossRef]

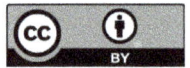

© 2019 by the author. Licensee MDPI, Basel, Switzerland. This article is an open access article distributed under the terms and conditions of the Creative Commons Attribution (CC BY) license (http://creativecommons.org/licenses/by/4.0/).

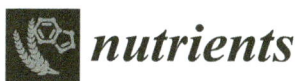

Review

Of Mice and Men—The Physiology, Psychology, and Pathology of Overhydration

Tamara Hew-Butler *, Valerie Smith-Hale, Alyssa Pollard-McGrandy and Matthew VanSumeren

Division of Kinesiology, Health and Sport Studies, Wayne State University, Detroit, MI 48202, USA
* Correspondence: tamara.hew-butler@wayne.edu; Tel.: +313-577-8130

Received: 30 May 2019; Accepted: 3 July 2019; Published: 7 July 2019

Abstract: The detrimental effects of dehydration, to both mental and physical health, are well-described. The potential adverse consequences of overhydration, however, are less understood. The difficulty for most humans to routinely ingest ≥2 liters (L)—or "eight glasses"—of water per day highlights the likely presence of an inhibitory neural circuit which limits the deleterious consequences of overdrinking in mammals but can be consciously overridden in humans. This review summarizes the existing data obtained from both animal (mostly rodent) and human studies regarding the physiology, psychology, and pathology of overhydration. The physiology section will highlight the molecular strength and significance of aquaporin-2 (AQP2) water channel downregulation, in response to chronic anti-diuretic hormone suppression. Absence of the anti-diuretic hormone, arginine vasopressin (AVP), facilitates copious free water urinary excretion (polyuria) in equal volumes to polydipsia to maintain plasma tonicity within normal physiological limits. The psychology section will highlight reasons why humans and rodents may volitionally overdrink, likely in response to anxiety or social isolation whereas polydipsia triggers mesolimbic reward pathways. Lastly, the potential acute (water intoxication) and chronic (urinary bladder distension, ureter dilation and hydronephrosis) pathologies associated with overhydration will be examined largely from the perspective of human case reports and early animal trials.

Keywords: hydration; dehydration; hypohydration; hyponatremia; polydipsia

1. Introduction

Hydration and the evolving search for an adequate universal daily water intake recommendation remains elusive [1] and somewhat contentious [2,3]. Most of the disagreement over an adequate index for fluid intake, however, likely revolves around the disparate and non-standardized metrics commonly utilized to define both normal and abnormal hydration status (HS) [4]. For example, the clinical definition of dehydration is cellular dehydration from extracellular hypertonicity [5,6] while scientists often use the term dehydration to describe the process of losing water [4]. Alternatively, the term hypohydration refers to a negative water balance [7] or state of water deficit [4]. Regardless of which hydration terminology is utilized to define HS, the vast majority of the scientific and lay literature highlights the well-recognized detrimental effects of dehydration and/or hypohydration on a variety of conditions such as kidney stones [3], obesity [8], recurrent urinary tract infections [9], cognition [10], and athletic performance [11].

At the opposite end of the hydration spectrum, a paucity of data exists on the topic of overhydration. In 1923, Rowntree published a series of animal and human data exploring the detrimental effects of "water intoxication" [12]. Rowntree successfully induced water intoxication (characterized by restlessness, lethargy, polyuria, diarrhea, salivation, frothing at the mouth, nausea, retching, vomiting, muscle twitching, seizures, coma and death) in dogs, cats, rabbits and guinea-pigs by rapidly administering tap or distilled water (50 mL/kg bodyweight every 30 min) rectally, intravenously, through a stomach tube and/or ureteral catheter to induce water overload [12]. Combined with similar human cases of water intoxication [13–17], it appears clear that extreme fluid administration in excess of excretion rates—or more modest intakes when coupled with pathological anti-diuretic hormone secretion—are indeed detrimental (and sometimes toxic) to health [12].

Thus, while the current evidence suggests that modest hypohydration and extreme overhydration have deleterious health consequences, the question remains whether modest overhydration is beneficial or detrimental to health. This review will explore the physiology, psychology, and pathology of overhydration. Both animal (mostly mice) and human studies will be detailed, with an emphasis placed upon the psychogenic polydipsia literature to more clearly evaluate: (1) long-term physiological changes associated with concomitant and sustained polyuria and (2) the putative neurogenic pathways which may differentially drive high (anxiolytic) versus low habitual fluid consumption. We will refer to the term polydipsia to represent excessive drinking (beyond regulatory need) without any known medical cause [18].

2. Physiology

As comprehensively described elsewhere [1,19–22], water balance is exquisitely regulated in all mammals (and some non-mammals) [22,23] in physiological defense of both osmotic balance (plasma tonicity) and circulatory volume. Plasma tonicity dictates cellular size, and is tightly regulated by a coordinated system of osmosensors, neural networks, endocrine mediators, and physiologically-driven behaviors which cooperatively serve to sustain extracellular fluid osmolality around a remarkably constant set-point of 300 mOsmol/kgH$_2$O [20] (or, plasma sodium concentration ~140 mmol/L) [21]. Central to this evolutionarily stable feedback-loop controlling osmotic regulation is the kidney, whose immediate ability to retain or excrete free water is vital to the overall maintenance of fluid homeostasis [19,24]. For clinical convenience, we will refer to a plasma sodium concentration ([Na$^+$]) between 135–145 mmol/L as the "normal" range for extracellular fluid osmolality/plasma tonicity since sodium is the main extracellular cation found within the plasma [21].

When modest amounts of water (or other hypotonic fluids) are ingested above osmotically-driven thirst stimulation (overhydration), osmoreceptors located within the highly vascularized circumventricular organs (CVO's) within the brain detect a (dilutional) decrease in plasma [Na$^+$] once water is absorbed into the circulation from the gastrointestinal (GI) tract [20,25]. These CVO's, located outside of the blood brain barrier, suppress both the release of the body's main anti-diuretic hormone, arginine vasopressin (AVP), from the posterior pituitary gland and suppress the sensation of osmotically-driven thirst to prevent further dilution of plasma [Na$^+$]. Oropharyngeal receptors, activated by physical contact with ingested fluids [26–28], as well as gastrointestinal sensors responding to stretch receptors sensing fullness [29–32] serve to terminate drinking behavior, perhaps as an anticipatory measure to prevent the pathophysiological consequences of overdrinking (i.e., cellular swelling). In fact, recent electrophysiological and optogenic studies performed on mice confirm the presence of a distinct neuronal network, mediated by cross-talk between the brain and gastrointestinal tract, through activation of the subfornical organ within the CVO [32]. The subfornical organ appears to coordinate a variety of neuronal inputs that anticipate the homeostatic consequences of food and fluid intake well before changes in plasma tonicity are observed [32,33].

Functional magnetic resonance imaging (fMRI) studies further suggest that the brain senses water intake in response to thirst as "pleasant", while overdrinking suppresses this hedonic response [34–36]. The alliesthesia associated with drinking while thirsty mainly activates the anterior midcingulate cortex and orbitofrontal cortex, suggesting that drinking to thirst is pleasurable and involuntary [35,36]. In contrast, continued drinking after thirst satiation (+1 L above thirst suppression) [34] activates brain areas associated with swallowing inhibition as well as cortical areas associated with unpleasantness ratings [34,35]. Activation of the motor cortex, striatum and thalamus suggests that voluntary motor activity is required to continue drinking above thirst satiation [34]. As such, drinking above thirst requires a threefold increase in volitional effort compared to drinking when thirsty [34]. Independent data collected from a clinical trial, where 316 participants with stage three chronic kidney disease were "coached" to increase daily water intake by 1–1.5 L/day, corroborate these fMRI findings and confirm that drinking above thirst is difficult and unpleasant [37]. The average increase in water intake in the participants randomized into the "coached hydration" group, could only increase their daily water intake by ~0.6 L relative to the control group [37]. Thus, the inability for free-living adults to voluntarily sustain even modest 500 mL (~2 cup) increases in daily water consumption (above thirst) underscores the strength of the central inhibitory pathways that serve to prevent the deleterious and life-threatening consequences of fluid overload.

Both thirst stimulation and AVP release are centrally coordinated in real-time by input largely from the cranial nerve system. As such, central integration of neuronal feedback from osmoreceptors (subfornical organ), baroreceptors (tenth cranial nerve), the mouth (fifth cranial nerve), tongue (seventh cranial nerve), oropharynx (ninth cranial nerve), and stomach (tenth cranial nerve) ultimately results in either the stimulation or suppression of AVP from the posterior pituitary gland [20,21,35]. AVP then regulates plasma [Na^+]/tonicity by retaining or excreting water within the kidney collecting duct. The permeability of the kidney collecting duct increases when AVP binds to the vasopressin-2 receptors (V2R), which stimulates the insertion of aquaporin 2 (AQP2) water channels into the lumen of the kidney collecting duct [19,24]. The insertion of these AQP2 water channels allows for water molecules (otherwise destined for urinary excretion) to be reabsorbed back into the circulation when plasma tonicity is high (or circulating plasma volume low) to conserve total body water. Conversely, with overdrinking, there is central inhibition of the AVP release, which withdraws AQP2 channels from the lumen of the kidney collecting duct; thereby promoting urinary free water excretion which matches fluid ingestion beyond physiological need.

It is important to emphasize that the neuroendocrine feedback loop coordinating fluid balance between the brain and kidney is highly conserved within the DNA (deoxyribonucleic acid) of vertebrate and invertebrate species dating back 700 million years [23]. Once released into the circulation, AVP can increase kidney collecting duct permeability within 40 s of activation of the V2R in rodent species [38]. Quantification studies of microdissected renal tubule segments, obtained from the middle part of rodent inner medullary collecting duct, estimate that there are ~12 million individual AQP2 water channels present within each kidney collecting duct cell [24]. Thus, the molecular strength and precision of the diuretic renal response to AVP suppression is powerful and allows for urinary excretion rates approximating 1 L/h, as seen in patients with diabetes insipidus [21] and compulsive water drinkers [39,40].

Interestingly enough, chronic overhydration (>3 days), triggers the downregulation of AQP2 water channels within the kidney collecting duct cells [19,24]. This phenomenon has been verified directly in a series of elegant studies performed on water-loaded rats and mice [19,24] and indirectly confirmed in human studies [41–44]. The sustained suppression of circulating AVP in response to overdrinking enhances urinary free water excretion and teleologically represents the most appropriate renal adaptation to a constant fluid intake load (polydipsia = polyuria). However, when high fluid intakes are suddenly curtailed [42–44], the downregulation of AQP2 water channels triggers a transient inability to reabsorb water molecules back through the kidney collecting duct in response to AVP V2R stimulation [19,24,45]. This renal insensitivity to AVP secretion augments urinary fluid losses (above intake), which is clinically characterized by an inability to concentrate urinary solutes [43,44,46,47] coupled with enhanced body water/weight loss [42]. This phenomenon of "water loading", popularized by combat sport athletes and body builders before competition as a method to "weigh-in light" [39,45], highlights the dynamic molecular adaptability within the kidney collecting duct cells in response to chronic (>3 days) changes in water intake that have been clearly demonstrated in rodent models [19,24,48–51]. A return to regulated drinking (osmotically-driven thirst stimulation) and concomitant AVP exposure will restore AQP2 expression within collecting duct epithelium by 3–5 days [48] and reverse the physiologic nephrogenic diabetes insipidus induced by chronic water loading in both mice and men [24].

3. Psychology

At the most extreme range of overhydration, compulsive water drinking has been recognized in emotionally disturbed individuals without neurogenic (i.e., inability of secrete AVP from the posterior pituitary) or nephrogenic (i.e., kidneys resistant to AVP stimulation) diabetes insipidus [47]. Sometimes referred to as "psychogenic polydipsia" [52,53], 80% of compulsive water drinkers represent neurotic females with a history of schizophrenia [40,54], depression [14,45], and/or anxiety [53,55]. Psychogenic polydipsia in schizophrenic patients was first identified in 1936 through investigation of profuse polyuria, which eventually ceased when the polydipsia was minimized [56].

To a more modest degree of drinking, social polydipsia—or overdrinking to achieve health benefits—has become popularized within western culture. The most common "one-size-fits-all" guideline suggests that all healthy humans need to drink at least eight glasses of water daily beyond fluids obtained through foods or other beverages. This popular recommendation persists despite equivocal evidence, which supports the claim that water intake maximizes skin heath, digestion, renal, sexual, or neurological function [3,57,58]. The continued success of this advice is evidenced by robust water bottle sales, which topped 2.78 billion dollars in 2018 within the United States alone [59]. At extreme levels (>5 L daily), social polydipsia may result in profound dilation of the bladder, ureters and kidneys [60] and at worst, water intoxication (i.e., overconsumption of fluids beyond excretion rates leading to the signs and symptoms of encephalopathy) [12]. Of note, updated (2017) guidelines put forth by the European Food Safety Authority (EFSA) now defines total water intake to include all beverages consumed plus the moisture contained in foods [61].

Drinking beyond the dictates of thirst has been popularized within athletic circles to prevent the detrimental effects of hypohydration on health and performance [11]. Although guidelines have evolved to drink to minimize body weight losses (<2%) [62], other drinking guidelines recommend drinking before the onset of thirst stimulation to maintain a dilute urine (urine specific gravity <1.020) [11]. Some athletes, unfortunately, have taken this advice to extreme levels (i.e., drinking 80–100 cups of fluid during a marathon footrace [63]) and have developed water intoxication [13,64]. Additionally, water loading has become a popular practice for combat sport athletes to enhance water weight losses before weigh-ins [42] while actors participating in pornographic films have begun water loading to enhance their squirting performance abilities [58]. The prevalence of symptomatic water intoxication in prolonged endurance races remains relatively rare (<1%), however [65].

Why otherwise healthy people, outside of sports or social reasons, habitually drink high volumes of fluid [66] above physiological need remains a curious and unanswered phenomenon. Studies performed in mice exposed to chronic stress [67,68] or raised in isolation [69,70], provide psychological insight into this peculiar finding. Male C57BL/6 mice subjected to chronic social defeat stress (i.e., exposure to bigger, meaner, "bully" mice) demonstrate a distinct phenotype characterized by enhanced fluid intake [67,70] and water retention [68]. Additionally, two-month old Sabra mice [70] and adolescent male Sprague-Dawley rats [69] reared (post-weaning) in isolation developed significant polydipsia compared with control animals. Follow-up molecular and electrophysiological studies implicate the mesolimbic dopamine circuit in the manifestation of polydipsia in response to loneliness and social anxiety [67].

One explanation as to why anxious mice develop polydipsia, is that water intake may somehow reduce dopaminergic neuron excitability within the ventral tegmental area (VTA), or the reward area, of the brain. Of note, schizophrenia has been linked to enhanced dopaminergic receptor excitability [67,71], which likely mediates polydipsia as either a reward-seeking [67] or anxiolytic [67,68,70] behavior. Further investigations on drug-induced polydipsia are required to tease out the potential neurochemical circuits linking dopamine, reward, and drinking. Drugs that demonstrate the most promising results, include: methamphetamines (which inhibit dopamine reuptake in the brain) [72] such as 3,4 methyldioxymethamphetamine (Ecstasy) [73], agonists, which downregulate dopamine receptor 2 (DRD2) [74], first and second generation antipsychotics [75], and antidepressant medications [76]. All these drugs have been linked to hyponatremia from non-osmotic AVP secretion, but their relationship to polydipsia is under-appreciated. Of note, a variety of drugs and excipients have been shown to affect hydration status by augmenting fluid losses, affecting thirst and/or appetite, increasing intestinal permeability and/or renal reabsorption rates [7].

Human observations corroborate these animal findings, as most psychogenic polydipsic patients report that drinking makes them feel better [77]. Patients with hallucinations also report that drinking fluids suppress the "voices" [78], further suggesting that the act of drinking activates neural circuits associated with primitive coping mechanisms [77]. Other investigators suggest that the anterior hippocampus and nucleus accumbens are involved in polydipsia as a reward-seeking behavior in psychiatric patients [77]. Alternatively, compulsive water drinking has been documented in non-neurotic individuals seeking to achieve a drunken-like state [14,55]. For example, a 16-year-old female drank copious amounts of water because it made her feel "funny and high, like after a beer" [55] while a 46-year-old man with a history of depression ran out of money to buy beer, so drank large amounts of water because it made him feel "slightly drunk" [14]. Therefore, coupled with evidence suggesting that drinking fluids improves cognition [10], it is possible that polydipsia activates a dopaminergic reward circuit that attenuates anxiety in susceptible individuals exposed to chronic stress and/or social isolation. A summary of this proposed relationship is detailed in Figure 1. Further investigation on the potential anxiolytic effects of polydipsia, especially in females, warrants further investigation with particular regards to whether this practice is adaptive or maladaptive over the long term.

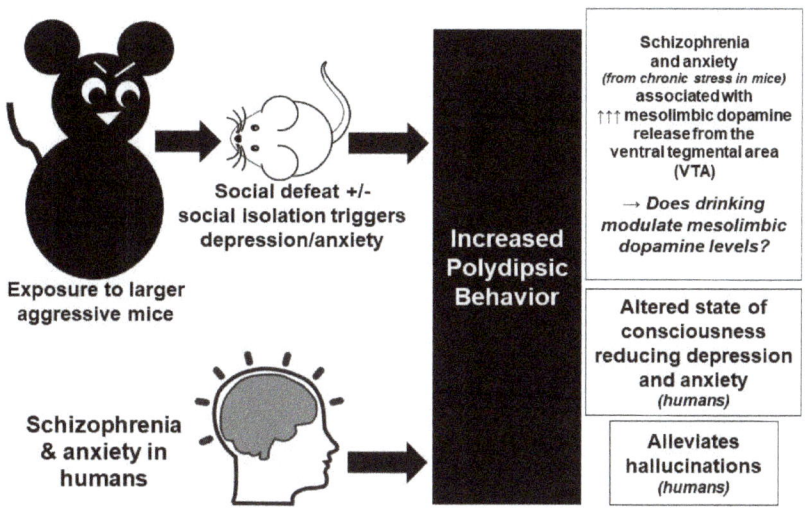

Figure 1. Summary of data obtained from mice and humans linking polydipsia to mesolimbic reward centers, which serve to reduce anxiety and/or signs and symptoms of psychiatric illness.

4. Pathology

As previously summarized, total body fluid regulation is exquisitely regulated in defense of plasma [Na$^+$]/tonicity and circulating volume. Accordingly, complications from overdrinking are rare. The most common (and dire) clinical consequence from overdrinking is water intoxication, which is biochemically defined as a plasma [Na$^+$] below the normal range set by the lab performing the test (usually a plasma [Na$^+$] < 135 mmol/L, which is called "hyponatremia", because hypo = low and natremia = blood sodium) [21]. As first described by Rowntree in 1923, the fatal consequences of water intoxication occur when fluid administration exceeds the capacity to excrete any fluid excess and exacerbated by AVP stimulation (water retention) [12]. Hyponatremia causes water to flow down an osmotic gradient from outside of cells to inside of cells and causes all cells within the body to swell. Hyponatremia is fatal when cerebral swelling in excess of 5–8% exceeds the rigid confines of the skull, resulting in brainstem herniation, cerebral hypoxia, and loss of vegetative functions [13,64].

Gross estimations suggest that an acute (<1 h) fluid intake around 3–4 L (~1 gallon) is enough to induce symptomatic hyponatremia in otherwise healthy individuals at rest [12,52]. Although maximal urine excretion rates allow humans to tolerate water intakes approximating 20 L per day without ill-effects [79], the actual fluid intake tolerance limit appears to be closer to 10 L per day in normal individuals [43,79]. De Wardener and Herxheimer each drank 10 L of water per day (250–500 mL every 30–60 min during waking hours) for 11 days and reported physical signs of headache, scotoma, skin coldness with pallor, and puffiness of the face [43]. These two subjects also reported that their lips felt dry (without the sensation of thirst), food was tasteless, emotional liability was high, and simple intellectual tasks became increasingly difficult during this period of enhanced water intake [43]. Of note, the pathogenic effects of overhydration are not isolated to oral intake. The first water intoxication fatality was reported in 1935, in a 50-year-old female who received 9 L of fluid over 24-h through the rectum (proctoclysis) following an otherwise uncomplicated gallbladder surgery [17]. Thus, it is difficult to commit to recommending a threshold volume of water that can be safely consumed (or administered) over time, since both the ~3 L per hour and ~10 L per day can be tolerated by some (especially athletes with high sweat rates [80]) but fatal to others. Of note, when non-osmotic AVP secretion is present, or when sodium losses are severe, modest water ingestion at rates of 1–2 L/h can induce symptomatic hyponatremia [13,21]. Non-osmotic stimuli to AVP secretion, sodium losses, a variety of drugs and excipients influencing hydration status, and type of fluids consumed are beyond the scope of this review and detailed elsewhere [7,81,82].

The body's appropriate fluid homeostatic response to polydipsia is polyuria (i.e., excessive urine production). For individuals with normal kidney function, any excess fluid that is ingested (beyond osmoregulatory need) is promptly excreted by the body. For example, the 10 L of water ingested by De Wardener and Herxheimer resulted in a daily urine output of 10 L [43]. Polyuria is also the characteristic feature of diabetes insipidus (both neurologic and nephrogenic), whereas chronic urinary free water excretion (from AVP suppression or renal insensitivity) is counterbalanced by osmotic thirst stimulation and concomitant water intake, which matches urinary fluid losses (to maintain plasma [Na^+] within the normal physiological range) [21,47,83]. As such, sustained polyuria has been shown to cause profound urinary tract changes such as bladder distension, dilation of the ureters, renal back pressure atrophy, hydronephrosis, traumatic rupture of the urinary tract, and renal failure [60,84–88]. One such case of (reversible) hydronephrosis occurred in an otherwise healthy 53-year-old female who drank 4.5–5.5 L of fluid daily over the subsequent three years to "stay healthy" and because "all her friends do so" [60]. Another possible mechanical consequence of polydipsia is gastric distension [89], which may be advantageous in those trying to lose weight (producing the sensation of stomach fullness ahead of meals) [8]. Figure 2 summarizes the acute and chronic physiological effects of overhydration while Figure 3 summarizes the acute and chronic physiological effects of water intake when hypohydrated.

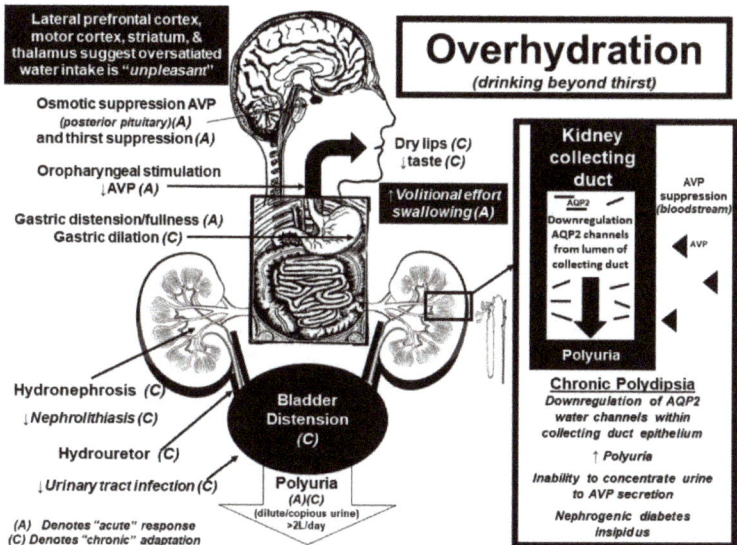

Figure 2. Summary diagram of acute (A) and chronic (C) physiological responses integrating potential pathologies and benefits associated with overdrinking in the satiated condition (above thirst stimulation).

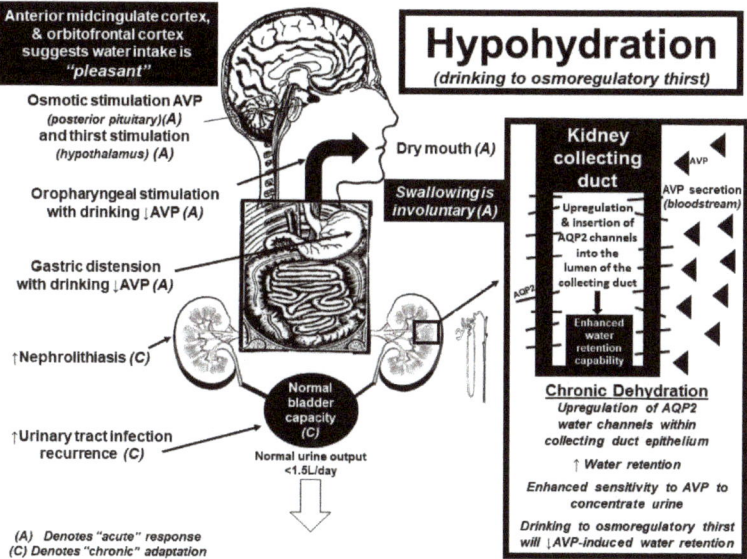

Figure 3. Summary diagram of acute (A) and chronic (C) physiological responses and potential pathologies associated with drinking to thirst when hypohydrated.

With specific regards to kidney function, individuals with a history of kidney stones (nephrolithiasis) have a reduced risk of recurrent stone formation if they consume more than 2 L of water per day [3,57]. One hypothesis is that increased water intake (>2 L/day for 12-months) reduces renal papillary density, which may precipitate calcium oxalate stone formation [90]. Conversely, excessive fluid intake may exacerbate proteinuria [91], have no effect [37] or accelerate [92] the progression of chronic renal disease.

It has been demonstrated in a randomized-control trial that premenopausal women with a history of recurrent urinary tract infections (UTI), who drink less than 1.5 L of water daily (low volume drinkers), can reduce the recurrence rate of UTI's from three to two episodes/year by increasing water consumption by +1.3 L/day [9]. However, increased fluid intake has not been equivocally shown to enhance skin complexion or kidney function [3,57], while data are unclear regarding constipation [57,93]. Data regarding the effect of water intake on weight loss are mixed. Some studies demonstrate positive associations between water intake, weight management and body composition [94–96], while others demonstrate an increase in energy intake when pre-meal water ingestion was removed [97,98]. Alternatively, a randomized control trial performed on obese and overweight adolescents did not demonstrate enhanced weight loss with increased water consumption [8].

It is important to note that water intake is not completely benign. Otherwise healthy individuals have died or developed significant brain swelling (hyponatremic encephalopathy) from drinking too much fluid to prevent kidney stones [99], sooth a toothache [100], dilute ingested poison [16], counter a UTI [101], treat gastroenteritis [15], and alleviate constipation [46,102], as shown in Table 1. These cases highlight the need to dampen overzealous (but well-intended) advice to "stay hydrated".

Table 1. Cases of hyponatremic encephalopathy (and death) in otherwise healthy people who overdrank to treat another medical condition (L = liters).

Subject	Amount of Fluid Consumed	Reason for Polydipsia	Report
Not described	3 L/20 min	Test skin elasticity	Rowntree 1923 [12]
16 yo female	20 L/day	Facial acne	Lee 1989 [55]
44 yo male	12 L/day	Kidney stones	Berry 1977 [99]
9.5 yo male	10–15 L/24 h	Soothe toothache	Pickering 1971 [100]
* 40 yo female	"plenty of water"	Dilute poison (ingested)	Sarvesvaran 1984 [16]
59 yo female	"plenty of water"	Urinary tract infection	Lee 2016 [101]
* 27 yo female	"lots of water"	Gastroenteritis	Sjoblom 1997 [15]
52 yo male	6 L/2 h + 1 L enema	Constipation	Swanson 1958 [102]
74 yo female	10–14 glasses water/day	Soften stool	Walls 1977 [46]

* fatality.

The potential for abnormal thirst regulation to contribute to pathological water consumption has been documented in a few select scenarios (one in humans and another in cattle). Compulsive water drinkers demonstrate abnormal thirst regulation, whereas the osmotic threshold for thirst stimulation is paradoxically lower than the osmotic threshold for AVP release [83]. Whether or not this reverse in osmotic thresholds for thirst and AVP stimulation is a cause or effect of psychogenic polydipsia remains unclear. Additionally, the animal studies suggest that most mammals will not voluntarily develop water intoxication, unless artificially induced in the laboratory to investigate hyponatremia [12,103]. The only confirmed exception are calves (and in rare instances, adult cattle) who develop fatal water intoxication only after given access to water following a period of water deprivation for reasons which remain unclear [104].

Finally, in contrast to the potential beneficial effects of polydipsia in healthy humans detailed elsewhere [1,4,57], fluid overload is conversely associated with an increase in mortality in unhealthy animals and humans. More specifically, hyponatremia is associated with an increased mortality rate in hospitalized dogs and cats [105]. Schizophrenic patients with polydipsia demonstrate a higher mortality rate [18] while fluid retention/overload predicts 30-day mortality rate in geriatric patients [106] while increasing morbidity and mortality in critically ill children [107]. One proposed mechanism to explain the increased mortality in compromised patients is a plausible relationship between fluid overload and inflammation, which has been observed in patients with chronic kidney disease [108,109]. Whether or not fluid overload or hyponatremia is a cause or result of disease progression remains unclear [110].

5. Conclusions

Studies performed in mice and men collectively suggest that modest overhydration results in modest urine production (which matches fluid intake volumes) in homeostatic defense of plasma tonicity and intracellular size. In the chronic condition (>3 days) sustained AVP suppression results in the downregulation of AQP2 water channels within the kidney collecting duct, which results in a transient (3–5 days) inability to concentrate urine or reabsorb kidney water back into the circulation in response to AVP stimulation. Complications from acute (>3 L/h) or chronic (5–10+ L/day) water intakes at rest are uncommon but may result in acute water intoxication or chronic urinary tract abnormalities such as urinary bladder distention, ureter dilation, and hydronephrosis. Modest overhydration (>2 L/day in sedentary individuals of average size in temperate environments) may prevent kidney stones in individuals with recurrent nephrolithiasis or reduce the number of urinary tract infections in susceptible premenopausal females. The anxiolytic effects of copious water intake on a subset of vulnerable individuals, with or without mental illness, has been demonstrated along with data suggesting that overhydration enhances cognitive function. Further studies assessing the benefits and detriments of water intake above thirst are required, as long as water intakes are not extreme and warnings of the potentially fatal consequences of water intoxication are duly noted.

Author Contributions: T.H.-B. contributed to the conceptualization, data curation, and writing–original draft preparation; T.H.-B., V.S.-H., A.P.-M. and M.V. contributed to the resources and writing–reviewing and editing of this manuscript.

Funding: This research received no external funding.

Conflicts of Interest: The authors declare no conflicts of interest.

References

1. Armstrong, L.E.; Johnson, E.C. Water Intake, Water Balance, and the Elusive Daily Water Requirement. *Nutrients* **2018**, *10*, 1928. [CrossRef]
2. McCartney, M. Margaret McCartney: Hydration, common sense, and evidence. *BMJ* **2017**, *359*, j4642. [CrossRef] [PubMed]
3. Valtin, H. "Drink at least eight glasses of water a day." Really? Is there scientific evidence for "8 × 8"? *Am. J. Physiol. Regul. Integr. Comp. Physiol.* **2002**, *283*, R993–R1004. [CrossRef] [PubMed]
4. Kavouras, S.A. Hydration, dehydration, underhydration, optimal hydration: Are we barking up the wrong tree? *Eur. J. Nutr.* **2019**, *58*, 471–473. [CrossRef] [PubMed]
5. McGee, S.; Abernathy, W.B.; Simel, D. IS This Patient Hypovolemic? *JAMA* **1999**, *281*, 1022–1029. [CrossRef] [PubMed]
6. Mange, K.; Matsuura, D.; Cizman, B.; Soto, H.; Ziyadeh, F.N.; Goldfarb, S.; Neilson, E.G. Language guiding therapy: The case of dehydration versus volume depletion. *Ann. Intern. Med.* **1997**, *127*, 848–853. [CrossRef]
7. Puga, A.M.; Lopez-Oliva, S.; Trives, C.; Partearroyo, T.; Varela-Moreiras, G. Effects of Drugs and Excipients on Hydration Status. *Nutrients* **2019**, *11*. [CrossRef]
8. Wong, J.M.W.; Ebbeling, C.B.; Robinson, L.; Feldman, H.A.; Ludwig, D.S. Effects of Advice to Drink 8 Cups of Water per Day in Adolescents with Overweight or Obesity: A Randomized Clinical Trial. *JAMA Pediatr.* **2017**, *171*, e170012. [CrossRef]
9. Hooton, T.M.; Vecchio, M.; Iroz, A.; Tack, I.; Dornic, Q.; Seksek, I.; Lotan, Y. Effect of Increased Daily Water Intake in Premenopausal Women with Recurrent Urinary Tract Infections: A Randomized Clinical Trial. *JAMA Intern. Med.* **2018**, *178*, 1509–1515. [CrossRef]
10. Wittbrodt, M.T.; Millard-Stafford, M. Dehydration Impairs Cognitive Performance: A Meta-analysis. *Med. Sci. Sports Exerc.* **2018**, *50*, 2360–2368. [CrossRef]
11. Sawka, M.N.; Burke, L.M.; Eichner, E.R.; Maughan, R.J.; Montain, S.J.; Stachenfeld, N.S. American College of Sports Medicine position stand. Exercise and fluid replacement. *Med. Sci. Sports Exerc.* **2007**, *39*, 377–390. [PubMed]
12. Rowntree, L.G. Water Intoxication. *Arch. Intern. Med.* **1923**, *32*, 157–174. [CrossRef]

13. Hew-Butler, T.; Rosner, M.H.; Fowkes-Godek, S.; Dugas, J.P.; Hoffman, M.D.; Lewis, D.P.; Maughan, R.J.; Miller, K.C.; Montain, S.J.; Rehrer, N.J.; et al. Statement of the Third International Exercise-Associated Hyponatremia Consensus Development Conference, Carlsbad, California, 2015. *Clin. J. Sport Med.* **2015**, *25*, 303–320. [CrossRef] [PubMed]
14. Singh, S.; Padi, M.H.; Bullard, H.; Freeman, H. Water intoxication in psychiatric patients. *Br. J. Psychiatry* **1985**, *146*, 127–131. [CrossRef] [PubMed]
15. Sjoblom, E.; Hojer, J.; Ludwigs, U.; Pirskanen, R. Fatal hyponatraemic brain oedema due to common gastroenteritis with accidental water intoxication. *Intensive Care Med.* **1997**, *23*, 348–350. [CrossRef] [PubMed]
16. Sarvesvaran, R. Dilute the poison—A case of fatal water intoxication. *Med. Sci. Law* **1984**, *24*, 92–94. [CrossRef] [PubMed]
17. Helwig, F.C.; Schutz, C.B.; Curry, D.E. Water Intoxication: Report of a fatal human case with clinical, pathologic and experimental studies. *JAMA* **1935**, *104*, 1569–1575. [CrossRef]
18. Hawken, E.R.; Crookall, J.M.; Reddick, D.; Millson, R.C.; Milev, R.; Delva, N. Mortality over a 20-year period in patients with primary polydipsia associated with schizophrenia: A retrospective study. *Schizophr. Res.* **2009**, *107*, 128–133. [CrossRef]
19. Knepper, M.A.; Kwon, T.H.; Nielsen, S. Molecular physiology of water balance. *N. Engl. J. Med.* **2015**, *372*, 1349–1358. [CrossRef]
20. Bourque, C.W. Central mechanisms of osmosensation and systemic osmoregulation. *Nat. Rev. Neurosci.* **2008**, *9*, 519–531. [CrossRef]
21. Verbalis, J.G. Disorders of body water homeostasis. *Best Pract. Res. Clin. Endocrinol. Metab.* **2003**, *17*, 471–503. [CrossRef]
22. Sterns, R.H. Disorders of plasma sodium. *N. Engl. J. Med.* **2015**, *372*, 55–65. [CrossRef] [PubMed]
23. Beets, I.; Temmerman, L.; Janssen, T.; Schoofs, L. Ancient neuromodulation by vasopressin/oxytocin-related peptides. *Worm* **2013**, *2*, e24246. [CrossRef] [PubMed]
24. Knepper, M.A. Molecular physiology of urinary concentrating mechanism: Regulation of aquaporin water channels by vasopressin. *Am. J. Physiol.* **1997**, *272*, F3–F12. [CrossRef] [PubMed]
25. McKinley, M.J.; Cairns, M.J.; Denton, D.A.; Egan, G.; Mathai, M.L.; Uschakov, A.; Wade, J.D.; Weisinger, R.S.; Oldfield, B.J. Physiological and pathophysiological influences on thirst. *Physiol. Behav.* **2004**, *81*, 795–803. [CrossRef] [PubMed]
26. Figaro, M.K.; Mack, G.W. Regulation of fluid intake in dehydrated humans: Role of oropharyngeal stimulation. *Am. J. Physiol.* **1997**, *272*, R1740–R1746. [CrossRef] [PubMed]
27. Salata, R.A.; Verbalis, J.G.; Robinson, A.G. Cold water stimulation of oropharyngeal receptors in man inhibits release of vasopressin. *J. Clin. Endocrinol. Metab.* **1987**, *65*, 561–567. [CrossRef]
28. Seckl, J.R.; Williams, T.D.; Lightman, S.L. Oral hypertonic saline causes transient fall of vasopressin in humans. *Am. J. Physiol.* **1986**, *251*, R214–R217. [CrossRef]
29. Rolls, B.J.; Wood, R.J.; Rolls, E.T.; Lind, H.; Lind, W.; Ledingham, J.G. Thirst following water deprivation in humans. *Am. J. Physiol.* **1980**, *239*, R476–R482. [CrossRef]
30. Phillips, P.A.; Rolls, B.J.; Ledingham, J.G.; Forsling, M.L.; Morton, J.J. Osmotic thirst and vasopressin release in humans: A double-blind crossover study. *Am. J. Physiol.* **1985**, *248*, R645–R650. [CrossRef]
31. Costill, D.L.; Kammer, W.F.; Fisher, A. Fluid ingestion during distance running. *Arch. Environ. Health* **1970**, *21*, 520–525. [CrossRef] [PubMed]
32. Zimmerman, C.A.; Lin, Y.C.; Leib, D.E.; Guo, L.; Huey, E.L.; Daly, G.E.; Chen, Y.; Knight, Z.A. Thirst neurons anticipate the homeostatic consequences of eating and drinking. *Nature* **2016**, *537*, 680–684. [CrossRef] [PubMed]
33. Zimmerman, C.A.; Huey, E.L.; Ahn, J.S.; Beutler, L.R.; Tan, C.L.; Kosar, S.; Bai, L.; Chen, Y.; Corpuz, T.V.; Madisen, L.; et al. A gut-to-brain signal of fluid osmolarity controls thirst satiation. *Nature* **2019**, *568*, 98–102. [CrossRef] [PubMed]
34. Saker, P.; Farrell, M.J.; Egan, G.F.; McKinley, M.J.; Denton, D.A. Overdrinking, swallowing inhibition, and regional brain responses prior to swallowing. *Proc. Natl. Acad. Sci. USA* **2016**, *113*, 12274–12279. [CrossRef] [PubMed]
35. Saker, P.; Farrell, M.J.; Adib, F.R.; Egan, G.F.; McKinley, M.J.; Denton, D.A. Regional brain responses associated with drinking water during thirst and after its satiation. *Proc. Natl. Acad. Sci. USA* **2014**, *111*, 5379–5384. [CrossRef] [PubMed]

36. Saker, P.; Farrell, M.J.; Egan, G.F.; McKinley, M.J.; Denton, D.A. Influence of anterior midcingulate cortex on drinking behavior during thirst and following satiation. *Proc. Natl. Acad. Sci. USA* **2018**, *115*, 786–791. [CrossRef] [PubMed]
37. Clark, W.F.; Sontrop, J.M.; Huang, S.H.; Gallo, K.; Moist, L.; House, A.A.; Cuerden, M.S.; Weir, M.A.; Bagga, A.; Brimble, S.; et al. Effect of Coaching to Increase Water Intake on Kidney Function Decline in Adults with Chronic Kidney Disease: The CKD WIT Randomized Clinical Trial. *JAMA* **2018**, *319*, 1870–1879. [CrossRef]
38. Wall, S.M.; Han, J.S.; Chou, C.L.; Knepper, M.A. Kinetics of urea and water permeability activation by vasopressin in rat terminal IMCD. *Am. J. Physiol.* **1992**, *262*, F989–F998. [CrossRef]
39. Goldman, M.B.; Luchins, D.J.; Robertson, G.L. Mechanisms of altered water metabolism in psychotic patients with polydipsia and hyponatremia. *N. Engl. J. Med.* **1988**, *318*, 397–403. [CrossRef]
40. Chinn, T.A. Compulsive water drinking. A review of the literature and an additional case. *J. Nerv. Ment. Dis.* **1974**, *158*, 78–80. [CrossRef]
41. Saito, T.; Ishikawa, S.; Ito, T.; Oda, H.; Ando, F.; Higashiyama, M.; Nagasaka, S.; Hieda, M.; Saito, T. Urinary excretion of aquaporin-2 water channel differentiates psychogenic polydipsia from central diabetes insipidus. *J. Clin. Endocrinol. Metab.* **1999**, *84*, 2235–2237. [CrossRef] [PubMed]
42. Reale, R.; Slater, G.; Cox, G.R.; Dunican, I.C.; Burke, L.M. The Effect of Water Loading on Acute Weight Loss Following Fluid Restriction in Combat Sports Athletes. *Int. J. Sport Nutr. Exerc. Metab.* **2018**, *28*, 565–573. [CrossRef] [PubMed]
43. De Wardener, H.E.; Herxheimer, A. The effect of a high water intake on the kidney's ability to concentrate the urine in man. 1957. *J. Am. Soc. Nephrol.* **2000**, *11*, 980–987.
44. Epstein, F.H.; Kleeman, C.R.; Hendrikx, A. The influence of bodily hydration on the renal concentrating process. *J. Clin. Investig.* **1957**, *36*, 629–634. [CrossRef]
45. Hariprasad, M.K.; Eisinger, R.P.; Nadler, I.M.; Padmanabhan, C.S.; Nidus, B.D. Hyponatremia in psychogenic polydipsia. *Arch. Intern. Med.* **1980**, *140*, 1639–1642. [CrossRef] [PubMed]
46. Walls, L.L.; Supinski, C.R.; Cotton, W.K.; McFadden, J.W. Compulsive water drinking: A review with report of an additional case. *J. Fam. Pract.* **1977**, *5*, 531–533. [PubMed]
47. Barlow, E.D.; De Wardener, H.E. Compulsive water drinking. *Q. J. Med.* **1959**, *28*, 235–258. [PubMed]
48. Kishore, B.K.; Terris, J.M.; Knepper, M.A. Quantitation of aquaporin-2 abundance in microdissected collecting ducts: Axial distribution and control by AVP. *Am. J. Physiol.* **1996**, *271*, F62–F70. [CrossRef]
49. Nielsen, S.; DiGiovanni, S.R.; Christensen, E.I.; Knepper, M.A.; Harris, H.W. Cellular and subcellular immunolocalization of vasopressin-regulated water channel in rat kidney. *Proc. Natl. Acad. Sci. USA* **1993**, *90*, 11663–11667. [CrossRef]
50. Lankford, S.P.; Chou, C.L.; Terada, Y.; Wall, S.M.; Wade, J.B.; Knepper, M.A. Regulation of collecting duct water permeability independent of cAMP-mediated AVP response. *Am. J. Physiol.* **1991**, *261*, F554–F566. [CrossRef]
51. Terris, J.; Ecelbarger, C.A.; Nielsen, S.; Knepper, M.A. Long-term regulation of four renal aquaporins in rats. *Am. J. Physiol.* **1996**, *271*, F414–F422. [CrossRef] [PubMed]
52. Dundas, B.; Harris, M.; Narasimhan, M. Psychogenic polydipsia review: Etiology, differential, and treatment. *Curr. Psychiatry Rep.* **2007**, *9*, 236–241. [CrossRef] [PubMed]
53. Williams, S.T.; Kores, R.C. Psychogenic polydipsia: Comparison of a community sample with an institutionalized population. *Psychiatry Res.* **2011**, *187*, 310–311. [CrossRef] [PubMed]
54. Gillum, D.M.; Linas, S.L. Water intoxication in a psychotic patient with normal renal water excretion. *Am. J. Med.* **1984**, *77*, 773–774. [CrossRef]
55. Lee, S.; Chow, C.C.; Koo, L.C. Altered state of consciousness in a compulsive water drinker. *Br. J. Psychiatry* **1989**, *154*, 556–558. [CrossRef] [PubMed]
56. Sleeper, F.H.; Jellinek, E.M. A comparitive physiologic, psychologic, and psychiatric study of polyuric and non-polyuric schizophrenic patients. *J. Nerv. Ment. Dis.* **1936**, *83*, 557–563. [CrossRef]
57. Liska, D.; Mah, E.; Brisbois, T.; Barrios, P.L.; Baker, L.B.; Spriet, L.L. Narrative Review of Hydration and Selected Health Outcomes in the General Population. *Nutrients* **2019**, *11*. [CrossRef]
58. Clark-Flory, T. 'It Is Definitely Pee': The Ecstatic, Pedialyte-Fueled Art of Performing Squirting in Porn. *Jezebel* 14 February 2019. Available online: https://jezebel.com/it-is-definitely-pee-the-ecstatic-pedialyte-fueled-ar-1832543103 (accessed on 28 May 2019).

59. Statista. Sales of the Leading Bottled Still Water Brands in the United States in 2018 (in Million U.S. Dollars). Available online: https://www.statista.com/statistics/188312/top-bottled-still-water-brands-in-the-united-states/ (accessed on 28 May 2019).
60. Maroz, N.; Maroz, U.; Iqbal, S.; Aiyer, R.; Kambhampati, G.; Ejaz, A.A. Nonobstructive hydronephrosis due to social polydipsia: A case report. *J. Med. Case Rep.* **2012**, *6*, 376. [CrossRef]
61. European Food Safety Authority (EFSA). Dietary reference values for nutrients: Summary report. *EFSA Support. Publ.* **2017**, *2017*, e15121. [CrossRef]
62. McDermott, B.P.; Anderson, S.A.; Armstrong, L.E.; Casa, D.J.; Cheuvront, S.N.; Cooper, L.; Kenney, W.L.; O'Connor, F.G.; Roberts, W.O. National Athletic Trainers' Association Position Statement: Fluid Replacement for the Physically Active. *J. Athl. Train.* **2017**, *52*, 877–895. [CrossRef]
63. Hew, T.D.; Chorley, J.N.; Cianca, J.C.; Divine, J.G. The incidence, risk factors, and clinical manifestations of hyponatremia in marathon runners. *Clin. J. Sport Med.* **2003**, *13*, 41–47. [CrossRef] [PubMed]
64. Ayus, J.C.; Varon, J.; Arieff, A.I. Hyponatremia, cerebral edema, and noncardiogenic pulmonary edema in marathon runners. *Ann. Intern. Med.* **2000**, *132*, 711–714. [CrossRef]
65. Noakes, T.D.; Sharwood, K.; Speedy, D.; Hew, T.; Reid, S.; Dugas, J.; Almond, C.; Wharam, P.; Weschler, L. Three independent biological mechanisms cause exercise-associated hyponatremia: Evidence from 2135 weighed competitive athletic performances. *Proc. Natl. Acad. Sci. USA* **2005**, *102*, 18550–18555. [CrossRef]
66. Johnson, E.C.; Munoz, C.X.; Jimenez, L.; Le, B.L.; Kupchak, B.R.; Kraemer, W.J.; Casa, D.J.; Maresh, C.M.; Armstrong, L.E. Hormonal and Thirst Modulated Maintenance of Fluid Balance in Young Women with Different Levels of Habitual Fluid Consumption. *Nutrients* **2016**, *8*. [CrossRef] [PubMed]
67. Krishnan, V.; Han, M.H.; Graham, D.L.; Berton, O.; Renthal, W.; Russo, S.J.; Laplant, Q.; Graham, A.; Lutter, M.; Lagace, D.C.; et al. Molecular adaptations underlying susceptibility and resistance to social defeat in brain reward regions. *Cell* **2007**, *131*, 391–404. [CrossRef]
68. Goto, T.; Kubota, Y.; Tanaka, Y.; Iio, W.; Moriya, N.; Toyoda, A. Subchronic and mild social defeat stress accelerates food intake and body weight gain with polydipsia-like features in mice. *Behav. Brain Res.* **2014**, *270*, 339–348. [CrossRef] [PubMed]
69. Hawken, E.R.; Delva, N.J.; Beninger, R.J. Increased drinking following social isolation rearing: Implications for polydipsia associated with schizophrenia. *PLoS ONE* **2013**, *8*, e56105. [CrossRef] [PubMed]
70. Gross, M.; Pinhasov, A. Chronic mild stress in submissive mice: Marked polydipsia and social avoidance without hedonic deficit in the sucrose preference test. *Behav. Brain Res.* **2016**, *298*, 25–34. [CrossRef] [PubMed]
71. Goldstein, M.; Deutch, A.Y. Dopaminergic mechanisms in the pathogenesis of schizophrenia. *FASEB J.* **1992**, *6*, 2413–2421. [CrossRef] [PubMed]
72. Martin-Gonzalez, E.; Prados-Pardo, A.; Mora, S.; Flores, P.; Moreno, M. Do psychoactive drugs have a therapeutic role in compulsivity? Studies on schedule-induced polydipsia. *Psychopharmacology (Berl)* **2018**, *235*, 419–432. [CrossRef] [PubMed]
73. Brvar, M.; Kozelj, G.; Osredkar, J.; Mozina, M.; Gricar, M.; Bunc, M. Polydipsia as another mechanism of hyponatremia after 'ecstasy' (3,4 methyldioxymethamphetamine) ingestion. *Eur. J. Emerg. Med.* **2004**, *11*, 302–304. [CrossRef] [PubMed]
74. Tsai, S.J. Dopamine receptor downregulation: An alternative strategy for schizophrenia treatment. *Med. Hypotheses* **2004**, *63*, 1047–1050. [CrossRef] [PubMed]
75. Falhammar, H.; Lindh, J.D.; Calissendorff, J.; Skov, J.; Nathanson, D.; Mannheimer, B. Antipsychotics and severe hyponatremia: A Swedish population-based case-control study. *Eur. J. Intern. Med.* **2019**, *60*, 71–77. [CrossRef] [PubMed]
76. Leth-Moller, K.B.; Hansen, A.H.; Torstensson, M.; Andersen, S.E.; Odum, L.; Gislasson, G.; Torp-Pedersen, C.; Holm, E.A. Antidepressants and the risk of hyponatremia: A Danish register-based population study. *BMJ Open* **2016**, *6*, e011200. [CrossRef] [PubMed]
77. Goldman, M.B. Brain circuit dysfunction in a distinct subset of chronic psychotic patients. *Schizophr. Res.* **2014**, *157*, 204–213. [CrossRef] [PubMed]
78. Forrer, G.R. Effect of oral activity on hallucinations. *AMA Arch. Gen. Psychiatry* **1960**, *2*, 100–103. [CrossRef] [PubMed]
79. Yonemura, K.; Hishida, A.; Miyajima, H.; Tawarahara, K.; Mizoguchi, K.; Nishimura, Y.; Ohishi, K. Water intoxication due to excessive water intake: Observation of initiation stage. *Jpn. J. Med.* **1987**, *26*, 249–252. [CrossRef] [PubMed]

80. Godek, S.F.; Bartolozzi, A.R.; Godek, J.J. Sweat rate and fluid turnover in American football players compared with runners in a hot and humid environment. *Br. J. Sports Med.* **2005**, *39*, 205–211. [CrossRef]
81. Hew-Butler, T.; Loi, V.; Pani, A.; Rosner, M.H. Exercise-Associated Hyponatremia: 2017 Update. *Front. Med. (Lausanne)* **2017**, *4*, 21. [CrossRef]
82. Hew-Butler, T. Arginine vasopressin, fluid balance and exercise: Is exercise-associated hyponatraemia a disorder of arginine vasopressin secretion? *Sports Med.* **2010**, *40*, 459–479. [CrossRef]
83. Thompson, C.J.; Edwards, C.R.; Baylis, P.H. Osmotic and non-osmotic regulation of thirst and vasopressin secretion in patients with compulsive water drinking. *Clin. Endocrinol. (Oxf.)* **1991**, *35*, 221–228. [CrossRef] [PubMed]
84. Blum, A.; Friedland, G.W. Urinary tract abnormalities due to chronic psychogenic polydipsia. *Am. J. Psychiatry* **1983**, *140*, 915–916. [PubMed]
85. Himeno, Y.; Ishibe, T. Bilaterally dilated upper urinary tract and bladder induced by diabetes insipidus. *Int. Urol. Nephrol.* **1990**, *22*, 129–132. [CrossRef] [PubMed]
86. Streitz, J.M., Jr.; Streitz, J.M. Polyuric urinary tract dilatation with renal damage. *J. Urol.* **1988**, *139*, 784–785. [CrossRef]
87. Zender, H.O.; Ruedin, P.; Moser, F.; Bolle, J.F.; Leski, M. Traumatic rupture of the urinary tract in a patient presenting nephrogenic diabetes insipidus associated with hydronephrosis and chronic renal failure: Case report and review of the literature. *Clin. Nephrol.* **1992**, *38*, 196–202. [PubMed]
88. Friedland, G.W.; Axman, M.M.; Russi, M.F.; Fair, W.R. Renal back pressure atrophy with compromised renal function due to diabetes insipidus. Case report. *Radiology* **1971**, *98*, 359–360. [CrossRef] [PubMed]
89. Sailer, C.; Winzeler, B.; Christ-Crain, M. Primary polydipsia in the medical and psychiatric patient: Characteristics, complications and therapy. *Swiss Med. Wkly.* **2017**, *147*, w14514.
90. Ferraro, P.M.; Vittori, M.; Macis, G.; D'Addessi, A.; Lombardi, G.; Palmisano, C.; Gervasoni, J.; Primiano, A.; Bassi, P.F.; Gambaro, G. Changes in renal papillary density after hydration therapy in calcium stone formers. *BMC Urol.* **2018**, *18*, 101. [CrossRef]
91. Clark, W.F.; Kortas, C.; Suri, R.S.; Moist, L.M.; Salvadori, M.; Weir, M.A.; Garg, A.X. Excessive fluid intake as a novel cause of proteinuria. *CMAJ* **2008**, *178*, 173–175. [CrossRef]
92. Hebert, L.A.; Greene, T.; Levey, A.; Falkenhain, M.E.; Klahr, S. High urine volume and low urine osmolality are risk factors for faster progression of renal disease. *Am. J. Kidney Dis.* **2003**, *41*, 962–971. [CrossRef]
93. Boilesen, S.N.; Tahan, S.; Dias, F.C.; Melli, L.; de Morais, M.B. Water and fluid intake in the prevention and treatment of functional constipation in children and adolescents: Is there evidence? *J. Pediatr. (Rio J.)* **2017**, *93*, 320–327. [CrossRef] [PubMed]
94. Dennis, E.A.; Dengo, A.L.; Comber, D.L.; Flack, K.D.; Savla, J.; Davy, K.P.; Davy, B.M. Water consumption increases weight loss during a hypocaloric diet intervention in middle-aged and older adults. *Obesity (Silver Spring)* **2010**, *18*, 300–307. [CrossRef] [PubMed]
95. Parretti, H.M.; Aveyard, P.; Blannin, A.; Clifford, S.J.; Coleman, S.J.; Roalfe, A.; Daley, A.J. Efficacy of water preloading before main meals as a strategy for weight loss in primary care patients with obesity: RCT. *Obesity (Silver Spring)* **2015**, *23*, 1785–1791. [CrossRef] [PubMed]
96. Vij, V.A.; Joshi, A.S. Effect of excessive water intake on body weight, body mass index, body fat, and appetite of overweight female participants. *J. Nat. Sci. Biol. Med.* **2014**, *5*, 340–344. [CrossRef] [PubMed]
97. Davy, B.M.; Dennis, E.A.; Dengo, A.L.; Wilson, K.L.; Davy, K.P. Water consumption reduces energy intake at a breakfast meal in obese older adults. *J. Am. Diet. Assoc.* **2008**, *108*, 1236–1239. [CrossRef] [PubMed]
98. Van Walleghen, E.L.; Orr, J.S.; Gentile, C.L.; Davy, B.M. Pre-meal water consumption reduces meal energy intake in older but not younger subjects. *Obesity (Silver Spring)* **2007**, *15*, 93–99. [CrossRef] [PubMed]
99. Berry, E.M.; Halon, D.; Fainaru, M. Iatrogenic polydipsia. *Lancet* **1977**, *2*, 937–938. [CrossRef]
100. Pickering, L.K.; Hogan, G.R. Voluntary water intoxication in a normal child. *J. Pediatr.* **1971**, *78*, 316–318. [CrossRef]
101. Lee, L.C.; Noronha, M. When plenty is too much: Water intoxication in a patient with a simple urinary tract infection. *BMJ Case Rep.* **2016**, *2016*. [CrossRef]
102. Swanson, A.G.; Iseri, O.A. Acute encephalopathy due to water intoxication. *N. Engl. J. Med.* **1958**, *258*, 831–834. [CrossRef]
103. Verbalis, J.G. Pathogenesis of hyponatremia in an experimental model of the syndrome of inappropriate antidiuresis. *Am. J. Physiol.* **1994**, *267*, R1617–R1625. [CrossRef] [PubMed]

104. Kawahara, N.; Ofuji, S.; Abe, S.; Tanaka, A.; Uematsu, M.; Ogata, Y. Water intoxication in adult cattle. *Jpn. J. Vet. Res.* **2016**, *64*, 159–164. [PubMed]
105. Ueda, Y.; Hopper, K.; Epstein, S.E. Incidence, Severity and Prognosis Associated with Hyponatremia in Dogs and Cats. *J. Vet. Intern. Med.* **2015**, *29*, 801–807. [CrossRef]
106. Johnson, P.; Waldreus, N.; Hahn, R.G.; Stenstrom, H.; Sjostrand, F. Fluid retention index predicts the 30-day mortality in geriatric care. *Scand. J. Clin. Lab. Investig.* **2015**, *75*, 444–451. [CrossRef] [PubMed]
107. Alobaidi, R.; Morgan, C.; Basu, R.K.; Stenson, E.; Featherstone, R.; Majumdar, S.R.; Bagshaw, S.M. Association Between Fluid Balance and Outcomes in Critically Ill Children: A Systematic Review and Meta-analysis. *JAMA Pediatr.* **2018**, *172*, 257–268. [CrossRef] [PubMed]
108. Dekker, M.J.E.; Konings, C.; Canaud, B.; van der Sande, F.M.; Stuard, S.; Raimann, J.G.; Ozturk, E.; Usvyat, L.; Kotanko, P.; Kooman, J.P. Interactions Between Malnutrition, Inflammation, and Fluid Overload and Their Associations with Survival in Prevalent Hemodialysis Patients. *J. Ren. Nutr.* **2018**, *28*, 435–444. [CrossRef] [PubMed]
109. Dekker, M.J.E.; van der Sande, F.M.; van den Berghe, F.; Leunissen, K.M.L.; Kooman, J.P. Fluid Overload and Inflammation Axis. *Blood Purif.* **2018**, *45*, 159–165. [CrossRef] [PubMed]
110. Hoorn, E.J.; Zietse, R. Hyponatremia and Mortality: How Innocent is the Bystander? *Clin. J. Am. Soc. Nephrol.* **2011**, *6*, 951–953. [CrossRef]

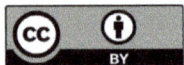

© 2019 by the authors. Licensee MDPI, Basel, Switzerland. This article is an open access article distributed under the terms and conditions of the Creative Commons Attribution (CC BY) license (http://creativecommons.org/licenses/by/4.0/).

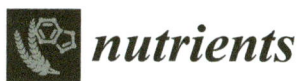

Review

Water Intake, Water Balance, and the Elusive Daily Water Requirement

Lawrence E. Armstrong [1] and Evan C. Johnson [2,*]

1. University of Connecticut, Human Performance Laboratory and Department of Nutritional Sciences, Storrs CT 06269-1110, USA; lawrence.armstrong@uconn.edu
2. University of Wyoming, Human Integrated Physiology Laboratory, Division of Kinesiology and Health, Laramie, WY 82071, USA
* Correspondence: evan.johnson@uwyo.edu; Tel: +307-766-5282

Received: 13 October 2018; Accepted: 27 November 2018; Published: 5 December 2018

Abstract: Water is essential for metabolism, substrate transport across membranes, cellular homeostasis, temperature regulation, and circulatory function. Although nutritional and physiological research teams and professional organizations have described the daily total water intakes (TWI, L/24h) and Adequate Intakes (AI) of children, women, and men, there is no widespread consensus regarding the human water requirements of different demographic groups. These requirements remain undefined because of the dynamic complexity inherent in the human water regulatory network, which involves the central nervous system and several organ systems, as well as large inter-individual differences. The present review analyzes published evidence that is relevant to these issues and presents a novel approach to assessing the daily water requirements of individuals in all sex and life-stage groups, as an alternative to AI values based on survey data. This empirical method focuses on the intensity of a specific neuroendocrine response (e.g., plasma arginine vasopressin (AVP) concentration) employed by the brain to regulate total body water volume and concentration. We consider this autonomically-controlled neuroendocrine response to be an inherent hydration biomarker and one means by which the brain maintains good health and optimal function. We also propose that this individualized method defines the elusive state of euhydration (i.e., water balance) and distinguishes it from hypohydration. Using plasma AVP concentration to analyze multiple published data sets that included both men and women, we determined that a mild neuroendocrine defense of body water commences when TWI is <1.8 L/24h, that 19–71% of adults in various countries consume less than this TWI each day, and consuming less than the 24-h water AI may influence the risk of dysfunctional metabolism and chronic diseases.

Keywords: water-electrolyte balance; drinking water; body water; water restriction

1. Introduction

Individuals with a normal P_{OSM} (e.g., 285–295 mOsm/kg) may be considered to be normally hydrated without regard to daily total water intake (TWI; [1]) or urinary biomarkers [2] because the brain actively regulates both total body water volume (within 0.5% day-to-day; [3]) and blood concentration (within a normal P_{OSM} range of 285–295 mOsm/kg; [4]) across a wide range of TWI (women, 1.3–6.1; men, 1.7–7.9 L/24h; [5,6]). Thus, an individual with suboptimal water intake may be evaluated to be euhydrated due to the defense of P_{OSM} through reduced urine production and other compensatory responses. However, there is no widespread consensus regarding a definition of euhydration. For example, the 2004 U.S. National Academy of Medicine (NAM) publication, which presented dietary reference intakes for water [6], included a lengthy review of water balance studies and water needs (i.e., using the stable isotope of water D_2O) of children and adults (Table 1). However, this report concluded that: (a) individual water requirements can vary greatly on a day-to-day basis because of differences in physical activity, climates, and dietary contents; and (b) there is no single daily water requirement for a given person. As a result, Adequate Intake (AI) volumes for water (i.e., which are not daily water requirements) were developed from median TWI values in the NHANES III survey database [5]. The 2010 European Food Safety Authority (EFSA) panel utilized a different approach when developing dietary reference intakes [7]. Water AI values for various life-stage groups (Table 1) were derived from three factors: observed intakes of European population groups, desirable urine osmolality values, and desirable TWI volumes per unit of dietary energy (Kcal) consumed. Similar to the NAM report (above), however, the EFSA report stated that a single water intake cannot meet the needs of everyone in any population group because the individual need for water is related to caloric consumption, the concentrating-diluting capacities of the kidneys, and water losses via excretion and secretion. This report defined the minimum water requirement in general terms as the amount of water that equals water losses and prevents adverse effects of insufficient water such as dehydration.

Table 1. Comparison of recommended Adequate Intakes [a] for water, published by European and American health organizations.

Life Stage & Sex	Age	European Food Safety Authority, Parma, Italy [b] 2010 (ml/day)	National Academy of Medicine, USA 2004 [b] (ml/day)
Infants	0–6 months	680 via milk	700
	6–12 months	800–1,000	800
Children	1–2 years	1100-1200	1300
	2–3 years	1300	
	4–8 years	1600	1700
	9–13 years, boys	2100	2400
	9–13 years, girls	1900	2100
	14–18 years, boys	2500	3300
	14–18 years, girls	2000	2300
Adults			
Men		2500	3700
Women		2000	2700
Pregnant Women	≥ 19 year	2300	3000
Lactating Women	≥ 19 year	2600–2700	3800
Elderly		same as adults	same as adults

[a] Adequate Intakes represent an amount that should meet the needs of almost everyone in a specific life-stage group who is healthy, consumes an average diet, and performs moderate levels of physical activity [6,7]; [b], values refer to total water intake (TWI = plain water + beverages + food moisture).

Neither the NAM nor the EFSA document presented a method to assess the human water requirement of individuals, or (b) neuroendocrine data to support daily AI values for water. However, it is widely accepted that the brain constantly acts to preserve homeostasis via neuroendocrine responses which defend set points of body water volume and concentration [8]. In contrast to the methods used in the NAM and EFSA reports, we propose that minimal/baseline fluid-electrolyte regulatory responses by the brain signal body water balance (i.e., euhydration), and that increased neuroendocrine responses (e.g., plasma AVP levels) represent the threshold at which the brain begins to defend body water volume and concentration (i.e., hypohydration). This is important because no measurement or biomarker has previously been proposed to define a state of euhydration (i.e., often defined loosely as normal total body water or water balance). Furthermore, we propose that neuroendocrine thresholds, in conjunction with TWI measurements, can reveal the water intake requirement of individuals in a specific life-stage group when the turnover of body water (e.g., intake versus loss) is relatively constant (i.e., no large activity-induced sweat loss), an average diet is consumed, and ample water is available to support *ad libitum* drinking. Sedentary adults whose free-living daily activities include working in an air-conditioned office and consuming a typical Western diet represent an example of such a group. We propose this individualized physiological measurement of neuroendocrine responses as a methodological alternative to AI values (Table 1).

Thus, the primary purpose of the present manuscript is not to modify current AIs but rather to provide novel additional perspectives regarding 24-h TWI, euhydration, and human water requirements. We have analyzed the relationship between 24-h TWI values and their corresponding plasma AVP levels from multiple research studies, and identified a plasma AVP concentration that approximates the neuroendocrine response threshold for water regulation in free-living adults. Interestingly, this AVP threshold is exceeded when 24-h TWI is <1.8 L/24h. The second purpose of the present manuscript is to increase awareness of the importance of daily water intake, because a considerable percentage of individuals in industrialized countries consume less than the 24-h water AI that is recommended for their life stage. Evidence for this purpose exists in a growing body of recent epidemiological studies that report statistically significant relationships between chronic low daily water consumption and disease states or metabolic dysfunction.

Because methods and terminology vary across publications, we emphasize the following important definitions. The term *water in beverages* refers to water + water in all other fluids (e.g., juice, tea, coffee, milk). The term *total water intake* refers to water + water in beverages + food moisture (e.g., fruit, soup). Distinct from the term *dehydration* (i.e., the process of losing water), the term *hypohydration* is presently defined as a steady-state condition of reduced total body water.

2. Representative Research Evidence

As shown in Table 2, a variety of methods and theoretical approaches have influenced our present understanding and theories regarding human water intake, euhydration, hypohydration, and water requirements. The range of measured or calculated variables includes dietary macronutrients, 24-h TWI (defined above), biomarkers of hydration status, water volumes (i.e., consumed, metabolized, excreted, turnover), and fluid-electrolyte regulating hormones. Not all these methods (column 1, Table 2) have contributed in meaningful ways to organizational recommendations regarding the daily water intake required for good health (Table 1). For example, the NAM recommendations [6] include consideration of large non-renal water losses via sweating, during labor or physical activity. This is a primary reason why 24-h TWI recommendations from European and U.S. organizations differ by 1.1–1.3 L/24h, in specific life stage and sex categories (Table 1). Table 3 describes eight components of 24-h water balance, shown as the headings for columns 2-9. All these components interact with each other in a network that includes the central nervous system (CNS), oropharyngeal region, gastrointestinal tract, kidneys, neuroendocrine system, cardiovascular system, skin, and respiratory organs; feedback from one organ system affects all others, directly and/or indirectly. The components of 24-h water balance in Table 3 have contributed to international recommendations regarding the daily water intake required for good health (Table 1). For example, the NAM recommendations [6] assimilated all water balance components in Table 3, and the recommendations of the EFSA (2010) [7] emphasized both desirable urine osmolality values and the observed TWI of specific groups.

A review of the hundreds of publications that contributed to our understanding of human water intake, euhydration, hypohydration, and water requirements is beyond the scope of this manuscript. However, the mean values (Table 3), measured variables, and reference citations (Tables 2 and 3), although not exhaustive, represent the nature and types of meaningful available evidence regarding human water needs.

Table 2. Investigational and theoretical approaches to assess human water intake, euhydration, hypohydration, and water requirements.

Methods	Variables Measured or Calculated	Relevance - Individuals	Relevance - Group	Critique	Representative Publications
Partitioning 24-h urine production into minimum urine volume [a] and free urine volume [b]	U_{VOL}, U_{MAX}, U_{VM}, U_{FUV}	X		U_{MAX} is determined via observations of a few males and was applied to individuals. U_{MAX} varies with age and had a large inter-subject variability.	[9]
Calculation of free water reserve [c] to determine individual 24-hour hydration status [d]	U_{VOL}, U_{MAX}, U_{VM}, U_{FWR}, U_{OSM}, U_{TOT}, NRWL		X	This population-based method updates the concepts of Gamble (above), does not determine the U_{MAX} of individuals, and estimates NRWL. In single (<24h) samples, confounding factors [e] may dominate and other hydration biomarkers are preferred.	[10–12]
Dietary recall to determine TWI	plain water, beverages, food moisture	X	X	Data are specific to the subject sample, and typically do not provide information regarding water balance or turnover.	[13–15]
Responses and hydration biomarkers of free-living LD [f] versus HD [f]	U_{OSM}, U_{SG}, U_{COL}, U_{VOL}, P_{OSM}, S_{OSM}, M_B		X	Studies assess the responses of adult groups who have habitually different TWIs.	[13,16–20]
Global, regional, and country water consumption recommendations	TWI (L/24 h)		X	Adequate intakes [g] for TWI are based on survey data median values.	[6,7,21]
Statistical categories of hydration status for free-living adults	U_{OSM}, U_{SG}, U_{COL}, U_{VOL}, P_{OSM}, M_B	X		Seven categories range from euhydrated to hypohydrated or hyperhydrated. Variables are expressed per single sample and 24-h collection.	[22,23]
Laboratory water turnover and movement, using the DLW technique or stable isotope of water [h]	$^2H_2^{18}O$, ^2H_2O, TBW, U_{VOL}, NRWL	X		Mean water turnover (L/24h) incorporates estimates of TWI, metabolic, transcutaneous, and inspired air water.	[22,24,25]
Water balance of free-living adults during daily activities	TBW, TWI, U_{OSM}, U_{VOL}, P_{OSM}, TPP, HCT, SR, M_B	X	X	Various methods are used to describe the water needs of specific life stage and sex groups.	[2,25,26]
Laboratory controlled experiments evaluating dehydration and rehydration	U_{OSM}, U_{SG}, U_{COL}, U_{VOL}, P_{OSM}, S_{OSM}, M_B,%ΔPV	X		Dehydration is accomplished via passive exposure to a hot environment, exercise, or water restriction. Rehydration is accomplished via water and beverage intake or intravenous fluid administration.	[27–32]
Laboratory investigations that focus on thirst sensations and drinking behavior	TWI, beverages, U_{OSM}, U_{VOL}, P_{OSM},%ΔPV, AVP	X			[33–35]
Laboratory comparison of beverages: rehydration efficacy	FC, U_{VOL}, BHI	X		Common beverages are evaluated to identify retention (relative to still water) in euhydrated, but not dehydrated, adults. The diuretic response is influenced by fluid characteristics including osmolality, energy density, and electrolyte content.	[36,37]
Plasma AVP or copeptin [i] responses	AVP, copeptin [i]		X	The hormone AVP maintains U_{VOL}, P_{OSM}, and body water balance within narrow limits, in conjunction with thirst.	[13,16,19,31]
Assessment of specific urine and plasma hydration biomarkers	U_{OSM}, U_{COL}, P_{OSM}, P_{OSM}:U_{SM} ratio	X	X	Most studies focus on the assessment of simple, practical hydration biomarkers for use during daily activities.	[16,18,38–41]
Field studies of hydration status during labor, exercise, or competition	TWI, SR, P_{OSM}, U_{OSM}, U_{SG}, U_{COL}, M_B	X		Research attempts to optimize health and performance.	[42–45]
Statistical and graphical determination of the probability of dehydration	P_{OSM}, U_{SG}, M_B		X	Predictions are based on a modest dehydration range (−2.1 to −3.5% M_B) in 6 men and 5 women.	[46]

Table 2. Cont.

Methods	Variables Measured or Calculated	Relevance Individuals	Relevance Group	Critique	Representative Publications
Calculated biological variation and diagnostic accuracy of dehydration biomarkers	P_{OSM}, S_{OSM}, U_{OSM}, U_{SG}, U_{COL}, M_B		X	Statistics evaluate biomarkers, on the basis of a functionally important range of -2.0 to -7.0% M_B, induced in 5 women and 13 men across × hours.	[47]
Theoretical consideration of intracellular and extracellular dehydration	P_{Na+}, P_{OSM}, S_{OSM}, U_{OSM}, U_{SG}, U_{COL}, M_B	X		Candidate biomarkers of dehydration must consider intracellular, extracellular, and mixed dehydration stimuli.	[48]

[a], minimum urine volume corresponds to the urine volume necessary to excrete urine solutes at maximum urine osmolality (defined as 1400 mOsm/kg); [b], free urine volume is a precursor to the modern concept of free water reserve (see Table 1); [c], free water reserve is calculated statistically as the virtual water volume that could be additionally reabsorbed at maximum osmolality, in all but 2% to 3% of healthy subjects at a specific life stage and sex; [d], collection of a 24-h urine sample, determination of urine volume and osmolality, and calculation of obligatory and free water volumes allow for the determination of individual 24-h hydration status, determined using statistical confidence intervals (Manz and Wentz, 2005 [11]); [e], e.g., meal timing and contents, physical activity; [f], LD and HD were defined slightly differently in each study (LD range, 1.0–1.6; HD range, 2.4–3.3 L/24h); [g], adequate water intake is not a requirement, but rather the TWI that meets the needs of almost everyone in a specific life stage and sex group, to prevent deleterious effects of dehydration (i.e., metabolic and functional abnormalities); [h], the DLW method is theoretically based on the differential turnover kinetics of the stable isotopes of oxygen (^{18}O) and hydrogen (^2H). After drinking a known mass of DLW ($^2H_2^{18}O$), ^2H is eliminated from body water as H_2O whereas ^{18}O is eliminated as H_2O and CO_2 (Racette et al., 1994 [49]). The accumulation of a stable isotope of water (^2H_2O) in plasma, saliva, urine, or sweat determines the rate of water movement throughout the body. [i], AVP is difficult to measure because of its brief half-life, whereas plasma copeptin is relatively stable and its concentration is strongly correlated to that of AVP. Abbreviations: AI, adequate intake; AVP, arginine vasopressin; DLW, doubly labeled water; HCT, hematocrit; HD, individuals who habitually consume a high daily water volume; LD, individuals who habitually consume a low daily water volume; M_B, body mass; NRWL, non-renal water loss as eccrine sweat, transdermal, respiratory and stool water; S_{OSM}, salivary osmolality; SR, sweat rate measured as M_B change; TBW, total body water; TWI, total water intake = (plain water + water in beverages + food moisture); T_{OSM}, tear osmolality; FC, fluid consumed during a defined time period; BHI, beverage hydration index, relative to water;%ΔPV, percent change of plasma volume; TPP, total plasma protein; U_{COL}, urine color [50]; U_{FUV}, free urine volume; U_{FWR}, free water reserve; U_{OSM}, urine osmolality; U_{TOT}, total excreted osmolar load; U_{SG}, urine specific gravity; U_{VM}, minimal urine volume; U_{VOL}, urine volume; U_{MAX}, maximal urine osmolality produced by the kidneys.;

Table 3. Dietary, physiological, metabolic, and behavioral components of human 24-h water balance.

	Total water intake [a] (L/24h)	Intracellular metabolic water production [b]	Total solute load [c] (mOsm/24h)	Urine osmolality [d] (mOsm/kg)	Maximal renal concentrating ability (mOsm/kg)	Urine volume (L/24h)	Non-renal water loss (L/24h) [e]	Free water reserve [f] (L/24h)
Functions and characteristics	Contributes to TBW	Product of human metabolism	Metabolized and digested products excreted in urine	Regulates TBW and ECV-ICV osmolality	Inherent quality of the kidneys	Regulates TBW and ECV-ICV osmolality	Excretory and secretory processes	Calculated index of euhydration, based on population statistics
Influential factors	Meal timing and contents, idiosyncratic thirst, physical activity, body size, cultural and learned preferences	Metabolic rate and substrates, physical activity, diet macronutrient and energy content, NES responses	Metabolic products, dietary contents, body size, idiosyncratic hunger, learned food preferences	TWI, MRCA, solute load, NRWL, physical activity, NES responses	Life-stage group, male or female sex	TWI, total solute load, NRWL, physical activity, NES responses	Diet, ventilatory rate, physical activity, body size	TWI, total solute load, NRWL, physical activity
Organs involved	GI, CNS, NES, mouth and throat	CNS, NES	GI, CNS, NES	Kidneys, CNS, NES	Kidneys, CNS, NES	GI, kidneys, CNS, NES	Skin, GI, respiratory organs	GI, kidneys, CNS, NES
Conscious or behavioral influence?	Yes, habitual 24-h water intake	No	Yes, solid food consumption	Yes, secondary to TWI and food contents	No	Yes, secondary to TWI and food contents	Yes, eccrine sweat loss during labor or exercise	Yes, secondary to water and food intake
Representative mean, median, or range of values for sedentary adults	♀, 1.8–2.0 and ♂, 1.9–2.4 (FR, UK); ♀&♂, 1.5–2.5 (13countries); ♀, 2.3 (range: 0.8–4.5) (USA); ♂, 3.0 (range: 1.4–7.7) and ♀, 2.5 (range: 1.2–4.6) (USA); ♀, 1.9 and ♂, 2.3 (GE); ♀&♂, 0.2–3.9 (FR) L/24h	♀, 0.2–0.3; ♂, 0.3–0.4; ♂, 0.4 L/24h	♀, 669–781 and ♂, 915–992 (GE); ♂, 951 (USA); ♀&♂, 362–1365 (4 countries); ♂, 750 (USA); ♀, 752 and ♂, 941 (GE) mOsm/24h	♀&♂, 120–1250 (FR); ♀&♂, 555 (UK) mOsm/kg	♀&♂, 1430 (UK) mOsm/kg; ♀&♂ range, 1100–1300 (GE); ♀&♂, 1010–1330 (USA)	♀&♂, 0.2–3.9 (FR); ♀&♂, 1.9 (n = 8, UK) L/24h	♂, 0.3–0.4 (UK); ♀, 0.5–0.7 and ♂, 0.7–1.3 (GE) L/24h	♀, 0.4–0.5 and ♂, 0.2–0.3 (GE); ♀, 0.5 and ♂, 0.3 (GE) L/24h
Reference citations	[1,11,14,15,25,38,51]	[25,52,53]	[1,11,12,41]	[38,54]	[1,54,55]	[38,54]	[1,24]	[1]

[a], TWI, total water intake = (plain water + water in beverages + food moisture); [b], water generated during substrate oxidation; [c], greatly influenced by diet composition; [d], in a 24-h sample; [e], NRWL includes eccrine sweat, transdermal, respiratory and stool water losses; [f], FWR = (24-h urine volume, L/day) − (obligatory urine volume, L/day). The latter term is the water volume necessary to excrete the 24-h solute load, hypothetically calculated as (830 mOsm/kg) − (3–4 mOsm/kg per year > 20 years of age) [1]. Hydration status is inadequate if FWR is negative. Abbreviations: TBW, total body water; NES, neuroendocrine system (central nervous system + hormones); ECV, extracellular volume; ICV, intracellular volume; MRCA, maximal renal concentrating ability; CNS, central nervous system (brain + spinal cord); GI, gastrointestinal organs; GE, Germany; FR, France; USA, United States of America.

3. Why are Human Water Requirements Elusive?

To maintain normal physiological functions (e.g.., blood pressure, pH, internal body temperature) and optimal health, and to deliver essential substances (e.g., oxygen, water, glucose, sodium, potassium) to cells, the CNS and neuroendocrine hormones act constantly to preserve internal homeostasis via a complex network of many organ and neural systems. Figure 1 presents several CNS-regulated variables which are relevant to body water balance. Each of these variables is simultaneously: (a) maintained (i.e., within the circulatory system or fluid compartments of the body) at a specific set point (e.g., a threshold beyond which the intensity of neuroendocrine responses increases); and (b) constantly changing throughout the human life span in response to water and food intake, urine production, and non-renal water losses. Because of these fluctuations, human body water regulation is also dynamic. Therefore, we utilize the phrase dynamic complexity to refer to a constantly changing, vastly integrated regulatory mechanism [56]. This dynamic complexity is amplified by interconnected fluid compartments (i.e., intracellular, interstitial, extracellular, circulatory), organ systems (Table 3), neural plasticity (i.e., adaptations), and interactions of the physical processes (i.e., osmotic and oncotic pressure, simple diffusion, active transport) which govern water and electrolyte movements throughout the body.

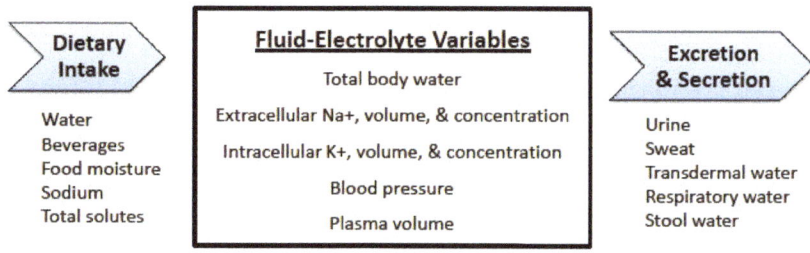

Figure 1. Variables that are regulated as part of body water homeostasis.

This dynamic complexity (Table 3, Figure 1) represents the primary reason why the daily water requirements of humans have not been determined to this date (Table 1). We provide the following evidence in support of this statement:

- The relative influence of physiological processes which maintain water balance (Table 3) varies with different life scenarios. During sedentary daily activities in a mild environment, renal responses and thirst are the primary homeostatic regulators. During continuous-intermittent labor, or prolonged exercise at low intensities (5–18h duration), renal responses and thirst have minor-to-large effects on water regulation, whereas sweat loss presents the foremost challenge to homeostasis [56].
- Large between- and within-subject variances (i.e., of the variables in Table 3) make it difficult to determine a water requirement for all persons within a life stage (Table 1). As an example, Figure 2 illustrates the large between-subject variance of habitual TWI that exists in healthy young women (range, <1.0 to >4.5 L/24h) [13]. A large range of habitual TWI (0.6–5.2 L/24h) has also been reported for women during pregnancy [57]. Similarly, the third National Health and Nutrition Examination Survey [5] reported that the 1st decile and 10th decile of the mean TWI were 1.7–7.9 L/24h for men (n = 3,091) and 1.3–6.1 L/24h for women (n = 2,801). An example of large within-subject variability is also seen in the day-to-day differences of sweat losses that are experienced by athletes [24]. Total sweat loss during sedentary work activity (e.g., 8h of computer programming in an air-conditioned environment) may amount to <0.2 L/24h, whereas the total sweat volume during a 164-km ultradistance cycling event often exceeds 9 L during a 9-h ride [42].

- The 24-h human water requirement varies with anthropomorphic characteristics, especially body mass. Large individuals require a greater daily TWI than small individuals [6].
- The daily water requirement of any life-stage group is influenced by dietary sodium, protein and total solute load, due to individual dietary preferences as well as traditional regional-cultural foods. For example, large differences of mean urine osmolality (U_{OSM}) have been reported for residents of Germany (860 mOsm/kg) and Poland (392 mOsm/kg). These differences are influenced by unique regional customs involving beverages (i.e., water, beer, wine) and food items [1] and the moisture content of solid foods; the latter factor varies among countries and demographic groups: the United States, 20–35% [2,51,58,59]; Germany, 27% [10]; the United Kingdom, 24–28%; and France, 35–38% [14].
- The principle that both water and beverages contribute to rehydration and the maintenance of body water has been fundamental in publications involving large populations [11,25], TWI differences in various countries [14,15], habitual low and high TWI consumers [16,17], water AI recommendations [6,7], the health effects of beverage consumption [60], young versus older adults [61], 12-h or 24-h water restriction [62,63], and experimental interventions which control and modify daily total water intake and beverage types [13,17,36,64]. However, small differences exist in the percentage of water retained (4-h post consumption), primarily due to beverage osmolality and the content of sodium chloride, protein, and/or energy [36,37].
- Intracellular water volume (~28 L in a 70 kg male) is considerably larger than extracellular water volume (~14 L) [65]. No hydration assessment technique measures intracellular water content or concentration directly [27].
- Although some authorities consider plasma osmolality (P_{OSM}) to be the best index of euhydration and hypohydration [2,6], P_{OSM} does not assess whole-body hydration validly in all settings, especially when TBW, water intake, and water loss are fluctuating [66]. Furthermore, P_{OSM} may not reflect widely accepted physiologic principles, as shown by decreased P_{OSM} (6 out of 39 subjects) after losing 3–8% of body mass via sweating [67], and increased P_{OSM} at rest (4 out of 30 values) 60 min after ingesting 500 ml of water [68]. These findings likely result from the large between- and within-subject variance that exists in P_{OSM} measurements [56].
- Arginine vasopressin (AVP) is the body's primary water-regulating hormone. It functions to maintain body water balance by keeping P_{OSM} within narrow limits and allowing the kidneys to alter water excretion in response to the body's needs, in conjunction with thirst [69]. Dehydration of a large enough volume to result in increased P_{OSM} is a stimulus for the release of AVP. Table 4 summarizes research publications that determined the plasma osmotic threshold (i.e., set point) for increased plasma AVP; most of these studies employed intravenous hypertonic saline infusions with serial blood samples. Across these studies, the mean osmotic threshold values range from 280–288 and individual values range from 276–291 mOsm/kg. This large range of P_{OSM} values illustrates dynamic complexity, in that the network of fluid-regulatory functions, and water movements between fluid compartments differ across experimental designs and between normal subjects (see column 1, Table 4). Table 5 further describes the complexity of AVP, in terms of its biological functions, factors that influence neurohypohysial AVP release, and diseases which are related to AVP dysfunction.
- Thirst is the primary means by which humans sense dehydration and hypohydration. Several factors influence the onset of thirst, including blood pressure, blood volume, AVP, and angiotensin II [8]. The primary stimulus for thirst, however, is P_{OSM}. Table 6 summarizes research studies which determined the plasma osmotic threshold for the appearance of thirst. Across these studies, the mean osmotic threshold values range from 286–298 and individual values range from 276–300 mOsm/kg. As with AVP (see previous item), this large range of P_{OSM} values illustrates dynamic complexity, in that the network of fluid-regulatory functions and water movements between fluid compartments differ across experimental designs and among normal subjects (Table 6). This range of P_{OSM} values also may explain part of the range in habitual TWI (Figure 2).

- Older adults (>65 years) experience reduced thirst and water intake, reduced maximal renal concentrating ability, greater plasma AVP concentration during water restriction, and reduced ability to excrete a water load when compared to younger adults [61,88,89]. Although the osmotic threshold for thirst apparently does not change during the aging process [88,90], older adults have a reduced autonomic baroreceptor capability to sense a depletion of blood volume [89,91]. In addition, older adults demonstrate changes in water satiation that hinder the ability to hydrate following an osmotic challenge. This deficiency has been linked to changes in cerebral blood flow and/or altered activation of the anterior midcingulate cortex area within the brain [92]. Thus, aging appears to be responsible for large between-subject variances (i.e., of the variables in Table 3) across age groups, which make it difficult to determine a universal water requirement for children, adults, and the elderly (Table 1).

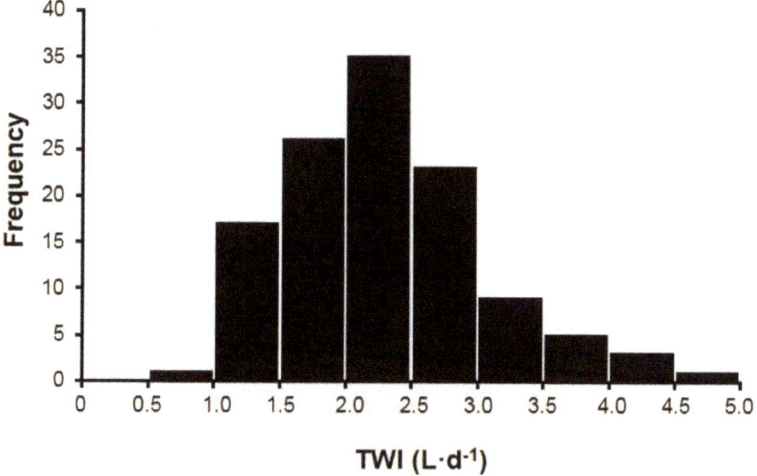

Figure 2. Frequency distribution of the habitual total water intake (TWI, 5-d mean values, n = 120) of healthy, college-aged women (n = 120). Reprinted with permission (Johnson et al., 2016 [13]).

Table 4. Plasma osmotic threshold [a] for plasma AVP increase.

Osmotic Threshold [b] (mOsm/kg)	Participants/Conditions	References
282 (280–285)	Normal adults (n = 6♂), dehydration via water restriction, upright posture	Moses and Miller, 1971 [70]
285 (284–286) [c]	Normal adults (n = 9♂), IV$_{HS}$	Moses and Miller, 1971 [70]
287 (286–288) [c]	Normal adults (n = 6♂), IV$_{HS}$	Moses and Miller, 1971 [70]
288 (287–289) [c]	Normal adults (n = 6♂), IV$_{HS}$, then IV$_{HS}$ plus dextran (expanded plasma volume)	Moses and Miller, 1971 [70]
280 (272–284) [c]	Normal adults (n = 25), recumbent rest, in three states: *ad libitum* fluid intake, acute water load (20 ml/kg) and water restriction	Robertson et al., 1973 [71]
280 (276–291) [c]	Normal adults (n = 9♂, 7♀), recumbent rest	Robertson et al., 1976 [72]
IV$_{HS}$, 287 (283–291) M, 286 (282–290)	Normal adults (3♀, 3♂), supine rest, IV$_{HS}$ (5%) and hypertonic mannitol (M, 20%)	Zerbe et al., 1983 [73]
285 (282–289)	Healthy adults (10♂), recumbent rest, IV$_{HS}$ and IV$_I$	Thompson et al., 1986 [74]
287 (286–288)	Healthy adults (7♂), recumbent rest, IV$_{HS}$	Thompson et al., 1988 [75]
287 (281–290)	Healthy adults (3♂, 4♀), recumbent rest, IV$_{HS}$	Thompson et al., 1991 [76]
MZ, 283 (277–290) DZ, 281 (274–285)	Healthy twins (7♂monozygotic pairs, 6♂dizygotic pairs), IV$_{HS}$	Zerbe et al., 1991 [77]

[a], refers to the plasma osmolality (i.e., determined statistically or graphically) at which plasma AVP concentration rises from baseline; [b], mean (range or 95% confidence interval); [c], data derived from a figure.

Table 5. Research findings that illustrate the dynamic complexity of AVP, a peptide hormone produced in the hypothalamus [a].

Biological functions
Regulates body water and sodium homeostasis by acting on renal nephrons to decrease urine volume and increase the concentration of urine
Maintains plasma osmolality within narrow limits
Encourages vasodilation in vascular smooth muscle cells by inducing NO production
Affects liver metabolism (e.g., gluconeogenesis, glycogenolysis)
Stimulates the pancreas to produce either insulin or glucagon, depending on blood glucose concentration
Factors which influence neurohypohysial AVP release and plasma AVP concentration
Plasma osmolality
Angiotensin II
Oropharyngeal environment
Water restriction and consumption
Osmolar content of diet, especially sodium
Hypoglycemia
Blood volume and pressure
Upright posture
Emotional stress
Exercise
Circadian rhythmicity
Hypoxia
Nausea
Pain
Diseases and disorders that involve AVP dysfunction
Diabetes insipidus and diabetes mellitus
Syndrome of inappropriate ADH excess (SIADH)
Sepsis
Severe bleeding, hemorrhage
Chronic hypernatremia
Primary polydipsia syndrome, compulsive water drinking
Kallmann's syndrome
Autosomal dominant polycystic kidney disease

[a], compiled from: [69,72,78–86].

Table 6. Plasma osmotic threshold [a] for appearance of the thirst sensation.

Mean (Range [b]) Osmotic Threshold (mOsm/kg)	Participants/Conditions	References
IV$_{HS}$, 298 (294–300) M, 296 (290–299)	Normal adults (n = 2–5 ♂&♀), supine rest, IV$_{HS}$ (5%) and hypertonic mannitol (M, 20%)	Zerbe et al., 1983 [73]
F, 297 (296–298) L, 293 (291–295)	Healthy women (n = 8) were tested in the follicular (F) and luteal (L) phases of the menstrual cycle, IV$_{HS}$	Spruce et al., 1985 [87]
287 (286–288)	Healthy males (n = 7), recumbent rest, IV$_{HS}$	Thompson et al., 1988 [75]
287 (282–291)	Healthy adults (3♂, 4♀), recumbent rest, IV$_{HS}$	Thompson et al., 1991 [76]
MZ, 286 (276–293) DZ, 289 (283–296)	Healthy twins (7♂ monozygotic pairs, 6♂ dizygotic pairs), IV$_{HS}$	Zerbe et al., 1991 [77]

[a], refers to the plasma osmolality (i.e., determined statistically or graphically) at which thirst is first perceived; [b], mean (range or 95% confidence interval); Abbreviations: IV$_{HS}$, intravenous hypertonic saline; IV$_I$, intravenous isotonic saline.

The preceding points of evidence exemplify the difficulties which the National Academy of Medicine, USA, and the European Food Safety Authority faced and which prompted them to establish Adequate Intakes (AI), which are not Recommended Dietary Allowances (requiring a higher level of evidence) or water requirements (Table 1). The NAM assumed the TWI AI volumes to be adequate, based on observed or experimentally determined approximations or estimates of water intake by a group of apparently healthy people [6]. The EFSA determined AIs on the basis of population statistics, utilizing calculated 'free water reserve' (ml/24h) [12]; this quantity is defined as the difference between the measured urine volume (ml/24h) and the calculated urine volume necessary to excrete all urine solutes (i.e., obligatory urine volume, mOsm/24-h) at the group mean value of maximum U_{OSM} [1,11]. Furthermore, both the NAM and EFSA noted that AI values for water apply only to moderate environmental temperatures and moderate physical activity levels, because non-renal water losses via sweating (see column 8 in Table 3) can exceed 8.0 L/24h when exercise-heat stress is extreme [7].

4. A Proposed Method to Assess Daily Water Requirements

We now propose a novel approach to the assessment of the daily water requirement of individuals in all life stages, which was not employed during the development of water AI values (Table 1). This method focuses on the thresholds and intensity of responses within the brain and neuroendocrine system (i.e., autonomic nerves and endocrine organs that release hormones to regulate water and electrolyte balance). Figure 3 provides a graphic representation of this technique. The central dashed line represents the set point (threshold) for each of the five regulated variables listed within the central rectangle; Tables 4 and 6 present set point values for a plasma AVP increase and the appearance of thirst. The regions to the left and right of the set point represent a water or sodium deficit, and water or sodium excess, respectively; the zones farthest to the left and right of the set point represent the greatest perturbations of each regulated variable due to change forces (e.g., dehydration, drinking, large dietary osmotic load). The block arrows to the left and right of the set point illustrate neuroendocrine responses which move each regulated variable toward the set point in an effort to restore altered homeostasis; examples include release of AVP, angiotension II, aldosterone, atrial natriuretic peptide, as well as blood vessel constriction or dilation, increased thirst, and water consumption (i.e., sensory and behavioral effects that are influenced by endocrine responses). The strongest neuroendocrine responses occur at the far left and far right of the threshold (labeled with the words deficit and excess). If all fluid-electrolyte regulatory variables are at or near the set point (or if all neuroendocrine responses are minimal), a state of euhydration exists because the brain is activating no compensatory responses; in contrast, when responses counteract water loss a state of dehydration or hypohydration exists. Measuring the intensity of neuroendocrine responses and identifying when set points have been exceeded allow for quantitative comparisons of values during controlled laboratory experiments. Alternatively, the area under the curve (i.e., response intensity plotted versus response duration) could be measured.

Figure 4 illustrates this approach to assessing individual daily water needs. In normal subjects, the increase in plasma AVP (panel A) is stimulated primarily by increased P_{OSM}. Increasing P_{OSM} signifies increasing perturbation of homeostasis; whereas an increasing plasma AVP concentration represents an increased intensity of neuroendocrine response and indicates that the brain is regulating body water via the kidneys. Thus, the data in the upper right quadrants of panel A and panel B correspond to intense neuroendocrine responses and a rigorous defense of total body water; the data in the lower left quadrants correspond to minimal-to-moderate defense of total body water.

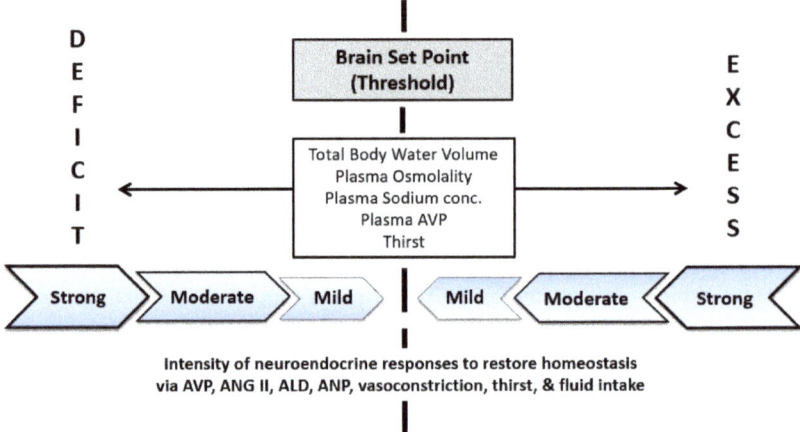

Figure 3. A proposed schematic of a method to assess human daily water requirements by measuring the intensity of neuroendocrine responses that are employed by the brain to defend homeostasis of body water volume and concentration. These responses and thresholds are inherent hydration biomarkers, and the means by which the brain maintains good health and optimal function. Abbreviations: AVP, arginine vasopressin; ANG II, angiotensin II; ALD, aldosterone; ANP, atrial naturietic peptide.

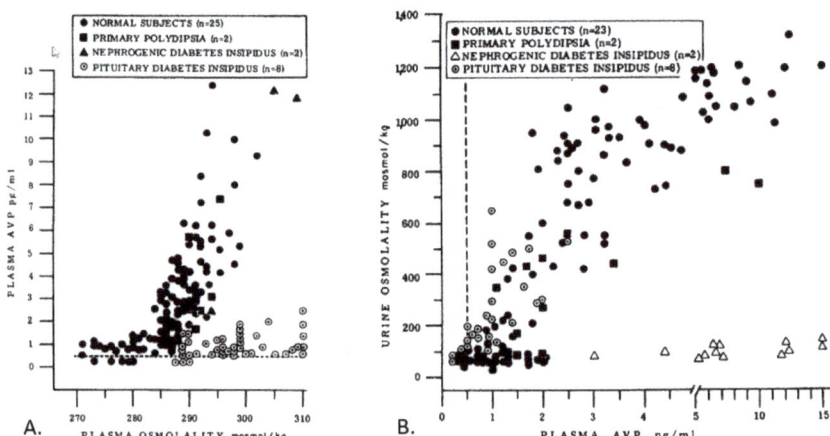

Figure 4. The relationship of plasma osmolality to plasma AVP (panel A), and the relationship of plasma AVP to urine osmolality (panel B). Reprinted with copyright from Robertson et al. [71]. Plasma was collected during recumbent rest in three states of water balance: ad libitum fluid intake, following an acute water load (20 ml/kg), and after acute periods of fluid restriction. The data represent healthy adults and patients with diverse types of polyuria (i.e., abnormally large urine volume and frequency). Dashed lines represent the sensitivity limit of the plasma AVP assay.

In normal adults, an increased intensity of neuroendocrine response (i.e., which defends the volume and concentration of total body water) results in decreased urine volume and increased urine osmolality, secondary to increased plasma AVP (Figure 4, panel B). As such, urinary variables (e.g., osmolality, specific gravity, 24-h urine volume) have been identified as valid hydration biomarkers in studies involving free-living pregnant women, nonpregnant women, and men [16,18,38,39,57]. Central, autonomically-controlled changes of plasma AVP concentration (i.e., at the border of euhydration and mild hypohydration; Figure 3) also act to maintain optimal health and functions in normal persons. In turn, AVP may be a prognostic indicator of various disease states (Table 7), including ischemic stroke, myocardial infarction, pneumonia, certain types of cancer, and septic shock [93–95].

Table 7. Effects of 12-h and 24-h water restriction [a] on plasma osmolality and AVP concentration.

Participants	Experimental Design Phase	Plasma Osmolality (mOsm/kg H$_2$O)	Plasma AVP (pg/ml)	Reference
8 ♀[b] (21–34 year)	Baseline, EU	289 ± 2	1.3 ± 0.6	Davison et al., AJP 1984 [62]
	12-h WR [c]	294 ± 2	2.9 ± 1.2	
5 ♂ & 3 ♀[b] (26–50 year)	Baseline, EU	292 ± 1	1.7 ± 0.2	Geelen et al., AJP 1984 [63]
	24-h WR [c]	302 ± 1	3.3 ± 0.5	
7 ♂ (20–31 year)	Baseline, EU	288 ± 1	1.0 ± 0.3	Phillips et al., NEJM 1984 [88]
	24-h WR [c,d]	291 ± 1	3.5 ± 0.3	
7 ♂ (67–75 year)	Baseline, EU	288 ± 1	1.8 ± 0.3	Phillips et al., NEJM 1984 [88]
	24-h WR [c,d]	296 ± 1	8.3 ± 0.3	

[a], diets included no water or beverages and dry food items; [b], nonpregnant women; [c], 24-h total water intake was not measured; [d], body mass loss was 1.8–1.9% of the baseline value; Abbreviations: AVP, arginine vasopressin; EU, euhydrated; WR, water restriction.

In terms of the water requirements of normal individuals, determining the intensity of the body's defense of total body water and tonicity (e.g., measuring changes of plasma AVP or regulated variables) provides a laboratory method to assess the intensity of homeostatic responses and the response thresholds which the brain employs. Once identified, these measurements could be compared to experimentally-controlled TWI volumes to determine the minimum 24-h TWI that generally elicits no neuroendocrine response above resting baseline levels (i.e., thereby representing euhydration or normal water balance). This method for assessing 24-h water balance also can be applied to the TWI of free-living adults. For example, in recent years several research teams have compared the physiological responses of habitual low-volume drinkers (LOW) to those of habitual high-volume drinkers (HIGH) [16–18,51]. Figure 5 depicts plasma the AVP concentrations of free-living LOW and HIGH during one morning laboratory visit on each of 8 days. The TWI levels of LOW (n = 14 ♀) and HIGH (n = 14 ♀) are described in the figure legend. The experimental design involved 3 d of baseline observations, 4 d of modified water intake (during which LOW consumed the TWI which HIGH habitually consumed, and vice versa), and 1 d of *ad libitum* water intake. The morning plasma AVP levels in Figure 5 were similar (LOW, 1.4–1.5 pg/ml; HIGH, 1.1–1.3 pg/ml) when both groups were consuming a similar high TWI (LOW, 3.5 L/24h; HIGH, 3.2 L/24h). Considering the plasma AVP threshold which indicates an obvious neuroendocrine response (~2.0 pg/ml [78]; Figure 4), LOW were above this threshold when consuming a TWI volume of 1.6–1.7 L/24h whereas HIGH were above this 2.0 pg/ml AVP threshold only when their TWI was modified to 2.0 L/24h on days 4–7. We interpret these data to mean that the brain did not attempt to conserve water when TWI was ≥3.2 L/24h, and that the water requirement of these healthy young women existed between 1.6 and 3.2 L/24h. Similar plasma AVP concentrations have been published in a study of LOW (TWI, 0.74 L/24h) and HIGH (TWI, 2.70 L/24h) by Perrier and colleagues [16]. Furthermore, a plasma AVP threshold <2.0 pg/ml corresponds closely with the euhydrated baseline values shown in Table 7 (1.0–1.8 pg/ml), as observed in four groups of men and women. However, when these test subjects underwent water restriction for 12h and 24h, a stronger neuroendocrine response was observed (i.e., representing hypohydration) as plasma AVP levels of 2.9–3.5 pg/ml in young adults and 8.3 pg/ml in older adults. In one Table 7 experiment [63], participants (5 ♂ & 3 ♀, 26–50 years) rehydrated with tap water (10 ml/kg, 620–870 ml) after a 24-h water restriction; 60 min after this water consumption, the average plasma AVP decreased from 3.3 to 1.5 pg/ml, suggesting that subjects had reached a state of euhydration.

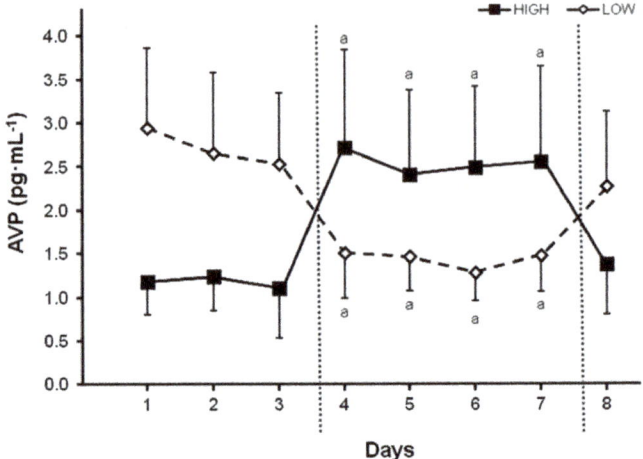

Figure 5. Morning plasma AVP concentrations of habitual high-volume drinkers (HIGH, 3.2 ± 0.6 L/24h, n = 14♀) and low-volume drinkers (LOW, 1.6 L/24h, n = 14♀) during ad libitum baseline (3 days), modified water intake (4 days; HIGH, 2.0 ± 0.2 and LOW, 3.5 ± 0.1 L/24h), and ad libitum recovery (1 day; HIGH, 3.2 ± 0.9 and LOW, 1.7 ± 0.5 L/24h). Different experimental phases are separated by vertical dotted lines. a, within-group significant difference from the 3-d baseline mean ($p < 0.001$). Reprinted with permission from Johnson et al., (2016) [13].

Utilizing a plasma AVP threshold of <2.0 pg/ml, this method could be employed to: (a) define and distinguish states of euhydration and hypohydration; and (b) evaluate the neuroendocrine response changes which occur with advanced age (Table 7; [61,88,91,96]) or any factor that potentiates the release of AVP into the circulation. Although a plasma AVP concentration is useful because it represents the sum of all factors that influence pituitary AVP release (Table 5) and AVP turnover in the circulation, we acknowledge that other hormonal/neurological biomarkers (e.g., angiotensin II, aldosterone) also play a role in water homeostasis. In addition, cases of over-hydration likely represent a limitation of this method. Excess body water may reduce plasma AVP to a level below the sensitivity of present-day technologies (i.e., most immunoassays detect AVP to ≥0.5 pg/ml; [69]), making it difficult to distinguish over-hydrated states from a normal euhydrated state (1.0–1.8 pg/ml; Table 7). One final limitation of this method is the circadian variation in AVP secretion. It would be imperative for any investigation utilizing this proposed method to ensure blood sampling at similar times if successive samples were taken as it has been demonstrated that AVP is both an outcome and input related to suprachiasmatic nucleus activity [97].

Plasma AVP concentration was selected as the primary outcome variable of this method because previous TWI investigations have also published AVP with no copeptin measurements. However, AVP has a short half-life and is difficult to isolate/analyze [69,98], whereas copeptin is stable at room temperature and is recognized as a diagnostic biomarker for various diseases [99,100]. Furthermore, several studies have reported a strong correlation between plasma AVP and copeptin levels in healthy individuals [98,101] and patients [102,103] across a wide range of P_{OSM}. Thus, it is very likely that copeptin will be measured in future investigations of neuroendocrine response intensity.

Currently, copeptin is just beginning to be used in clinical settings during randomized control trials evaluating changes in water intake and disease [104,105]. Clinical settings are ideal because copeptin measurement, although less prone to errors compared to AVP, still requires specialized and expensive equipment (i.e., B·R·A·H·M·S KRYPTOR random-access immunoassay analyzer, ThermoFisher Scientific). Copeptin is also utilized in hospital settings for the evaluation of heart failure [106]. Therefore, many researchers in the clinical setting already have access to copeptin analysis equipment. It is hoped that in the coming years this type of equipment will become a mainstay within hydratrion physiology laboratories, or advances in assay techniques will make copeptin quantification more accessible for all levels of researchers.

To our knowledge, only one study has assessed changes of plasma copeptin concentrations in normal adults during water restriction [107]. Resting euhydrated plasma copeptin values (i.e., representing no neuroendocrine response by the brain to conserve water) were 18.5 ± 6.8 pg/ml (4.6 ± 1.7 pmol/L; 8 ♀, 8 ♂) at baseline, and increased to 37.0 ± 20.9 pg/ml (9.2 ± 5.2 pmol/L) after a 28-h water restriction period that induced a 1.7% body mass loss. To determine a plasma copeptin threshold similar to the plasma AVP threshold of 2.0 pg/ml (see above), additional experiments similar to those in Table 7 are required.

5. Neuroendocrine Responses across a Range of TWIs

Figure 6 provides evidence regarding the daily water requirement of humans. Compiling a range of data from six studies that reported 22 different observation days [10,13,16,18,54,64], we plotted the relationships between TWI and the primary brain-regulated variable (P_{OSM}), the neuroendocrine response (plasma AVP) to changes of P_{OSM}, and the resulting changes in urine volume and concentration. The R^2 value for each relationship describes the amount of variance in the four variables that is explained by TWI values. Clearly, P_{OSM} is not strongly related to TWI ($R^2 = 0.18$, $p < 0.05$) because blood concentration is regulated by the brain within a narrow normal limit [4], across a wide range of TWI [6]; as reported in previous publications [16,18], P_{OSM} does not serve as a valid indicator of either TWI or water requirement in free-living adults. This fact opposes the theory that all individuals with normal P_{OSM} levels are similar [2,108], even if their 24-h TWI is low.

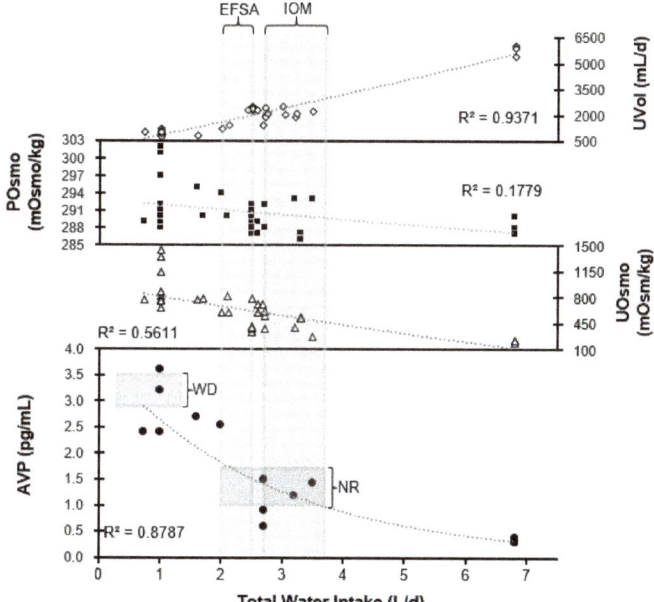

Figure 6. Urine volume (U_{VOL}), plasma osmolality (P_{OSM}), urine osmolality (U_{OSM}, 24h), and plasma AVP plotted against daily total water intake. EFSA and NAM water Adequate Intakes are shown as the vertical shaded column. AVP concentrations associated with water restriction (WR) and baseline resting total water intake (B) (Table 7) appear as horizontal shaded rows. All data points are group mean values (SD not shown) from investigations that measured TWI.

The relationship between TWI and urine osmolality in Figure 6 appears to be moderately strong ($R^2 = 0.56$, $p < 0.001$), but not very strong because of the simultaneous influence of dietary osmolar load on U_{OSM}. In contrast, the relationship between TWI and urine volume is very strong ($R^2 = 0.94$, $p < 0.001$). However, plasma AVP concentration is the only variable in Figure 6 that directly represents the intensity of neuroendocrine responses across a wide range of TWI (0.7–6.8 L/24h). As such, this relationship ($R^2 = 0.88$) provides evidence of the TWI volume that is required to maintain water and electrolyte homeostasis. Recalling that a plasma AVP concentration of ≥ 2.0 pg/ml indicates an obvious neuroendocrine response by the brain ([78]; Figure 4), and that the normal resting level (shaded zone labeled WR) of plasma AVP lies below 2.0 pg/ml, the line of best fit for the relationship between TWI and plasma AVP in Figure 6 shows that a plasma AVP concentration of 2.0 pg/ml is equivalent to a TWI of 1.8 L/24h. Approximately 40% of young healthy college-aged women in the USA (Figure 2), 19–24% of men and women in Great Britain [109], and 68–71% of men and women in Spain [110] consume less than this volume of water each day. In Figure 6, a TWI of 1.8 L/24h is equivalent to a urine volume of ~1400 mL/24h and a 24-h urine osmolality of ~770 mOsm/kg. Furthermore, a TWI of 1.8 L/24h is similar to the much-debated recommendation to drink "8 × 8" each day, which refers to consuming eight 8 oz glasses of water (1.89 L/24h) [108,111], and to the recommended daily AI of water for women (2.0 L/24h, Table 1) established by the European Food Safety Authority [7]. The two vertical shaded zones in Figure 6 display the EFSA and NAM daily water AI ranges for men and women; all of these AI correspond to plasma AVP levels <2.0 pg/ml and a minimal/baseline neuroendocrine defense of total body water and tonicity (Table 7). The daily water AI range of the NAM corresponds to plasma AVP levels well below 2.0 pg/ml, likely because the NAM proposed that human water requirements should not be based on a "minimal" intake [6], as this might eventually lead to a deficit and possible adverse performance and health consequences [2].

Figure 6 also depicts plasma AVP levels during the four 12-h and 24-h water restriction experiments (see the horizontal shaded zone labeled WR) that are described in Table 7. At the end of these water restriction periods, group mean plasma AVP concentrations ranged from 2.9–3.5 pg/ml, representing a mild-to-moderate neuroendocrine response (Figures 3 and 4). Interestingly, this range of concentrations (representing hypohydration of approximately 1% of body mass) is similar to the plasma AVP levels reported for individuals who habitually consume a low daily TWI of 0.7 L/24h (2.4 pg/ml; [16]), 1.0 L/24h (2.5–3.6 pg/ml; [54]), and 1.6 L/24h (2.5–2.9 pg/ml; Figure 5; [13]). This suggests that women who consume a TWI of 0.7–1.6 L/24h (i.e., ~20–30% of young healthy women; Figure 2)—well below the AI recommended by EFSA and NAM (Table 1)—experience a chronic mild-to-moderate neuroendocrine defense of total body water. This observation is significant because numerous investigations and letters to the editor have proposed that chronically elevated plasma AVP and angiotensin II levels may be related to negative health outcomes (e.g., cardiovascular disease, obesity, diabetes, cancer morbidity and mortality) [69,96,112] as well as the progression of disease states (e.g., salt-sensitive hypertension, chronic kidney disease, and diabetic nephropathy [113]). Other investigators have: (a) utilized plasma copeptin concentrations (i.e., part of the molecular pre-prohormone of AVP) to detect myocardial ischemia and other diseases (Figure 4; [8,69,114]); and (b) supported the use of AVP receptor antagonists to treat specific cardiovascular pathologies, suggesting dysfunctional body water regulation [115,116]. A 6-week study, involving 82 healthy adults (50% ♀) in three TWI groups (1.43, 1.83, and 2.42 L/24h), provided promising evidence (i.e., increasing the daily TWI of the two LOW groups to match 2.42 L/24h) of reduced circulating copeptin levels [19]. This study suggests that the reduction of plasma AVP via increased TWI offers a safe, cost-effective, and easy-to-implement primary preventive intervention that should be evaluated in large future clinical trials [117].

6. Evidence for a Role of 24-h TWI in Reducing Disease Risk

As noted above, a surprising number of adults in developed countries do not meet water AI recommendations (Table 1). This fact is significant in terms of long-term health outcomes because a growing body of epidemiological evidence shows that chronically elevated plasma AVP (likely due to an insufficient daily TWI) is related to cardiovascular, obesity and cancer morbidity and mortality, as well as the regulation of glucose metabolism. Unfortunately, controlled, randomized clinical trials (spanning multiple years or decades), which focus on the relationship between chronic low water volume intake and development of diseases, do not exist for three reasons [118]. First, lengthy controlled studies suffer from participant attrition and noncompliance because it is difficult for any person to maintain a constant hydration state or 24-h TWI across years of life. Second, multiple personal characteristics, dietary habits, or lifestyle behaviors may concurrently encourage disease development. Third, because of the large number of confounding dietary, behavioral, and genetic factors related to the development of the above diseases, the number of subjects required for adequately-powered statistical analyses which isolate the effects of water is large and the research is costly. Therefore, researchers must focus on the mechanisms that regulate body water (Figures 1 and 4) to investigate potential relationships between chronic low TWI and the development of diseases.

Recent epidemiological studies (n = 3000–4000 Scandinavian adults) have reported statistically significant associations between high plasma AVP (or its surrogates, including low daily TWI, low urine flow rate, high P_{OSM}, or copeptin) [69] and the incidence of type 2 diabetes, metabolic syndrome, end-stage renal disease, cardiovascular disease, and premature death [117,119–122]. Furthermore, during the past 25 years, several observational studies have reported that increased daily TWI reduces the risk of kidney stone formation and stone recurrence [118,123–128] preserves kidney function in chronic kidney disease [129], and retards cyst growth in polycystic kidney disease [130]. If these findings are supported by future controlled intervention studies, it is possible that increased daily water consumption will be recognized as a safe, cost-effective, simple primary preventive intervention for some kidney diseases [117,131]. However, establishing such relationships will be challenging (i.e., for the reasons noted in the preceding paragraph) [118], and will likely be specific to each type of kidney disease/dysfunction. For example, at least one recent randomized clinical trial found no benefit of coaching chronic kidney disease patients to increase their 24-h TWI, even though coaching resulted in a 24-h urine volume that was +0.6 L/day greater than an uncoached control group (p < 0.001) [104]. Thus, because epidemiological and observational studies do not allow for cause-and-effect inferences, randomized clinical trials and experimental studies employing animal models are needed to further evaluate mechanisms such as the contribution of AVP to renal, cardiovascular, and metabolic disorders [113].

7. AVP Influences Glucose Metabolism

The first observations regarding the association between "pituitary extract" and antidiuresis occurred more than a century ago [132], after which AVP synthesis and its mechanistic description became the subjects of the 1955 Nobel Prize in Chemistry [133]. Two decades later, medical professionals hypothesized that the excess water loss (i.e., polyuria) observed in people with type 2 diabetes mellitus resulted from decreased secretion of AVP. Contrary to their inclination, researchers testing this hypothesis observed that the plasma AVP concentration was markedly *elevated* in hyperglycemic patients [134]. These researchers, along with many during subsequent decades, hypothesized that increased plasma AVP was an ineffective effort to conserve water in the face of an overwhelming solute diuresis caused by glucose in urine (i.e., glucosuria). To our knowledge, this theory persisted until 2010, when epidemiological findings reversed the relationship between AVP and glucose regulation, from one of result to cause [135]. Based on an apparent dose-response relationship between copeptin and severity of the metabolic syndrome [136], the important work of Enhörning and colleagues [135] described a significant positive association between the baseline plasma copeptin concentration of healthy adults and their odds of developing impaired fasting glucose and/or diabetes during the five-year observation period. Shortly thereafter, it was confirmed that an inverse relationship existed between self-reported water intake and the development of hyperglycemia, during a nine-year longitudinal surveillance study [137]. These two investigations were theoretically connected by the fact that AVP is secreted in response to high plasma osmolality (i.e., low water intake) and acts via V2 receptors in renal nephrons, increasing translocation of the aquaporin 2 channel and facilitating increased water reabsorption [138]. Thus, chronically low water intake is associated with elevated plasma AVP [16], both of which predict the development of impaired glucose regulation.

Historically, low daily water intake, in the absence of symptoms and outside of athletic pursuits, has been considered to be innocuous because theoretically it was balanced by increased AVP secretion, enhanced renal water reabsorption, increased water consumption, and maintenance of water balance [108]. However, the examination of cellular receptors sensitive to AVP yielded insights into possible mechanisms responsible for the above results. Distinct from V2 membrane receptors, V1a receptors are expressed in the kidney, liver, vascular smooth muscle, blood platelets, and brain [69]. In the liver, V1a stimulation by AVP initiates calcium signaling reactions which increase glycogenolysis and blood glucose, directly in hepatocytes and indirectly via vasoconstriction-mediated ischemia [139]. Indeed, multiple animal investigations and human genetic studies have described the role of V1a receptors in glucose regulation and dysfunction [140–142].

Independently, V1b receptors are concentrated within the hypothalamic-pituitary-adrenocortical (HPA) axis, where they enhance ACTH and cortisol release, and the physiological effects of CRH, when stimulated by AVP. The downstream effect of increased plasma glucocorticoids is increased hepatic gluconeogenesis and decreased insulin sensitivity [143]. The role of AVP in glucocorticoid release is supported by observational data which show that individuals who consume low daily TWI exhibit increased plasma concentrations of both AVP and cortisol [16]. Additionally, men with type 2 diabetes exhibited deteriorated glucose control and increased plasma cortisol following three days of water restriction [144]. Thus, mounting evidence suggests that a link exists between AVP and glucose regulation. Our understanding of this relationship will expand in coming years.

8. Summary

Despite numerous efforts to define a state of euhydration and determine the daily water requirements of children, men, women, and older adults, no empirical research provides definitive answers and no universal consensus exists. The dynamic complexity of the water regulatory network, and inter-individual differences, are the primary reasons why widespread consensus regarding the daily water requirements has not been reached to this date. In the preceding paragraphs, we have proposed a novel experimental approach that offers an alternative to water AI survey data and the potential to determine 24-h water requirements of individuals. This approach involves the assessment of the intensity of neuroendocrine responses during euhydration and following experimental perturbations of essential regulated variables. Although future researchers may choose a different regulated variable, we focused on plasma AVP as the primary hydration biomarker to determine the intensity of neuroendocrine responses to a range of TWIs (Figure 6). A plasma AVP concentration < 2.0 pg/ml represents a baseline euhydrated state (i.e., the brain is not attempting to conserve water), whereas plasma AVP ≥2.0 pg/ml indicates dehydration or hypohydration because the brain is acting to conserve water ([78]; Figure 4). These concentrations provide a previously unpublished definition of each term. Our examination of data from multiple research studies (Figure 6) demonstrates that a plasma AVP concentration of 2.0 pg/ml is equivalent to a TWI of 1.8 L/24h. Observational studies demonstrate that 19–71% of adults in various countries consume this volume of water or less each day [13,109,110]. This is significant because increasing evidence shows that chronically elevated plasma AVP (likely due to an insufficient daily TWI) could contribute to a number of negative health outcomes. A TWI of 1.8 L/24h also questions the theory that all individuals with normal P_{OSM} levels are similar [2,108], even if their 24-h TWI is low. Fortunately, the chronic reduction of plasma AVP by consuming a daily TWI that maintains plasma AVP <2.0 pg/ml suggests a safe, cost-effective, and easy-to-implement primary preventive intervention that can be evaluated in future long-term clinical trials.

Author Contributions: L.E.A. and E.C.J. worked together on the generation, editing, table design and figure creation for this manuscript.

Acknowledgments: The authors would like to thank Professor Ivan Tack, M.D., Ph.D., Toulouse School of Medicine, Toulouse, France for sharing insights regarding the central regulation of renal function and Hillary Yoder, M.S. for providing clerical assistance with the production of the manuscript.

Conflicts of Interest: Lawrence Armstrong has previously served as a Scientific Advisory Board member, paid consultant, and has received research funding from Danone Nutricia Research, France. He presently serves as a member of the Board of Trustees, Drinking Water Research Foundation, Alexandria, VA and is also a paid consultant to the Foundation. Evan Johnson has previously received funding for research investigations from Danone Nutricia Research, France, and served as a paid consultant to Dr. Armstrong during the preparation of this paper for the Drinking Water Research Foundation, Alexandria, VA, USA.

References

1. Manz, F.; Wentz, A. 24-h hydration status: Parameters, epidemiology and recommendations. *Eur. J. Clin. Nutr.* **2003**, *57*, S101–S108. [CrossRef] [PubMed]
2. Sawka, M.N.; Cheuvront, S.N.; Carter, R. Human water needs. *Nutr. Rev.* **2005**, *63*, S303–S309. [CrossRef]
3. Greenleaf, J.E. Problem: Thirst, drinking behavior, and involuntary dehydration. *Med. Sci. Sports Exerc.* **1992**, *24*, 645–656. [CrossRef] [PubMed]
4. Kratz, A.; Ferraro, M.; Sluss, P.M.; Lewandrowski, K.B. Laboratory Reference Values. *N. Engl. J. Med.* **2004**, *35*, 1548–1563. [CrossRef] [PubMed]
5. The third national health and nutrition examination survey (NHANES III 1988–1994). Available online: https://wwwn.cdc.gov/nchs/data/nhanes3/3a/VIFSE-acc.pdf (accessed on 25 May 2018).
6. Institute of Medicine. *Dietary reference intakes for water, potassium, sodium, chloride, and sulfate*; Institute of Medicine: Washington, DC, USA, 2004.
7. EFSA Panel on Dietic Products, Nutrition, and Allergies (NDA). Scientific opinion on dietary reference values for water. *EFSA J.* **2010**, *8*, 1459–1507.
8. Thornton, S.N. Thirst and hydration: Physiology and consequences of dysfunction. *Physiol. Behav.* **2010**, *100*, 15–21. [CrossRef]
9. Gamble, J. *Chemical Anatomy, Physiology and Pathology of Extracellular Fluid: A Lecture Syllabus*; Harvard University Press: Cambridge, MA, USA, 1947.
10. Manz, F.; Johner, S.A.; Wentz, A.; Boeing, H.; Remer, T. Water balance throughout the adult life span in a German population. *Br. J. Nutr.* **2012**, *107*, 1673–1681. [CrossRef]
11. Manz, F.; Wentz, A. Hydration status in the United States and Germany. *Nutr. Rev.* **2005**, *63*, S55–S62. [CrossRef]
12. Manz, F.; Wentz, A.; Sichert-Hellert, W. The most essential nutrient: Defining the adequate intake of water. *J. Pediatr.* **2002**, *141*, 587–592. [CrossRef]
13. Johnson, E.C.; Muñoz, C.X.; Jimenez, L.; Le Bellego, L.; Kupchak, B.R.; Kraemer, W.J.; Casa, D.J.; Maresh, C.M.; Armstrong, L.E. Hormonal and thirst modulated maintenance of fluid balance in young women with different levels of habitual fluid consumption. *Nutrients* **2016**, *8*, 302. [CrossRef]
14. Guelinckx, I.; Tavoularis, G.; König, J.; Morin, C.; Gharbi, H.; Gandy, J. Contribution of water from food and fluids to total water intake: Analysis of a French and UK population surveys. *Nutrients* **2016**, *8*, 630. [CrossRef] [PubMed]
15. Guelinckx, I.; Ferreira-Pêgo, C.; Moreno, L.A.; Kavouras, S.A.; Gandy, J.; Martinez, H.; Bardosono, S.; Abdollahi, M.; Nasseri, E.; Jarosz, A.; et al. Intake of water and different beverages in adults across 13 countries. *Eur. J. Nutr.* **2015**, *54*, 45–55. [CrossRef] [PubMed]
16. Perrier, E.; Vergne, S.; Klein, A.; Poupin, M.; Rondeau, P.; Le Bellego, L.; Armstrong, L.E.; Lang, F.; Stookey, J.; Tack, I. Hydration biomarkers in free-living adults with different levels of habitual fluid consumption. *Br. J. Nutr.* **2013**, *109*, 1678–1687. [CrossRef] [PubMed]
17. Pross, N.; Demazières, A.; Girard, N.; Barnouin, R.; Metzger, D.; Klein, A.; Perrier, E.; Guelinckx, I. Effects of changes in water intake on mood of high and low drinkers. *PLoS ONE* **2014**, *9*, e94754. [CrossRef]
18. Perrier, E.; Demazières, A.; Girard, N.; Pross, N.; Osbild, D.; Metzger, D.; Guelinckx, I.; Klein, A. Circadian variation and responsiveness of hydration biomarkers to changes in daily water intake. *Eur. J. Appl. Physiol.* **2013**, *113*, 2143–2151. [CrossRef]
19. Lemetais, G.; Melander, O.; Vecchio, M.; Bottin, J.H.; Enhörning, S.; Perrier, E.T. Effect of increased water intake on plasma copeptin in healthy adults. *Eur. J. Nutr.* **2018**, *57*, 1883–1890. [CrossRef]

20. Pross, N.; Demazières, A.; Girard, N.; Barnouin, R.; Santoro, F.; Chevillotte, E.; Klein, A.; Le Bellego, L. Influence of progressive fluid restriction on mood and physiological markers of dehydration in women. *Br. J. Nutr.* **2013**, *109*, 313–321. [CrossRef]
21. National Health and Medical Research Council. National Health and Medical Research Council of Australia. In *Australian Dietary Guidlines*; National Health and Medical Research Council: Canberra, Australia, 2013.
22. Armstrong, L.E.; Pumerantz, A.C.; Fiala, K.A.; Roti, M.W.; Kavouras, S.A.; Casa, D.J.; Maresh, C.M. Human hydration indices: Acute and longitudinal reference values. *Int. J. Sport Nutr. Exerc. MeTable* **2010**, *20*, 145–153. [CrossRef]
23. Armstrong, L.E.; Johnson, E.C.; Muñoz, C.X.; Swokla, B.; Le Bellego, L.; Jimenez, L.; Casa, D.J.; Maresh, C.M. Hydration biomarkers and dietary fluid consumption of women. *J. Acad. Nutr. Diet.* **2012**, *112*, 1056–1061. [CrossRef]
24. Leiper, J.B.; Pitsiladis, Y.; Maughan, R.J. Comparison of water turnover rates in men undertaking prolonged cycling exercise and sedentary men. *Int. J. Sports Med.* **2001**, *22*, 181–185. [CrossRef]
25. Raman, A.; Schoeller, D.A.; Subar, A.F.; Troiano, R.P.; Schatzkin, A.; Harris, T.; Bauer, D.; Bingham, S.A.; Everhart, J.E.; Newman, A.B.; et al. Water turnover in 458 American adults 40–79 year of age. *Am. J. Physiol. Renal Physiol.* **2004**, *286*, F394–F401. [CrossRef] [PubMed]
26. McKenzie, A.L.; Armstrong, L.E. Monitoring body water balance in pregnant and nursing women: The validity of urine color. *Ann. Nutr. Metab.* **2017**, *70*, 18–22. [CrossRef] [PubMed]
27. Armstrong, L.E.; Kenefick, R.W.; Castellani, J.W.; Riebe, D.; Kavouras, S.A.; Kuznicki, J.T.; Maresh, C.M. Bioimpedance spectroscopy technique: Intra-, extracellular, and total body water. *Med. Sci. Sports Exerc.* **1997**, *29*, 1657–1663. [CrossRef] [PubMed]
28. Davis, J.M.; Burgess, W.A.; Slentz, C.A.; Bartoli, W.P.; Pate, R.R. Effects of ingesting 6% and 12% glucose/electrolyte beverages during prolonged intermittent cycling in the heat. *Eur. J. Appl. Physiol. Occup. Physiol.* **1988**, *57*, 563–569. [CrossRef] [PubMed]
29. Sawka, M.N.; Young, A.J.; Francesconi, R.P.; Muza, S.R.; Pandolf, K.B. Thermoregulatory and blood responses during exercise at graded hypohydration levels. *J. Appl. Physiol.* **1985**, *59*, 1394–1401. [CrossRef] [PubMed]
30. Armstrong, L.E.; Maresh, C.M.; Gabaree, C.V.; Hoffman, J.R.; Kavouras, S.A.; Kenefick, R.W.; Castellani, J.W.; Ahlquist, L.E. Thermal and circulatory responses during exercise: Effects of hypohydration, dehydration, and water intake. *J. Appl. Physiol.* **1997**, *82*, 2028–2035. [CrossRef] [PubMed]
31. Kenefick, R.W.; Maresh, C.M.; Armstrong, L.E.; Castellani, J.W.; Riebe, D.; Echegaray, M.E.; Kavorous, S.A. Plasma vasopressin and aldosterone responses to oral and intravenous saline rehydration. *J. Appl. Physiol.* **2000**, *89*, 2117–2122. [CrossRef] [PubMed]
32. Muñoz, C.X.; Johnson, E.C.; Demartini, J.K.; Huggins, R.A.; McKenzie, A.L.; Casa, D.J.; Maresh, C.M.; Armstrong, L.E. Assessment of hydration biomarkers including salivary osmolality during passive and active dehydration. *Eur. J. Clin. Nutr.* **2013**, *67*, 1257–1263. [CrossRef]
33. Rolls, E.T.; Rolls, B.J.; Rowe, E.A. Sensory-specific and motivation-specific satiety for the sight and taste of food and water in man. *Physiol. Behav.* **1983**, *30*, 185–192. [CrossRef]
34. Geelen, G.; Greenleaf, J.E.; Keil, L.C. Drinking-induced plasma vasopressin and norepinephrine changes in dehydrated humans. *J. Clin. Endocrinol. Metab.* **1996**, *81*, 2131–2135.
35. Engell, D.B.; Maller, O.; Sawka, M.N.; Francesconi, R.N.; Drolet, L.; Young, A.J. Thirst and fluid intake following graded hypohydration levels in humans. *Physiol. Behav.* **1987**, *40*, 229–236. [CrossRef]
36. Maughan, R.J.; Watson, P.; Cordery, P.A.; Walsh, N.P.; Oliver, S.J.; Dolci, A.; Rodriguez-Sanchez, N.; Galloway, S.D. A randomized trial to assess the potential of different beverages to affect hydration status: Development of a beverage hydration index. *Am. J. Clin. Nutr.* **2016**, *103*, 717–723. [CrossRef] [PubMed]
37. Evans, G.H.; James, L.J.; Shirreffs, S.M.; Maughan, R.J. Optimizing the restoration and maintenance of fluid balance after exercise-induced dehydration. *J. Appl. Physiol.* **2017**, *122*, 945–951. [CrossRef]
38. Perrier, E.T.; Buendia-Jimenez, I.; Vecchio, M.; Armstrong, L.E.; Tack, I.; Klein, A. Twenty-four-hour urine osmolality as a physiological index of adequate water intake. *Dis. Markers* **2015**, *2015*, 231063. [CrossRef] [PubMed]
39. McKenzie, A.L.; Muñoz, C.X.; Armstrong, L.E. Accuracy of urine color to detect equal to or greater than 2% body mass loss in men. *J Athl. Train* **2015**, *50*, 1306–1309. [CrossRef] [PubMed]
40. Romano, G.; Bortolotti, N.; Falleti, E.; Favret, G.; Gonano, F.; Bartoli, G.E. The influence of furosemide on free water clearance. *Panminerva. Med.* **1999**, *41*, 103–108. [PubMed]

41. Armstrong, L.E.; Johnson, E.C.; McKenzie, A.L.; Muñoz, C.X. Interpreting common hydration biomarkers on the basis of solute and water excretion. *Eur. J. Clin. Nutr.* **2013**, *67*, 249–253. [CrossRef] [PubMed]
42. Armstrong, L.E.; Johnson, E.C.; Ganio, M.S.; Judelson, D.A.; Vingren, J.L.; Kupchak, B.R.; Kunces, L.J.; Muñoz, C.X.; McKenzie, A.L.; Williamson, K.H. Effective body water and body mass changes during summer ultra-endurance road cycling. *J. Sports Sci.* **2015**, *33*, 125–135. [CrossRef] [PubMed]
43. Maughan, R.J.; Shirreffs, S.M.; Merson, S.J.; Horswill, C.A. Fluid and electrolyte balance in elite male football (soccer) players training in a cool environment. *J. Sports Sci.* **2005**, *23*, 73–79. [CrossRef] [PubMed]
44. Rehrer, N.J.; Burke, L.M. Sweat losses during various sports. *Aust. J. Nutr. Diet.* **1996**, *53*, S13–S16.
45. Adolph, E.F. *Physiology of Man in the Desert*; Adolf, E.F., Ed.; Interscience Pub.: Cummings Park, MA, USA, 1947.
46. Cheuvront, S.N.; Fraser, C.G.; Kenefick, R.W.; Ely, B.R.; Sawka, M.N. Reference change values for monitoring dehydration. *Clin. Chem. Lab. Med.* **2011**, *49*, 1033–1037. [CrossRef] [PubMed]
47. Cheuvront, S.N.; Ely, B.R.; Kenefick, R.W.; Sawka, M.N. Biological variation and diagnostic accuracy of dehydration assessment markers. *Am. J. Clin. Nutr.* **2010**, *92*, 565–573. [CrossRef] [PubMed]
48. Cheuvront, S.N.; Kenefick, R.W. Dehydration: Physiology, assessment, and performance effects. *Compr Physiol* **2014**, *4*, 257–285. [PubMed]
49. Racette, S.B.; Schoeller, D.A.; Luke, A.H.; Shay, K.; Hnilicka, J.; Kushner, R.F. Relative dilution spaces of ^{2}H- and ^{18}O-labeled water in humans. *Am. J. Physiol.* **1994**, *267*, E585–E590. [CrossRef] [PubMed]
50. Armstrong, L.E.; Maresh, C.M.; Castellani, J.; Bergeron, M.; Kenefick, R.; La Gasse, K.; Riebe, D. Urinary indices of hydration status. *Int. J. Sport Nutr.* **1994**, *4*, 265–279. [CrossRef] [PubMed]
51. Johnson, E.C.; Muñoz, C.X.; Le Bellego, L.; Klein, A.; Casa, D.J.; Maresh, C.M.; Armstrong, L.E. Markers of the hydration process during fluid volume modification in women with habitual high or low daily fluid intakes. *Eur. J. Appl. Physiol.* **2015**, *115*, 1067–1074. [CrossRef]
52. Maughan, R.J.; Shirreffs, S.M.; Leiper, J.B. Errors in the estimation of hydration status from changes in body mass. *J. Sports Sci.* **2007**, *25*, 797–804. [CrossRef]
53. Hoyt, R.W.; Honig, A. Environmental influences on body fluid balance during exercise: Altitude. In *Body Fluid Balance: Exercise and Sport*; Buskirk, E., Puhl, S.M., Eds.; CRC: Boca Raton, FL, USA, 1996; pp. 183–196.
54. Shore, A.C.; Markandu, N.D.; Sagnella, G.A.; Singer, D.R.; Forsling, M.L.; Buckley, M.G.; Sugden, A.L.; MacGregor, G.A. Endocrine and renal response to water loading and water restriction in normal man. *Clin. Sci.* **1988**, *75*, 171–177. [CrossRef]
55. Miles, B.E.; Paton, A.; De Wardener, H.E. Maximum urine concentration. *Br. Med. J.* **1954**, *2*, 901–905. [CrossRef] [PubMed]
56. Armstrong, L.E. Assessing hydration status: The elusive gold standard. *J. Am. Coll. Nutr.* **2007**, *26*, 575s–584s. [CrossRef] [PubMed]
57. McKenzie, A.L.; Perrier, E.T.; Guelinckx, I.; Kavouras, S.A.; Aerni, G.; Lee, E.C.; Volek, J.S.; Maresh, C.M.; Armstrong, L.E. Relationships between hydration biomarkers and total fluid intake in pregnant and lactating women. *Eur. J. Nutr.* **2017**, *56*, 2161–2170. [CrossRef] [PubMed]
58. Grandjean, A.C.; Reimers, K.J.; Haven, M.C.; Curtis, G.L. The effect on hydration of two diets, one with and one without plain water. *J. Am. Coll. Nutr.* **2003**, *22*, 165–173. [CrossRef]
59. Tucker, M.A.; Ganio, M.S.; Adams, J.D.; Brown, L.A.; Ridings, C.B.; Burchfield, J.M.; Robinson, F.B.; McDermott, J.L.; Schreiber, B.A.; Moyen, N.E.; et al. Hydration status over 24-H is not affected by ingested beverage composition. *J. Am. Coll. Nutr.* **2015**, *34*, 318–327. [CrossRef] [PubMed]
60. Popkin, B.M.; Armstrong, L.E.; Bray, G.M.; Caballero, B.; Frei, B.; Willett, W.C. A new proposed guidance system for beverage consumption in the United States. *Am. J. Clin. Nutr.* **2006**, *83*, 529–542. [CrossRef]
61. Rolls, B.J.; Phillips, P.A. Aging and disturbances of thirst and fluid balance. *Nutr. Rev.* **1990**, *48*, 137–144. [CrossRef] [PubMed]
62. Davison, J.M.; Gilmore, E.A.; Durr, J.; Robertson, G.L.; Lindheimer, M.D. Altered osmotic thresholds for vasopressin secretion and thirst in human pregnancy. *Am. J. Physiol.* **1984**, *246*, F105–F109. [CrossRef] [PubMed]
63. Geelen, G.; Keil, L.C.; Kravik, S.E.; Wade, C.E.; Thrasher, T.N.; Barnes, P.R.; Pyka, G.; Nesvig, C.; Greenleaf, J.E. Inhibition of plasma vasopressin after drinking in dehydrated humans. *Am. J. Physiol.* **1984**, *247*, R968–R971. [CrossRef] [PubMed]

64. Stookey, J.D.; Hamer, J.; Killilea, D.W. Change in hydration indices associated with an increase in total water intake of more than 0.5 L/day, sustained over 4 weeks, in healthy young men with initial total water intake below 2 L/day. *Physiol. Rep.* **2017**. [CrossRef]
65. Silverthorn, D.U. *Human Physiology: An integrated approach*, 5th ed.; Silverthorn, D.U., Ed.; Pearson/Benjamin Cummings: San Franciso, CA, USA, 2009.
66. Armstrong, L.E.; Maughan, R.J.; Senay, L.C.; Shirreffs, S.M. Limitations to the use of plasma osmolality as a hydration biomarker. *Am. J. Clin. Nutr.* **2013**, *98*, 503–504. [CrossRef]
67. Sawka, M.N.; Montain, S.J.; Latzka, W.A. Body fluid balance during exercise-heat exposure. In *Body Fluid Balance: Exercise and Sport*; CRC Press: Boca Raton, FL, USA, 1996; pp. 139–157.
68. Sollanek, K.J.; Kenefick, R.W.; Cheuvront, S.N.; Axtell, R.S. Potential impact of a 500-mL water bolus and body mass on plasma osmolality dilution. *Eur. J. Appl. Physiol.* **2011**, *111*, 1999–2004. [CrossRef]
69. Bankir, L.; Bichet, D.G.; Morgenthaler, N.G. Vasopressin: Physiology, assessment and osmosensation. *J. Intern. Med.* **2017**, *282*, 284–297. [CrossRef] [PubMed]
70. Moses, A.M.; Miller, M. Osmotic threshold for vasopressin release as determined by saline infusion and by dehydration. *Neuroendocrinology* **1971**, *7*, 219–226. [CrossRef] [PubMed]
71. Robertson, G.L.; Mahr, E.A.; Athar, S.; Sinha, T. Development and clinical application of a new method for the radioimmunoassay of arginine vasopressin in human plasma. *J. Clin. Invest.* **1973**, *52*, 2340–2352. [CrossRef] [PubMed]
72. Robertson, G.L.; Shelton, R.L.; Athar, S. The osmoregulation of vasopressin. *Kidney Int.* **1976**, *10*, 25–37. [CrossRef] [PubMed]
73. Zerbe, R.L.; Robertson, G.L. Osmoregulation of thirst and vasopressin secretion in human subjects: Effect of various solutes. *Am. J. Physiol.* **1983**, *244*, E607–E614. [CrossRef] [PubMed]
74. Thompson, C.J.; Bland, J.; Burd, J.; Baylis, P.H. The osmotic thresholds for thirst and vasopressin release are similar in healthy man. *Clin. Sci.* **1986**, *71*, 651–656. [CrossRef] [PubMed]
75. Thompson, C.J.; Davis, S.N.; Butler, P.C.; Charlton, J.A.; Baylis, P.H. Osmoregulation of thirst and vasopressin secretion in insulin-dependent diabetes mellitus. *Clin. Sci.* **1988**, *74*, 599–606. [CrossRef] [PubMed]
76. Thompson, C.J.; Edwards, C.R.W.; Baylis, P.H. Osmotic and non-osmotic regulation of thirst and vasopressin secretion in patients with compulsive water drinking. *Clin. Endocrinol.* **1991**, *35*, 221–228. [CrossRef]
77. Zerbe, R.L.; Miller, J.Z.; Robertson, G.L. The reproducibility and heritability of individual differences in osmoregulatory function in normal human subjects. *J. Lab. Clin. Med.* **1991**, *117*, 51–59.
78. Vokes, T. Water homeostasis. *Annu. Rev. Nutr.* **1987**, *7*, 383–406. [CrossRef]
79. Halter, J.B.; Goldberg, A.P.; Robertson, G.L.; Porte, D., Jr. Selective osmoreceptor dysfunction in the syndrome of chronic hypernatremia. *J. Clin. Endocrinol. MeTable* **1977**, *44*, 609–616. [CrossRef] [PubMed]
80. Hochberg, Z.; Moses, A.M.; Miller, M.; Benderli, A.; Richman, R.A. Altered osmotic threshold for vasopressin release and impaired thirst sensation: Additional abnormalities in Kallmann's syndrome. *J. Clin. Endocrinol. Metab.* **1982**, *55*, 779–782. [CrossRef] [PubMed]
81. Katz, F.H.; Smith, J.A.; Lock, J.P.; Loeffel, D.E. Plasma vasopressin variation and renin activity in normal active humans. *Horm. Res.* **1979**, *10*, 289–302. [CrossRef] [PubMed]
82. Melander, O. Vasopressin: Novel roles for a new hormone-Emerging therapies in cardiometabolic and renal diseases. *J. Intern. Med.* **2017**, *282*, 281–283. [CrossRef] [PubMed]
83. Moses, A.M.; Miller, M.; Streeten, D.H. Quantitative influence of blood volume expansion on the osmotic threshold for vasopressin release. *J. Clin. Endocrinol. Metab.* **1967**, *27*, 655–662. [CrossRef] [PubMed]
84. Robertson, G.L.; Athar, S. The interaction of blood osmolality and blood volume in regulating plasma vasopressin in man. *J. Clin. Endocrinol. Metab.* **1976**, *42*, 613–620. [CrossRef] [PubMed]
85. Schrier, R.W.; Berl, T.; Anderson, R.J. Osmotic and nonosmotic control of vasopressin release. *Am. J. Physiol.* **1979**, *236*, F321–F332. [CrossRef] [PubMed]
86. Zerbe, R.L.; Robertson, G.L. Osmotic and nonosmotic regulation of thirst and vasopressin secretion. In *Clinical Disorders of Fluid and Electrolyte Metabolism*, 5th ed.; Narins, R., Ed.; McGraw Hill: New York, NY, USA, 1994; Volume 5, pp. 81–100.
87. Spruce, B.A.; Baylis, P.H.; Burd, J.; Watson, M.J. Variation in osmoregulation of arginine vasopressin during the human menstrual cycle. *Clin. Endocrinol.* **1985**, *22*, 37–42. [CrossRef]
88. Phillips, P.A.; Rolls, B.J.; Ledingham, J.G.; Forsling, M.L.; Morton, J.J.; Crowe, M.J.; Wollner, L. Reduced thirst after water deprivation in healthy elderly men. *N. Engl. J. Med.* **1984**, *311*, 753–759. [CrossRef]

89. Kenney, W.L.; Chiu, P. Influence of age on thirst and fluid intake. *Med. Sci. Sports Exerc.* **2001**, *33*, 1524–1532. [CrossRef]
90. Davies, I.; O'Neill, P.A.; McLean, K.A.; Catania, J.; Bennett, D. Age-associated alterations in thirst and arginine vasopressin in response to a water or sodium load. *Age Ageing* **1995**, *24*, 151–159. [CrossRef]
91. Stachenfeld, N.S.; DiPietro, L.; Nadel, E.R.; Mack, G.W. Mechanism of attenuated thirst in aging: Role of central volume receptors. *Am. J. Physiol.* **1997**, *272*, R148–R157. [CrossRef] [PubMed]
92. Farrell, M.J.; Zamarripa, F.; Shade, R.; Phillips, P.A.; McKinley, M.; Fox, P.T.; Blair-West, J.; Denton, D.A.; Egan, G.F. Effect of aging on regional cerebral blood flow responses associated with osmotic thirst and its satiation by water drinking: A PET study. *Proc. Natl. Acad. Sci. U.S.A.* **2008**, *8*, 382–387. [CrossRef]
93. Morgenthaler, N.G.; Struck, J.; Jochberger, S.; Dünser, M.W. Copeptin: Clinical use of a new biomarker. *Trends Endocrinol. Metab.* **2008**, *19*, 43–49. [CrossRef]
94. Katan, M.; Christ-Crain, M. The stress hormone copeptin: A new prognostic biomarker in acute illness. *Swiss Med. Wkly.* **2010**, *140*, w13101. [CrossRef] [PubMed]
95. Munro, A.H.G.; Crompton, G.K. Inappropriate antidiuretic hormone secretion in oat-cell carcinoma of bronchus Aggravation of hyponatraemia by intravenous cyclophosphamide. *Thorax* **1972**, *27*, 40–642. [CrossRef]
96. Thornton, S.N. Angiotensin, the hypovolaemia hormone, aggravates hypertension, obesity, diabetes and cancer. *J. Intern. Med.* **2009**, *265*, 616–617. [CrossRef]
97. Eric, L. Bittman Vasopressin: More than just an output of the circadian pacemaker? Focus on "Vasopressin receptor V1a regulates circadian rhythms of locomotor activity and expression of clock-controlled genes in the suprachiasmatic nuclei". *Am. J. Physiol. Regul. Integr. Comp. Physiol.* **2009**, *296*, R821–R823.
98. Morgenthaler, N.G.; Struck, J.; Alonso, C.; Bergmann, A. Assay for the measurement of copeptin, a stable peptide derived from the precursor of vasopressin. *Clin. Chem.* **2006**, *52*, 112–119. [CrossRef]
99. Roussel, R.; Fezeu, L.; Marre, M.; Velho, G.; Fumeron, F.; Jungers, P.; Lantieri, O.; Balkau, B.; Bouby, N.; Bankir, L.; et al. Comparison between copeptin and vasopressin in a population from the community and in people with chronic kidney disease. *J. Clin. Endocrinol. Metab.* **2014**, *99*, 4656–4663. [CrossRef]
100. Morgenthaler, N.G. Copeptin: A biomarker of cardiovascular and renal function. *Congest. Heart Fail.* **2010**, *16*, S37–S44. [CrossRef] [PubMed]
101. Balanescu, S.; Kopp, P.; Gaskill, M.B.; Morgenthaler, N.G.; Schindler, C.; Rutishauser, J. Correlation of plasma copeptin and vasopressin concentrations in hypo-, iso-, and hyperosmolar States. *J. Clin. Endocrinol. Metab.* **2011**, *96*, 1046–1052. [CrossRef] [PubMed]
102. Westermann, I.; Dünser, M.W.; Haas, T.; Jochberger, S.; Luckner, G.; Mayr, V.D.; Wenzel, V.; Stadlbauer, K.H.; Innerhofer, P.; Morgenthaler, N.; et al. Endogenous vasopressin and copeptin response in multiple trauma patients. *Shock* **2007**, *28*, 644–649. [CrossRef] [PubMed]
103. Ettema, E.M.; Heida, J.; Casteleijn, N.F.; Boesten, L.; Westerhuis, R.; Gaillard, C.; Gansevoort, R.T.; Franssen, C.F.M.; Zittema, D. The effect of renal function and hemodialysis treatment on plasma vasopressin and copeptin levels. *Kidney Int. Rep.* **2017**, *2*, 410–419. [CrossRef] [PubMed]
104. Clark, W.F.; Sontrop, J.M.; Huang, S.H.; Gallo, K.; Moist, L.; House, A.A.; Cuerden, M.S.; Weir, M.A.; Bagga, A.; Brimble, S.; et al. Effect of coaching to increase water intake on kidney function decline in adults with chronic kidney disease: The CKD WIT randomized clinical trial. *JAMA* **2018**, *319*, 1870–1879. [CrossRef] [PubMed]
105. Enhörning, S.; Tasevska, I.; Roussel, R.; Bouby, N.; Persson, M.; Burri, P.; Bankir, L.; Melander, O. Effects of hydration on plasma copeptin, glycemia and gluco-regulatory hormones: A water intervention in humans. *Eur J. Nutr.* **2017**. [CrossRef]
106. Balling, L.; Gustafsson, F. Copeptin as a biomarker in heart failure. *Biomark Med.* **2014**, *8*, 841–854. [CrossRef]
107. Szinnai, G.; Morgenthaler, N.G.; Berneis, K.; Struck, J.; Muller, B.; Keller, U.; Christ-Crain, M. Changes in plasma copeptin, the c-terminal portion of arginine vasopressin during water deprivation and excess in healthy subjects. *J. Clin. Endocrinol. Metab.* **2007**, *92*, 3973–3978. [CrossRef]
108. Valtin, H. "Drink at least eight glasses of water a day." Really? Is there scientific evidence for "8 × 8"? *Am. J. Physiol. Regul. Integr. Comp. Physiol.* **2002**, *283*, R993–R1004. [CrossRef]
109. Gibson, S.; Shirreffs, S.M. Beverage consumption habits "24/7" among British adults: Association with total water intake and energy intake. *Nutr. J.* **2013**, *12*, 9. [CrossRef]

110. Nissensohn, M.; Sánchez-Villegas, A.; Ortega, R.M.; Aranceta-Bartrina, J.; Gil, A.; Gonzalez-Gross, M.; Varela-Moreiras, G.; Serra-Majem, L. Beverage consumption habits and association with total water and energy intakes in the Spanish Population: Findings of the ANIBES study. *Nutrients* **2016**, *8*, 232. [CrossRef]
111. Chang, A.; Kramer, H. Fluid intake for kidney disease prevention: An urban myth? *Clin. J. Am. Soc. Nephrol.* **2011**, *6*, 2558–2560. [CrossRef] [PubMed]
112. Bouby, N.; Clark, W.F.; Roussel, R.; Taveau, C.; Wang, C.J. Hydration and kidney health. *Obes. Facts.* **2014**, *7*, 19–32. [CrossRef] [PubMed]
113. Bankir, L.; Bouby, N.; Ritz, E. Vasopressin: A novel target for the prevention and retardation of kidney disease? *Nat. Rev. Nephrol.* **2013**, *9*, 223–239. [CrossRef]
114. Staub, D.; Morgenthaler, N.G.; Buser, C.; Breidthardt, T.; Potocki, M.; Noveanu, M.; Reichlin, T.; Bergmann, A.; Mueller, C. Use of copeptin in the detection of myocardial ischemia. *Clin. Chim. Acta* **2009**, *399*, 69–73. [CrossRef]
115. Schrier, R.W.; Masoumi, A.; Elhassan, E. Role of vasopressin and vasopressin receptor antagonists in type I cardiorenal syndrome. *Blood Purif.* **2009**, *27*, 28–32. [CrossRef] [PubMed]
116. Decaux, G.; Soupart, A.; Vassart, G. Non-peptide arginine-vasopressin antagonists: The vaptans. *Lancet* **2008**, *371*, 1624–1632. [CrossRef]
117. Melander, O. Vasopressin, from regulator to disease predictor for diabetes and cardiometabolic risk. *Ann. Nutr. Metab.* **2016**, *68*, 24–28. [CrossRef]
118. Armstrong, L.E. Challenges of linking chronic dehydration and fluid consumption to health outcomes. *Nutr. Rev.* **2012**, *70*, S121–S127. [CrossRef]
119. Enhörning, S.; Bankir, L.; Bouby, N.; Struck, J.; Hedblad, B.; Persson, M.; Morgenthaler, N.G.; Nilsson, P.M.; Melander, O. Copeptin, a marker of vasopressin, in abdominal obesity, diabetes and microalbuminuria: The prospective Malmo Diet and Cancer Study cardiovascular cohort. *Int. J. Obes.* **2013**, *37*, 598–603.
120. Enhörning, S.; Hedblad, B.; Nilsson, P.M.; Engström, G.; Melander, O. Copeptin is an independent predictor of diabetic heart disease and death. *Am. Heart J.* **2015**, *169*, 549–556. [CrossRef]
121. Tasevska, I.; Enhörning, S.; Christensson, A.; Persson, M.; Nilsson, P.M.; Melander, O. Increased levels of copeptin, a surrogate marker of arginine vasopressin, are associated with an increased risk of chronic kidney disease in a general population. *Am. J. Nephrol.* **2016**, *44*, 22–28. [CrossRef]
122. Velho, G.; El Boustany, R.; Lefèvre, G.; Mohammedi, K.; Fumeron, F.; Potier, L.; Bankir, L.; Bouby, N.; Hadjadj, S.; Marre, M.; et al. Plasma Copeptin, Kidney Outcomes, Ischemic Heart Disease, and All-Cause Mortality in People With Long-standing Type 1 Diabetes. *Diabetes Care* **2016**, *39*, 2288–2295. [CrossRef]
123. Borghi, L.; Meschi, T.; Amato, F.; Briganti, A.; Novarini, A.; Giannini, A. Urinary volume, water and recurrences in idiopathic calcium nephrolithiasis: A 5-year randomized prospective study. *J. Urol.* **1996**, *155*, 839–843. [CrossRef]
124. Borghi, L.; Meschi, T.; Schianchi, T.; Allegri, F.; Guerra, A.; Maggiore, U.; Novarini, A. Medical treatment of nephrolithiasis. *Endocrinol. Metab. Clin. North Am.* **2002**, *31*, 1051–1064. [CrossRef]
125. Borghi, L.; Meschi, T.; Schianchi, T.; Briganti, A.; Guerra, A.; Allegri, F.; Novarini, A. Urine volume: Stone risk factor and preventive measure. *Nephron* **1999**, *81*, 31–37. [CrossRef]
126. Siener, R.; Hesse, A. Fluid intake and epidemiology of urolithiasis. *Eur. J. Clin. Nutr.* **2003**, *57*, S47–S51. [CrossRef]
127. Siener, R.; Schade, N.; Nicolay, C.; von Unruh, G.E.; Hesse, A. The efficacy of dietary intervention on urinary risk factors for stone formation in recurrent calcium oxalate stone patients. *J. Urol.* **2005**, *173*, 1601–1605. [CrossRef]
128. Wenzel, U.O.; Hebert, L.A.; Stahl, R.A.; Krenz, I. My doctor said I should drink a lot! Recommendations for fluid intake in patients with chronic kidney disease. *Clin. J. Am. Soc. Nephrol.* **2006**, *1*, 344–346. [CrossRef]
129. Wang, C.J.; Grantham, J.J.; Wetmore, J.B. The medicinal use of water in renal disease. *Kidney Int.* **2013**, *84*, 45–53. [CrossRef]
130. Clark, W.F.; Sontrop, J.M.; Huang, S.H.; Moist, L.; Bouby, N.; Bankir, L. Hydration and Chronic Kidney Disease Progression: A Critical Review of the Evidence. *Am. J. Nephrol.* **2016**, *43*, 281–292. [CrossRef]
131. Sontrop, J.M.; Dixon, S.N.; Garg, A.X.; Buendia-Jimenez, I.; Dohein, O.; Huang, S.H.; Clark, W.F. Association between water intake, chronic kidney disease, and cardiovascular disease: A cross-sectional analysis of NHANES data. *Am. J. Nephrol.* **2013**, *37*, 434–442. [CrossRef]
132. Farini, F. Diabete insipido ed opoterapia. *Gazz. Osped. Clin.* **1913**, *34*, 1135–1139.

133. Ragnarsson, U. The nobel trail of Vincent du Vigneaud. *J. Pept. Sci.* **2007**, *13*, 431–433. [CrossRef]
134. Zerbe, R.L.; Vinicor, F.; Robertson, G.L. Plasma vasopressin in uncontrolled diabetes mellitus. *Diabetes* **1979**, *28*, 503–508. [CrossRef]
135. Enhörning, S.; Wang, T.J.; Nilsson, P.M.; Almgren, P.; Hedblad, B.; Berglund, G.; Struck, J.; Morgenthaler, N.G.; Bergmann, A.; Lindholm, E.; et al. Plasma copeptin and the risk of diabetes mellitus. *Circulation* **2010**, *121*, 2102–2108.
136. Saleem, U.; Khaleghi, M.; Morgenthaler, N.G.; Bergmann, A.; Struck, J.; Mosley, T.H., Jr.; Kullo, I.J. Plasma carboxy-terminal provasopressin (copeptin): A novel marker of insulin resistance and metabolic syndrome. *J. Clin. Endocrinol. Metab.* **2009**, *94*, 2558–2564. [CrossRef]
137. Roussel, R.; Fezeu, L.; Bouby, N.; Balkau, B.; Lantieri, O.; Alhenc-Gelas, F.; Marre, M.; Bankir, L. Low water intake and risk for new-onset hyperglycemia. *Diabetes Care* **2011**, *34*, 2551–2554. [CrossRef]
138. Nielsen, S.; Chou, C.L.; Marples, D.; Christensen, E.I.; Kishore, B.K.; Knepper, M.A. Vasopressin increases water permeability of kidney collecting duct by inducing translocation of aquaporin-CD water channels to plasma membrane. *Proc. Natl. Acad. Sci. USA* **1995**, *92*, 1013–1017. [CrossRef]
139. Nakamura, K.; Velho, G.; Bouby, N. Vasopressin and metabolic disorders: Translation from experimental models to clinical use. *J. Intern. Med.* **2017**, *282*, 298–309. [CrossRef]
140. Taveau, C.; Chollet, C.; Bichet, D.G.; Velho, G.; Guillon, G.; Corbani, M.; Roussel, R.; Bankir, L.; Melander, O.; Bouby, N. Acute and chronic hyperglycemic effects of vasopressin in normal rats: Involvement of V1A receptors. *Am. J. Physiol. Endocrinol. Metab.* **2017**, *312*, E127–E135. [CrossRef] [PubMed]
141. Taveau, C.; Chollet, C.; Waeckel, L.; Desposito, D.; Bichet, D.G.; Arthus, M.F.; Magnan, C.; Philippe, E.; Paradis, V.; Foufelle, F.; et al. Vasopressin and hydration play a major role in the development of glucose intolerance and hepatic steatosis in obese rats. *Diabetologia* **2015**, *58*, 1081–1090. [CrossRef] [PubMed]
142. Enhörning, S.; Leosdottir, M.; Wallstrom, P.; Gullberg, B.; Berglund, G.; Wirfalt, E.; Melander, O. Relation between human vasopressin 1a gene variance, fat intake, and diabetes. *Am. J. Clin. Nutr.* **2009**, *89*, 400–406. [CrossRef] [PubMed]
143. Kuo, T.; McQueen, A.; Chen, T.C.; Wang, J.C. Regulation of glucose homeostasis by glucocorticoids. *Adv. Exp. Med. Biol.* **2015**, *872*, 99–126.
144. Johnson, E.C.; Bardis, C.N.; Jansen, L.T.; Adams, J.D.; Kirkland, T.W.; Kavouras, S.A. Reduced water intake deteriorates glucose regulation in patients with type 2 diabetes. *Nutr. Res.* **2017**, *43*, 25–32. [CrossRef]

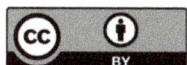

© 2018 by the authors. Licensee MDPI, Basel, Switzerland. This article is an open access article distributed under the terms and conditions of the Creative Commons Attribution (CC BY) license (http://creativecommons.org/licenses/by/4.0/).

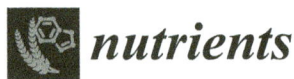

Article

The Utility of Thirst as a Measure of Hydration Status Following Exercise-Induced Dehydration

William M. Adams [1],*, Lesley W. Vandermark [2], Luke N. Belval [3] and Douglas J. Casa [4]

1. Department of Kinesiology, University of North Carolina at Greensboro, 1408 Walker Avenue, 237L Coleman Building, Greensboro, NC 27412, USA
2. Department of Health, Human Performance, & Recreation, University of Arkansas, HPER 310D, Fayetteville, AR 72701, USA; lwvander@uark.edu
3. Institute for Exercise and Environmental Medicine, Texas Health Presbyterian Hospital Dallas and University of Texas Southwestern Medical Center, 7232 Greenville Ave, Dallas, TX 75231, USA; LukeBelval@texashealth.org
4. Korey Stringer Institute, Human Performance Laboratory, Department of Kinesiology, University of Connecticut, 2095 Hillside Rd, Unit 1110, Storrs, CT 06269, USA; douglas.casa@uconn.edu
* Correspondence: wmadams@uncg.edu; Tel.: +1-336-256-1455; Fax: +1-336-334-3238

Received: 20 September 2019; Accepted: 1 November 2019; Published: 7 November 2019

Abstract: The purpose of this study was to examine the perception of thirst as a marker of hydration status following prolonged exercise in the heat. Twelve men (mean ± SD; age, 23 ± 4 y; body mass, 81.4 ± 9.9 kg; height, 182 ± 9 cm; body fat, 14.3% ± 4.7%) completed two 180 min bouts of exercise on a motorized treadmill in a hot environment (35.2 ± 0.6 °C; RH, 30.0 ± 5.4%), followed by a 60 min recovery period. Participants completed a euhydrated (EUH) and hypohydrated (HYPO) trial. During recovery, participants were randomly assigned to either fluid replacement (EUH$_{FL}$ and HYPO$_{FL}$; 10 min ad libitum consumption) or no fluid replacement (EUH$_{NF}$ and HYPO$_{NF}$). Thirst was measured using both a nine-point scale and separate visual analog scales. The percent of body mass loss (%BML) was significantly greater immediately post exercise in HYPO (HYPO$_{FL}$, 3.0% ± 1.2%; HYPO$_{NF}$, 2.6% ± 0.6%) compared to EUH (EUH$_{FL}$, 0.2% ± 0.7%; EUH$_{NF}$, 0.6% ± 0.5%) trials ($p < 0.001$). Following recovery, there were no differences in %BML between HYPO$_{FL}$ and HYPO$_{NF}$ ($p > 0.05$) or between EUH$_{FL}$ and EUH$_{NF}$ ($p > 0.05$). Beginning at minute 5 during the recovery period, thirst perception was significantly greater in HYPO$_{NF}$ than EUH$_{FL}$, EUH$_{NF}$, and HYPO$_{FL}$ ($p < 0.05$). A 10 min, ad libitum consumption of fluid post exercise when hypohydrated (%BML > 2%), negated differences in perception of thirst between euhydrated and hypohydrated trials. These results represent a limitation in the utility of thirst in guiding hydration practices.

Keywords: fluid replacement; hypohydration; assessment; perception; exercise

---

1. Introduction

The complexities surrounding the turnover of body water complicates any single measure of hydration status qualifying as a standard for assessment [1]. Methods for assessing hydration status utilize urinary and hematologic measures, among others; however, these methods are not without limitations regarding accuracy and applicability in all settings [1–4]. Furthermore, many of these assessment methods require expensive laboratory instrumentation and/or expertise in these techniques, limiting real-world applicability for all persons.

Thirst, defined as a desire to consume fluids as a result of a body water deficit, is a subjective perception controlled by both neuroendocrine responses to maintain fluid homeostasis [5–7] and psychosocial influences [8]. The physiological onset of thirst, occurring with fluid losses of a magnitude of 1–2% body mass loss [6,9] is influenced by hyperosmolality, hormonal responses (arginine vasopressin

(AVP) and angiotensin II (Ang II)), and peripheral osmoreceptors [10–12], but is highly variable within individuals [5]. In addition, non-homeostatic influences, such as beverage taste, availability, individual drinking habits, and timing with meals, dictate daily fluid intake [8].

Current recommendations advocate for using thirst to guide hydration practices during exercise to reduce the risk of exertional hyponatremia [13]; however, recommendations by the American College of Sports Medicine [14] and the National Athletic Trainers' Association [15] encourage individualized replacement of fluid losses to prevent dehydration-mediated loss of >2% of body mass during exercise. Evidence suggests that relying solely on thirst as a means of replacing fluid losses during exercise, especially in hot environmental conditions, may prevent the full restoration of body water losses, leading to involuntary dehydration [6]. Armstrong et al. [16] has suggested that thirst may provide an inexpensive means of assessing hydration status upon waking in the morning, but differences in thirst perception were negated following the consumption of a bolus of fluid, despite hypohydration equaling 2% body mass loss. Similar findings were observed when ad libitum consumption of water was allowed following high intensity intermittent exercise; however, body water deficits were only 1.3% of body mass [17].

An assessment of thirst's tracking of hydration status has previously been performed during exercise and at rest. However, few studies have investigated the efficacy of thirst as a potential marker of hydration status when a bolus of water was provided following exercise-induced dehydration upon a magnitude of ~3% body mass loss. Therefore, the purpose of this study was to examine the perception of thirst as a marker of hydration status following prolonged exercise in the heat. It was hypothesized that when a bolus of fluid was consumed following exercise-induced dehydration, thirst sensation would be attenuated despite a sustained level of dehydration above the threshold (~2% body mass loss from dehydration) in which thirst is present.

2. Materials and Methods

2.1. Design

Participants completed two testing sessions in a randomized, counter-balanced manner. We randomly assigned participants to testing sessions, designed to manipulate participants' hydration states following exercise: euhydrated (EUH) and hypohydrated (HYPO). The EUH trial consisted of a euhydrated arrival to the laboratory, followed by minimal fluid losses throughout the duration of exercise dictated by participant's individual fluid needs. The HYPO trial was designed to achieve a state of hypohydration of roughly 3% body mass loss and was achieved via 14 h fluid restriction prior to arrival to the laboratory and throughout the bout of exercise. Following exercise, participants completed a 60 min bout of recovery in the heat, where they were randomly allocated to either a fluid replacement group or fluid restriction group. All exercise sessions occurred at the same time of day, ±1 h, and were separated by a minimum of 72 h to minimize the circadian variability of the physiological variables of interest and allow for appropriate recovery from the previous sessions, respectively. Exercise and recovery took place in a climate-controlled environmental chamber (Model 200, Minus-Eleven, Inc., Malden, MA, USA) with conditions being: ambient temperature, 35.2 ± 0.6 °C; RH, 30.0% ± 5.4%; wet bulb globe temperature, 26.6 ± 1.1 °C. Additionally, all exercise sessions took place during the winter months in Connecticut, USA to ensure that none of the participants were heat acclimated.

2.2. Participants

Twelve recreationally active men between the ages of 18 and 35 volunteered to participate in this study (mean ± SD; age, 23 ± 4 y; body mass, 81.4 ± 9.9 kg; height, 182 ± 9 cm; body fat, 14.3% ± 4.7%). All participants reported exercising a minimum of 4–5 d·wk^{-1} for at least 30 min per session. Participants were excluded if they reported any chronic health problems, such as cardiovascular, metabolic, or respiratory disease; current illness or musculoskeletal injury; or a previous history of exertional heat illness within the last 3 y. Participants provided written and informed consent to participate in this study, which was approved by the University of Connecticut's Institutional Review Board (protocol number: H15-154) and in accordance with the Declaration of Helsinki.

2.3. Procedures

Familiarization Session. Prior to the exercise sessions, participants completed a familiarization session for them to become acquainted with the laboratory and testing procedures. The familiarization session was scheduled as close to the scheduled testing session times as possible, to ensure minimal variability in reference hydration values due to circadian rhythm. To ensure participants arrived euhydrated, they were asked to consume 500 mL of water prior to going to bed the night before and upon waking in the morning. Hydration status was measured upon arrival to the laboratory using urine specific gravity ($U_{SG} \leq 1.020$) (refractometer, model A300CL; Atago Inc., Tokyo, Japan) and urine color ($U_{COL} \leq 4$) via urine color chart [18]. Participants arriving to the laboratory for the EUH trial with a $U_{SG} > 1.020$ were instructed to consume an additional 500 mL of fluid prior to the start of exercise. Participants arriving to the laboratory for the HYPO trial with a $U_{SG} > 1.020$ were not provided fluid, as the purpose of the HYPO trial was to induce a state of hypohydration prior to the start of exercise.

Each participant's height was measured using a standard stadiometer and their body fat was calculated via three-site skinfold measurements of the chest, abdomen, and thigh using calibrated calipers (Lange Skinfold Caliper; Beta Technology Inc., Santa Cruz, CA, USA) [19]. Participants were instructed on the insertion of the rectal thermometer (Model 401, Measurement Specialties, Hampton, VA, USA), which was used for the monitoring of body temperature during the exercise sessions. They were also familiarized to the perceptual scales that they were asked about during the exercise sessions: the thirst perception (TH) and thirst sensation scales (TSS), described below.

Each participant's sweat rate was measured to determine their fluid needs during the EUH exercise trial. A nude body mass (NBM) was measured to the nearest 0.1 kg using a calibrated scale (Defender 5000, OHAUS, Parsippany, NJ, USA) before entering the environmental chamber. Upon entering the chamber, they stood for 15 min to become equilibrated to the environmental conditions prior to exercise. Exercise consisted of walking on a motorized treadmill at a speed ranging from 5.6 to 6.4 km·h^{-1} at a 2% gradient for a total of 30 min. Participants were instructed to set a speed equivalent to a "fast walk" that they would be able to sustain for up to 3 h. The speed selected during the familiarization session remained the same for both exercise sessions. Following exercise, participants provided another NBM to determine sweat rate by assessing body mass change. Body water losses were used to quantify the prescribed fluid replacement during exercise of the EUH trial; 0.001 kg equaled 1 mL.

Testing Sessions. For all testing sessions, participants were instructed to conduct their normal daily routine (e.g., exercise, food and fluid intake), so as to not deviate from their individual norm. Participants were asked to consume an additional 500 mL of water the night prior and the morning of the EUH trial to ensure a state of euhydration. For the HYPO trial, participants were asked to restrict fluid intake (including fluid heavy foods) for 14 h prior to their arrival to the laboratory. Participants were scheduled for the same time of day for each of their trials to minimize any effects of circadian rhythms on physiologic function.

Upon arrival to the laboratory for the EUH and HYPO trials, we obtained the following measures; NBM, U_{SG}, and U_{COL}. Following a 15 min equilibration in the environmental chamber, pre-exercise (PRE_{EX}) measures of rectal temperature (T_{REC}), heart rate (HR) (Race Trainer, Timex Group USA, Middlebury, CT, USA), body mass, TH, and TSS were obtained. A blood sample, with participants in a seated position, was also drawn at this time for the assessment of serum osmolality prior to exercise. Participants then began exercise, consisting of six 30 min bouts of exercise, each involving a 25 min walk at the speed at which participants performed the sweat rate assessment test, followed by a 5 min rest. During the 5 min rest period, participants stepped off the treadmill, removed their shoes and t-shirt, toweled off as much as possible and provided a body mass measure to track body mass loss over the course of exercise. Before commencing the next bout of exercise, T_{REC}, HR, RPE, and TH were measured. During the EUH trial, participants consumed equal boluses of water during each 25 min exercise bout at a volume matching their calculated sweat rate for that time period. During the HYPO trial, participants were restricted from water throughout exercise.

Following the 3 h bout of exercise, participants stepped off the treadmill, provided body mass, T_{REC}, HR, TH, and TSS post-exercise ($POST_{EX}$) measures, and sat in a chair to begin a 60 min period of recovery. During recovery, participants were randomly assigned to one of two recovery conditions; fluid replacement (FL; EUH_{FL} and $HYPO_{FL}$) or no fluid replacement (NF; EUH_{NF} and $HYPO_{NF}$). Participants remained in the same recovery group for both trials. For EUH_{FL} and $HYPO_{FL}$ conditions, participants were given a bolus of water equaling their total body mass losses that occurred during exercise. The participants were allotted 10 min to consume the water and were permitted to consume the water ad libitum. After 10 min, any remaining water was taken from the participants and they remained in a seated position for the next 50 min. Following the completion of the recovery portion of the trial, T_{REC} and HR were measured and TH and TSS were assessed for a post-recovery ($POST_{REC}$) time point. Prior to exiting the environmental chamber, a $POST_{REC}$ blood sample was obtained for assessment of serum osmolality. Participants then exited the environmental chamber and provided final NBM, U_{SG}, and U_{COL} measures.

2.4. Thirst Assessment

TH was measured using nine-point (1–9) Likert scale that provided verbal anchors of 1, "Not Thirsty at All"; 3, "A Little Thirsty"; 5, "Moderately Thirsty"; 7, "Very Thirsty"; and 9, "Very, Very Thirsty" [20]. Participants were asked, "How thirsty are you right now?" when shown the scale, and they provided a numerical answer based on their perceived feeling of thirst.

The second measure of thirst assessment, TSS, was measured using a 100 mm visual analog scale, for which participants were asked, "How thirsty do you feel right now?" (not at all thirsty–very thirsty); "How pleasant would it be to drink some water right now?" (very unpleasant–very pleasant); "How dry does your mouth feel right now?" (not at all dry–very dry); "How would you describe the taste in your mouth?" (normal–very unpleasant); "How full does your stomach feel right now?" (not at all full–very full); "How sick to your stomach do you feel right now?" (not at all sick–very sick) [21,22]. All six visual analog scales were on one piece of paper and each 100 mm line was anchored using the aforementioned words/phrases in parentheses above. Participants were asked to mark on each line their responses to each question.

2.5. Hematological Measures

Five milliliters of blood was drawn from an antecubital vein into a collection tube without additive (BD Vacutainer, Becton Dickinson Company, Franklin Lakes, NJ, USA) and allowed to clot at room temperature. Samples were then centrifuged at 3000 rpm at 4 °C and assessed in triplicate for serum osmolality using the freezing point depression method (Model 3320, Advanced Instruments, Norwood, MA, USA).

2.6. Statistical Analysis

All statistical analyses were performed using SPSS Statistical Software version 21 (IBM Corporation, Armonk, NY, USA). Tests for normality were conducted using the Shapiro–Wilk tests with any non-normally distributed data being analyzed by the appropriate non-parametric tests. All values are presented as means ± standard deviations unless otherwise noted. In addition, comparisons between variables are presented as mean differences (MD) and 95% confidence intervals (95%CI). Effect size (ES) was also calculated using Cohen's d, for which d = 0.2 was considered a small effect, d = 0.5 was considered a medium effect, and d = 0.8 was considered a large effect. A priori power analysis (G*Power 3.1, Düsseldorf, DE) computing an F test for repeated measures ANOVA with within–between interaction for two groups (NF and FL) across 20 timepoints with an alpha level of 0.05, power of 0.8, and a medium effect size of d = 0.5 yielded a total sample size of 8. A sample size of 12 (n = 6 were each assigned to each of NF and FL groups) was used to ensure a power of >0.8.

Three-way (condition × trial × time) repeated-measures ANOVAs were used to assess differences in dependent variables (TH, TSS, body mass, serum osmolality, HR, and T_{REC}) between conditions (FL and NF), trials (EUH and HYPO), across time. With significant three-way interactions, follow-up post hoc testing utilizing appropriate two-way ANOVAs were utilized. Significance was set a priori at $p < 0.05$.

Post hoc power analysis comparing TH (comparison of pooled means during recovery) yielded a power-achieved of $\beta = 0.997$, confirming that the sample size selected was appropriate for the analysis. Post hoc power analysis comparing the TSS measures of thirstiness, pleasantness, dryness, taste, fullness, and sickness yielded power measures of $\beta = 0.579$, $\beta = 0.338$, $\beta = 0.516$, $\beta = 0.415$, $\beta = 0.453$, and $\beta = 0.435$, respectively.

3. Results

Figure 1A depicts the change in TH throughout exercise and recovery and Figure 1B depicts the delta change (recovery–exercise) in pooled means for TH. There was a significant three-way interaction for TH between EUH_{FL}, EUH_{NF}, $HYPO_{FL}$, and $HYPO_{NF}$ ($p = 0.015$). Follow-up testing revealed that, during recovery, mean TH was significantly greater in $HYPO_{NF}$ than EUH_{FL} ($p < 0.001$, ES = 6.44), EUH_{NF} ($p < 0.001$, ES = 5.05), and $HYPO_{FL}$ ($p = 0.002$, ES = 3.70) (Figure 1A).

Figure 2 portrays the separate measures assessed in TSS at the PRE_{EX}, $POST_{EX}$, and $POST_{REC}$ time point. There were no significant differences in feelings of thirstiness ($p = 0.052$), pleasantness toward drinking water ($p = 0.211$), dryness in the mouth ($p = 0.072$), taste in the mouth ($p = 0.12$), fullness ($p = 0.099$), and sickness ($p = 0.145$) between trial, recovery condition, and time; however, it can be observed that feelings of thirstiness and dryness in the mouth trended toward significance in this three-way interaction. Despite no significant three-way interactions, there were significant trial × time interactions for thirstiness ($p = 0.004$), pleasantness in the mouth ($p = 0.034$), dryness in the mouth ($p = 0.002$), and fullness ($p = 0.034$). Specifically, thirstiness was significantly greater at $POST_{EX}$ (ES = 5.81) and $POST_{REC}$ (ES = 3.48) in the HYPO trial ($POST_{EX}$, 69.5 ± 9.0; $POST_{REC}$, 51.9 ± 14.1) than EUH trial ($POST_{EX}$, 23.1 ± 6.8; $POST_{REC}$, 15.5 ± 4.4). Pleasantness in the mouth was significantly greater (greater unpleasant feeling) at $POST_{EX}$ (ES = 8.01) and $POST_{REC}$ (ES = 3.95) in the HYPO trial ($POST_{EX}$, 84.9 ± 5.9; $POST_{REC}$, 67.3 ± 10.6) than in the EUH trial ($POST_{EX}$, 36.4 ± 6.2; $POST_{REC}$, 32.1 ± 6.8). Dryness in the mouth was significantly greater at $POST_{EX}$ (ES = 6.48) and $POST_{REC}$ (ES = 3.18) in the HYPO trial ($POST_{EX}$, 70.3 ± 5.9; $POST_{REC}$, 60.6 ± 12.3) than in the EUH trial ($POST_{EX}$, 26.2 ± 7.6; $POST_{REC}$, 29.2 ± 6.6). Lastly, participants experienced significantly greater fullness at $POST_{EX}$ (ES = 2.93) in the EUH trial (39.5 ± 9.0) compared to the HYPO trial (16.9 ± 6.1).

The hypohydrated trials ($HYPO_{FL}$ and $HYPO_{NF}$) resulted in significantly greater levels of dehydration at $POST_{EX}$ and $POST_{REC}$ than the euhydrated trials (EUH_{FL} and EUH_{NF}), as measured by the percentage of body mass loss (%BML) ($p < 0.001$) (Table 1). Fluid replacement after exercise did not influence %BML between HYPO trials ($HYPO_{FL}$, 2.1% ± 1.1%; $HYPO_{NF}$, 2.6% ± 0.6%) or EUH trials (EUH_{FL}, 0.2% ± 0.7%; EUH_{NF}, 0.6% ± 0.5%) at $POST_{REC}$, respectively ($p = 0.330$) (Table 1). Serological and urinary hydration measures are shown in Table 2. Changes in T_{REC} ($p = 0.052$) and HR ($p = 0.067$) trended toward statistical significance (Figure 3).

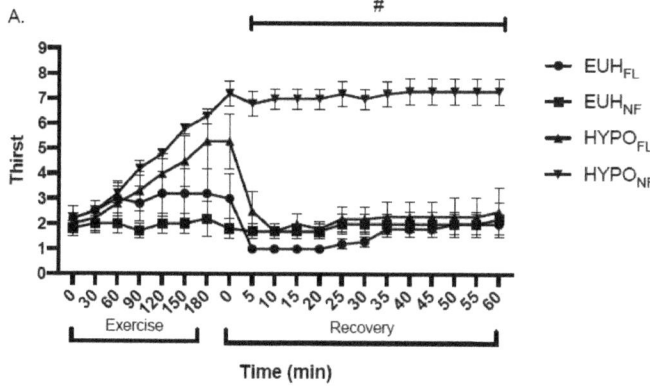

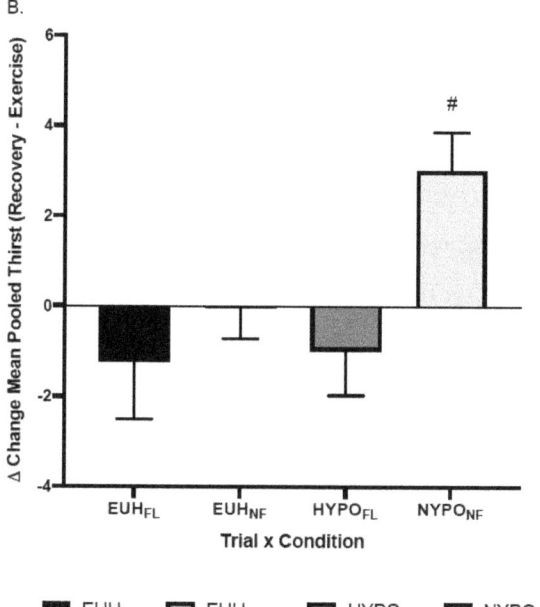

Figure 1. (**A**) Thirst perception throughout exercise and post-exercise recovery and (**B**) delta change (recovery–exercise) of pooled means in thirst perception (TH) by trial × condition. # indicates a significant difference between $HYPO_{FL}$ and $HYPO_{NF}$, EUH_{FL}, and EUH_{NF}, $p < 0.05$. EUH_{FL} = minimized fluid losses during exercise and remaining losses replaced during recovery; EUH_{NF} = minimized fluid losses during exercise and did not replace losses during recovery; $HYPO_{FL}$ = fluid restricted during exercise and losses replaced during recovery; $HYPO_{NF}$ = fluid restricted during exercise and losses not replaced during recovery.

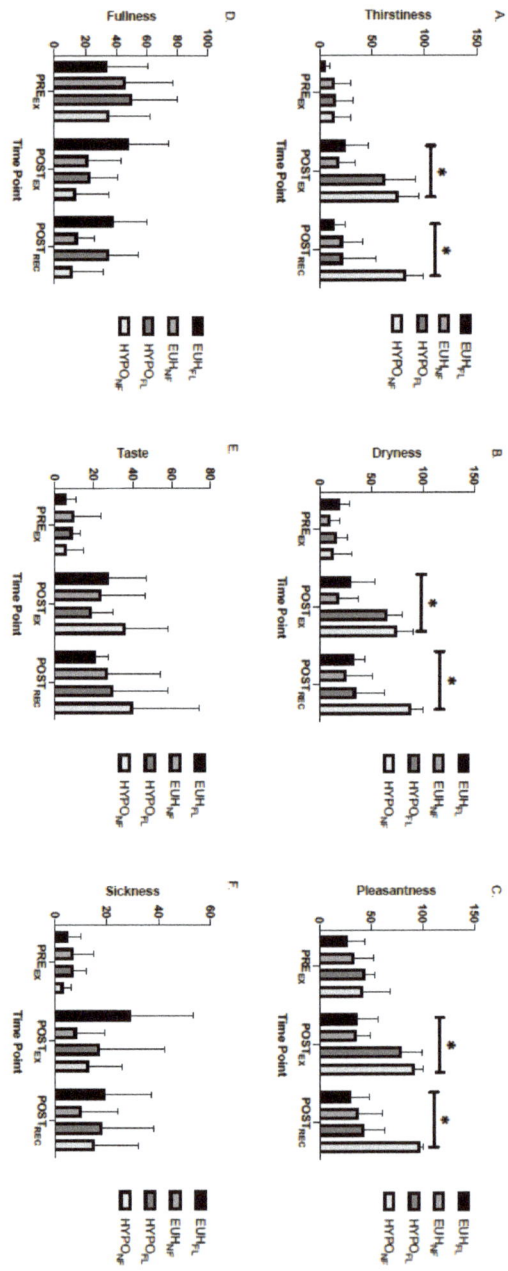

Figure 2. Perceptions of (**A**) thirstiness, (**B**) dryness, (**C**) pleasantness, (**D**) fullness, (**E**) taste, and (**F**) sickness in EUH_{FL} EUH_{NF} $HYPO_{FL}$ and $HYPO_{NF}$ groups. * indicates a significant difference between the HYPO trial ($HYPO_{FL}$ and $HYPO_{NF}$) and EUH trial (EUH_{FL} and EUH_{NF}); $p < 0.05$. EUH_{FL} = minimized fluid losses during exercise and remaining losses replaced during recovery; EUH_{NF} = minimized fluid losses during exercise and did not replace losses during recovery; $HYPO_{FL}$ = fluid restricted during exercise and losses replaced during recovery; $HYPO_{NF}$ = fluid restricted during exercise and losses not replaced during recovery.

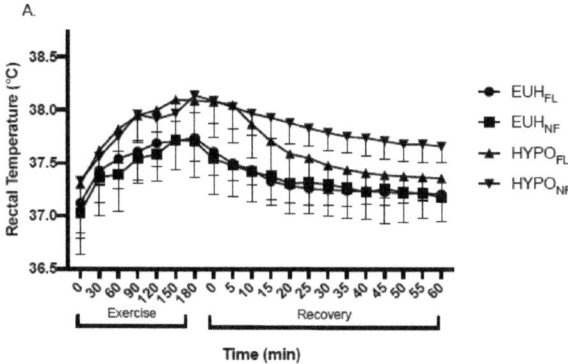

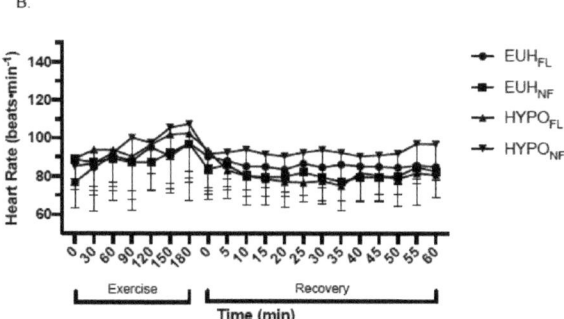

Figure 3. Changes in (**A**) rectal temperature and (**B**) heart rate during exercise and recovery in EUH$_{FL}$, EUH$_{NF}$, HYPO$_{FL}$, and HYPO$_{NF}$ groups. EUH$_{FL}$ = minimized fluid losses during exercise and remaining losses replaced during recovery; EUH$_{NF}$ = minimized fluid losses during exercise and did not replace losses during recovery; HYPO$_{FL}$ = fluid restricted during exercise and losses replaced during recovery; HYPO$_{NF}$ = fluid restricted during exercise and losses not replaced during recovery.

Table 1. Body mass changes by condition.

Condition	PRE$_{EX}$ Mass (kg)	POST$_{EX}$ Mass (kg)	POST$_{EX}$ %BML (%)	POST$_{REC}$ Mass (kg)	POST$_{REC}$ %BML (%)	POST$_{REC}$ Fluid Consumed (mL)	% BML Replaced (%)
EUH$_{FL}$	77.0 ± 10.9	76.8 ± 10.2	0.2 ± 0.7	76.9 ± 11.1	0.2 ± 0.7	337.5 ± 48.3	57.4 ± 13.2
EUH$_{NF}$	85.9 ± 6.3	85.4 ± 6.7	0.6 ± 0.7	85.4 ± 6.3	0.6 ± 0.5	0 ± 0	0 ± 0
HYPO$_{FL}$	76.4 ± 11.3	74.1 ± 11.0	3.0 ± 1.2 $^{\alpha,\beta}$	74.8 ± 11.4	2.1 ± 1.1 $^{\alpha,\beta}$	1100.0 ± 155.0	55.3 ± 15.6
HYPO$_{NF}$	86.4 ± 6.5	84.1 ± 6.1	2.6 ± 0.6 $^{\chi,\delta}$	84.1 ± 6.5	2.6 ± 0.6 $^{\chi,\delta}$	0 ± 0	0 ± 0

α = HYPO$_{FL}$ significantly different than EUH$_{FL}$, $p < 0.05$; β = HYPO$_{FL}$ significantly different than EUH$_{NF}$, $p < 0.05$; χ = HYPO$_{NF}$ significantly different than EUH$_{FL}$, $p < 0.05$; δ = HYPO$_{NF}$ significantly different than EUH$_{NF}$, $p < 0.05$.

Table 2. Serological and urinary hydration variables.

Variable	Condition	PRE$_{EX}$	POST$_{REC}$
Serum Osmolality (mOsm·kg^{-1})	EUH$_{FL}$	295 ± 2	296 ± 3
	EUH$_{NF}$	290 ± 5	291 ± 5
	HYPO$_{FL}$	296 ± 8	310 ± 6 ^{β,*}
	HYPO$_{NF}$	294 ± 3	304 ± 3 ^{δ,*}
Urine Specific Gravity (AU)	EUH$_{FL}$	1.012 ± 0.009	1.009 ± 0.004
	EUH$_{NF}$	1.018 ± 0.005	1.017 ± 0.007
	HYPO$_{FL}$	1.014 ± 0.008	1.017 ± 0.004
	HYPO$_{NF}$	1.021 ± 0.007	1.020 ± 0.005

PRE$_{EX}$, prior to commencement of exercise; POST$_{REC}$, 60 min post exercise. β = HYPO$_{FL}$ significantly different than EUH$_{NF}$, $p < 0.05$; δ = HYPO$_{NF}$ significantly different than EUH$_{NF}$, $p < 0.05$; * = POST significantly greater than PRE, $p < 0.05$.

4. Discussion

This study evaluated the use of thirst as a marker of hydration following exercise-induced dehydration. Subjective sensations of thirst (TH and TSS) were significantly elevated immediately following an exercise bout that induced a level of hypohydration of 2.8% ± 0.9% body mass loss (combined mean of HYPO$_{FL}$ and HYPO$_{NF}$ groups). Our hypothesis was supported in that when HYPO$_{FL}$ was permitted to consume water ad libitum during the initial 10 min of a 60 min bout of recovery following exercise, subjective feelings of thirst (TH) were minimized throughout and at the completion of recovery to levels similar to the EUH$_{FL}$ and EUH$_{NF}$ groups, despite %BML remaining >2% (Figure 1A). Measures of thirstiness and dryness in the mouth, as measured by TSS, approached statistical significance ($p = 0.052$ and $p = 0.072$, respectively), with HYPO$_{FL}$ exhibiting a reduction in thirst and dryness in the mouth following 60 min of recovery (Figure 2).

The role of oropharyngeal receptors in attenuating thirst has been extensively studied in both human [11,17,23–26] and animal models [27–30]. Figaro and Mack [11] showed that oropharyngeal receptors played an immediate role in inhibiting thirst, and thus, fluid intake, without influencing plasma osmolality when fluid was extracted immediately from the stomach after consumption. In addition, Mears et al. [17] found that thirst, which was stimulated by a rise in serum osmolality following a bout of high intensity interval exercise, rapidly declined upon the consumption of fluid immediately after exercise. Thirst also remained elevated when fluid consumption was delayed for 30 min or prohibited at any point during recovery, despite a decline in serum osmolality. Our findings support these results and the role that oropharyngeal receptors play in reducing the thirst sensation, despite a sustained elevation of serum osmolality, in that the sensation of thirst was immediately reduced in HYPO$_{FL}$ once fluid was permitted and remained at levels similar to EUH$_{FL}$ and EUH$_{NF}$ (Figures 1A and 2), despite a sustained elevation in serum osmolality levels compared to baseline (+14 mOsm·kg^{-1}). This is evident in Figure 1B, where the delta change of pooled means for TH between recovery and exercise shows a negative delta change for EUH$_{FL}$, EUH$_{NF}$, and HYPO$_{FL}$ compared to HYPO$_{NF}$; this figure shows that sensations of thirst for the former conditions are lower across the recovery period on average than what appeared during exercise.

Interestingly, unlike the work by Figaro and Mack [11] and Mears et al. [17], we did not see a decline in serum osmolality when ad libitum fluid intake was permitted. We postulate that this may be due to the total volume of water consumed. In the Figaro and Mack [11] and Mears et al. [17] studies, participants replaced ~67–86% and 63–82% of the water lost during exercise, respectively. In our study, participants in HYPO$_{FL}$ only replaced ~55% of what they lost, which may have influenced the amount of water absorbed into the vasculature during recovery. As we did not measure serum osmolality immediately following exercise or throughout the recovery portion of the trial, nor did we measure the amount of fluid absorbed from the gastrointestinal tract during recovery, we are unable to develop a further rationale as to why we did not observe a change in serum osmolality. We postulate that the total volume of water consumed during the initial 10 min of recovery was not large enough to result in a change in serum osmolality.

The role of one's mouth's state may be an important factor when considering fluid replacement following exercise eliciting levels of dehydration that exceed 2% BML, a level of dehydration that has been shown to adversely affect physiological function [31–34] and exercise performance [4,35–37]. Our findings, in support of prior literature [10,21,26], show that individuals will have a reduced drive for consuming fluids once sensations of thirst, dryness in the mouth, and unpleasantness in the mouth are rectified and prior to completing fluid replacement; this incomplete fluid replacement has commonly been termed "involuntary" or "voluntary" dehydration [6,38]. Specifically, in our study, thirst, mouth dryness, and ratings of unpleasantness in the mouth in $HYPO_{FL}$ were lower at $POST_{REC}$ than $POST_{EX}$ (Figure 3), despite a level of hypohydration of 2.1% ± 1.1%, a level of body mass loss where thirst is typically induced [6,9]. Despite not being statistically significant, thirst ($p = 0.052$) and dryness in the mouth ($p = 0.072$) exhibited a large effect for $HYPO_{NF}$ at $POST_{REC}$ when compared to $HYPO_{FL}$ (ES = 7.15 and 6.3, respectively), EUH_{FL} (ES = 7.49 and 6.02, respectively), and EUH_{NF} (ES = 5.6 and 5.61, respectively) conditions.

We observed that within the first 10 min of recovery, participants in $HYPO_{FL}$ consumed approximately 55% of total fluid losses incurred during exercise, which is consistent with prior literature [11,17]. It must be noted, however, that we only permitted participants 10 min to consume water, which may have prevented additional consumption to offset fluid losses. Interestingly, Evans et al. [39] assessed ad libitum intake of fluids at 15 min increments for 2 h following exercise; their findings show that after 15 min of ad libitum fluid consumption, roughly 25–30% of fluid losses were replaced. Speculating as to the reason for this discrepancy, knowledge from the participants of how long they had access to fluid in the current study may have prompted them to consume more fluid than they would have if allotted more time overall to consume fluids. Despite this, we believe that if our participants were permitted to consume water throughout the entire 60 min recovery period, they would not fully replace fluid losses. Work by Maughan et al. [40–42] and Shirreffs et al. [43,44] suggest that following exercise, especially when there is limited time before the next bout, a strategic approach to rapid rehydration based on individual losses must be utilized to optimize the potential for rehydration. Relying solely on thirst alone would not be appropriate in this scenario, especially if fluid losses exceed ~3% of body mass, as shown in our study.

To contextualize the aforementioned into real-world context, allowing participants to consume fluids during the first 10 min of a post-exercise recovery period, may mimic what could occur in a sport. For example, sports such as soccer and rugby, require athletes to perform continuous exercise, with the elite levels of these sports preventing the number of substitutions permitted; this could create a scenario in which athletes enter the half-time portion of a competition (typically 10–15 min in length) hypohydrated to ~2% BML, especially if competition is being performed in hot conditions. If provided ad libitum access to fluids, based on our findings, these athletes would consume fluids to quench their thirst, and if only using thirst as a measure of preparedness for the second half of competition, would enter the latter half of the event hypohydrated to a level that may result in marked performance deficits. While our study did not examine whether thirst would remain attenuated if a second bout of exercise ensued based on the aforementioned example, our findings would support the recommendation that individualized fluid replacement strategies are optimal for minimizing the extent of fluid losses during exercise.

This study is not without limitations. We only tested male participants in this study, which may not be generalizable to females, particularly given the physiological changes that occur during the menstrual cycle that may influence hydration state and thirst [45]. Furthermore, we only permitted participants to consume water ad libitum for a 10 min block of time immediately post exercise. Without permitting ad libitum consumption of water for the entire duration of post-exercise recovery, we were unable to determine if fluid consumption would have continued to further correct fluid losses.

Additionally, given the influence of increasing the osmolarity of the fluid that is being consumed and the attenuation in the decline of thirst, we are unable to make a determination of how the osmolarity of fluid following exercise-induced hypohydration may have further augmented the replacement of fluids. Evans et al. [39] found no difference of ad libitum fluid ingested when comparing hypertonic 10%, 2%, and 0% glucose solutions; however, since an equal concentration of sodium was included in each beverage, it is unknown if differences would have been found if plain water was also ingested. Furthermore, the thirst scales utilized, TH [20] and TSS [21,22], have not been validated to date; there is no existing evidence that has compared changes in plasma osmolality to the thirst scales utilized for this study. While this prevents us from making conclusions based on perceptual scales validated against physiological measures, in utilizing a randomized cross-over design where participants completed both a euhydrated and hypohydrated trial under the same environmental conditions and exercise stress, we feel that the within-person changes in the thirst scales tested allows for consistency in these measures. Our post hoc power analysis revealed that we were underpowered for the TSS measures, which may explain why we observed non-significant findings for thirstiness, dryness in the mouth, pleasantness in the mouth, and fullness. Lastly, by not utilizing an exercise duration and/or intensity that may mimic various settings (athletic, occupational, and military settings) we are not able to make conclusive statements surrounding the use of thirst in guiding fluid replacement following the cessation of exercise.

5. Conclusions

In conclusion, our findings indicate that when a bolus of fluid is provided immediately following exercise-induced dehydration, the sensation of thirst rapidly declines to levels observed in euhydrated individuals for up to 60 min following exercise, despite a level of dehydration exceeding 2% body mass loss. The prolonged inhibition of thirst when less fluid was consumed than total water losses may prevent one's ability to rehydrate rapidly following prolonged exercise. These findings support the recommendation that individuals may benefit from knowing their fluid needs and that fluid replacement should be individualized based on fluid losses and subsequent fluid need. Future research should consider examining the types of fluids consumed and allowing participants consume fluids ad libitum at their discretion following exercise-induced dehydration. This would further expand on the utility of thirst as a tool to guide fluid replacement following exercise-induced dehydration and provide for more refined, data-informed recommendations being derived.

Author Contributions: W.M.A., L.W.V. and D.J.C. conceptualized the design and methodology of this study. W.M.A., L.W.V., and L.N.B. were responsible for the data curation. W.M.A. was responsible for the initial analysis and writing of the original draft of this manuscript. L.W.V., L.N.B., and D.J.C. were responsible for critically reviewing and revising the manuscript. W.M.A., L.W.V., L.N.B., and D.J.C. provided final approval of the manuscript prior to submission.

Funding: This study was funded in part by Nix, Inc.

Acknowledgments: The authors would like to thank Rachel Vanscoy, MS, ATC, Sarah Attanasio, MS, ATC, and Elizabeth L. Adams, for their assistance with this study.

Conflicts of Interest: The authors declare no conflicts of interest for the submitted work. In addition, the sponsor had no role in the design, execution, interpretation, or writing of the study.

References

1. Armstrong, L.E. Hydration assessment techniques. *Nutr. Rev.* **2005**, *63* (Suppl. 1), S40–S54. [CrossRef] [PubMed]
2. Armstrong, L.E. Assessing Hydration Status: The Elusive Gold Standard. *J. Am. Coll. Nutr.* **2007**, *26*, 575S–584S. [CrossRef] [PubMed]
3. Cheuvront, S.N.; Ely, B.R.; Kenefick, R.W.; Sawka, M.N. Biological variation and diagnostic accuracy of dehydration assessment markers. *Am. J. Clin. Nutr.* **2010**, *92*, 565–573. [CrossRef] [PubMed]

4. Cheuvront, S.N.; Kenefick, R.W. Dehydration: Physiology, Assessment, and Performance Effects. *Compr. Physiol.* **2014**, *4*, 257–285.
5. Cheuvront, S.N.; Kenefick, R.W.; Charkoudian, N.; Sawka, M.N. Physiologic basis for understanding quantitative dehydration assessment. *Am. J. Clin. Nutr.* **2013**, *97*, 455–462. [CrossRef]
6. Greenleaf, J.E. Problem: Thirst, drinking behavior, and involuntary dehydration. *Med. Sci. Sports Exerc.* **1992**, *24*, 645–656. [CrossRef]
7. McKinley, M.J.; Johnson, A.K. The Physiological Regulation of Thirst and Fluid Intake. *Physiology* **2004**, *19*, 1–6. [CrossRef]
8. Stanhewicz, A.E.; Kenney, W.L. Determinants of water and sodium intake and output. *Nutr. Rev.* **2015**, *73*, 73–82. [CrossRef]
9. Wolf, A. *Thirst; Physiology of the Urge to Drink and Problems of Water Lack*; Charles C Thomas Publisher: Springfield, IL, USA, 1950.
10. Brunstrom, J.M.; Tribbeck, P.M.; Macrae, A.W. The role of mouth state in the termination of drinking behavior in humans. *Physiol. Behav.* **2000**, *68*, 579–583. [CrossRef]
11. Figaro, M.K.; Mack, G.W. Regulation of fluid intake in dehydrated humans: Role of oropharyngeal stimulation. *Am. J. Physiol. Integr. Comp. Physiol.* **1997**, *272*, R1740–R1746. [CrossRef]
12. Seckl, J.R.; Williams, T.D.M.; Lightman, S.L. Oral hypertonic saline causes transient fall of vasopressin in humans. *Am. J. Physiol.* **1986**, *251*, R214–R217. [CrossRef] [PubMed]
13. Hew-Butler, T.; Rosner, M.H.; Fowkes-Godek, S.; Dugas, J.P.; Hoffman, M.D.; Lewis, D.P.; Maughan, R.J.; Miller, K.C.; Montain, S.J.; Rehrer, N.J.; et al. Statement of the 3rd International Exercise-Associated Hyponatremia Consensus Development Conference, Carlsbad, California, 2015. *Br. J. Sports Med.* **2015**, *49*, 1432–1446. [CrossRef] [PubMed]
14. Sawka, M.N.; Burke, L.M.; Eichner, E.R.; Maughan, R.J.; Montain, S.J.; Stachenfeld, N.S. American College of Sports Medicine position stand. Exercise and fluid replacement. *Med. Sci. Sports Exerc.* **2007**, *39*, 377–390. [PubMed]
15. McDermott, B.P.; Anderson, S.A.; Armstrong, L.E.; Casa, D.J.; Cheuvront, S.N.; Cooper, L.; Kenney, W.L.; O'Connor, F.G.; Roberts, W.O. National Athletic Trainers' Association Position Statement: Fluid Replacement for the Physically Active. *J. Athl. Train.* **2017**, *52*, 877–895. [CrossRef] [PubMed]
16. Armstrong, L.E.; Ganio, M.S.; Klau, J.F.; Johnson, E.C.; Casa, D.J.; Maresh, C.M. Novel hydration assessment techniques employing thirst and a water intake challenge in healthy men. *Appl. Physiol. Nutr. Metab.* **2014**, *39*, 138–144. [CrossRef]
17. Mears, S.A.; Watson, P.; Shirreffs, S.M. Thirst responses following high intensity intermittent exercise when access to ad libitum water intake was permitted, not permitted or delayed. *Physiol. Behav.* **2016**, *157*, 47–54. [CrossRef]
18. Armstrong, L.E.; Maresh, C.M.; Castellani, J.W.; Bergeron, M.F.; Kenefick, R.W.; Lagasse, K.E.; Riebe, D. Urinary Indices of Hydration Status. *Int. J. Sport Nutr.* **1994**, *4*, 265–279. [CrossRef]
19. Jackson, A.S.; Pollock, M.L. Generalized equations for predicting body density of men. *Br. J. Nutr.* **1978**, *40*, 497–504. [CrossRef]
20. Engell, D.B.; Maller, O.; Sawka, M.N.; Francesconi, R.N.; Drolet, L.; Young, A.J. Thirst and fluid intake following graded hypohydration levels in humans. *Physiol. Behav.* **1987**, *40*, 229–236. [CrossRef]
21. Rolls, B.J.; Wood, R.J.; Rolls, E.T.; Lind, H.; Lind, W.; Ledingham, J.G. Thirst following water deprivation in humans. *Am. J. Physiol. Integr. Comp. Physiol.* **1980**, *239*, R476–R482. [CrossRef]
22. Phillips, P.A.; Rolls, B.J.; Ledingham, J.G.G.; Forsling, M.L.; Morton, J.J.; Crow, M.J.; Wollner, L. Reduced thirst after water deprivation in healthy elderly men. *N. Engl. J. Med.* **1984**, *311*, 753–759. [CrossRef] [PubMed]
23. Salata, R.A.; Verbalis, J.G.; Robinson, A.G. Cold Water Stimulation of Oropharyngeal Receptors in Man Inhibits Release of Vasopressin. *J. Clin. Endocrinol. Metab.* **1987**, *65*, 561–567. [CrossRef] [PubMed]
24. O'Obika, L.F.; O'Okpere, S.; O'Ozoene, J.; Amabebe, E. The role of oropharnyegal receptors in thirst perception after dehydration and rehydration. *Niger. J. Physiol. Sci.* **2014**, *29*, 37–42.
25. Arnaoutis, G.; Kavouras, S.A.; Christaki, I.; Sidossis, L.S. Water Ingestion Improves Performance Compared with Mouth Rinse in Dehydrated Subjects. *Med. Sci. Sports Exerc.* **2012**, *44*, 175–179. [CrossRef] [PubMed]
26. Phillips, P.A.; Rolls, B.J.; Ledingham, J.G.; Morton, J.J. Body fluid changes, thirst and drinking in man during free access to water. *Physiol. Behav.* **1984**, *33*, 357–363. [CrossRef]

27. Thrasher, T.N.; Nistal-Herrera, J.F.; Keil, L.C.; Ramsay, D.J. Satiety and inhibition of vasopressin secretion after drinking in dehydrated dogs. *Am. J. Physiol. Metab.* **1981**, *240*, E394–E401. [CrossRef] [PubMed]
28. Appelgren, B.H.; Thrasher, T.N.; Keil, L.C.; Ramsay, D.J. Mechanism of drinking-induced inhibition of vasopressin secretion in dehydrated dogs. *Am. J. Physiol. Integr. Comp. Physiol.* **1991**, *261*, R1226–R1233. [CrossRef]
29. Thornton, S.N.; Baldwin, B.A.; Forsling, M.L. Drinking and vasopressin release following central injections of angiotensin II in minipigs. *Q. J. Exp. Physiol. Transl. Integr.* **1989**, *74*, 211–214. [CrossRef]
30. Blair-West, J.R.; Gibson, A.P.; Woods, R.L.; Brook, A.H. Acute reduction of plasma vasopressin levels by rehydration in sheep. *Am. J. Physiol.* **1985**, *248*, R68–R71. [CrossRef]
31. Sawka, M.N.; Young, A.J.; Francesconi, R.P.; Muza, S.R.; Pandolf, K.B. Thermoregulatory and blood responses during exercise at graded hypohydration levels. *J. Appl. Physiol.* **1985**, *59*, 1394–1401. [CrossRef]
32. Montain, S.J.; Coyle, E.F. Influence of graded dehydration on hyperthermia and cardiovascular drift during exercise. *J. Appl. Physiol.* **1992**, *73*, 1340–1350. [CrossRef] [PubMed]
33. Adams, W.M.; Mazerolle, S.M.; Casa, D.J.; Huggins, R.A.; Burton, L. The Secondary School Football Coach's Relationship with the Athletic Trainer and Perspectives on Exertional Heat Stroke. *J. Athl. Train.* **2014**, *49*, 469–477. [CrossRef] [PubMed]
34. Huggins, R.; Martschinske, J.; Applegate, K.; Armstrong, L.; Casa, D. Influence of Dehydration on Internal Body Temperature Changes During Exercise in the Heat: A Meta-Analysis. *Med. Sci. Sports Exerc.* **2012**, *44*, 791.
35. Casa, D.J.; Stearns, R.L.; Lopez, R.M.; Ganio, M.S.; McDermott, B.P.; Yeargin, S.W.; Yamamoto, L.M.; Mazerolle, S.M.; Roti, M.W.; Armstrong, L.E.; et al. Influence of Hydration on Physiological Function and Performance During Trail Running in the Heat. *J. Athl. Train.* **2010**, *45*, 147–156. [CrossRef] [PubMed]
36. Adams, J.D.; Sekiguchi, Y.; Suh, H.G.; Seal, A.D.; Sprong, C.A.; Kirkland, T.W.; Kavouras, S.A. Dehydration Impairs Cycling Performance, Independently of Thirst: A Blinded Study. *Med. Sci. Sports Exerc.* **2018**. [CrossRef] [PubMed]
37. Armstrong, L.E.; Costill, D.L.; Fink, W.J. Influence of diuretic-induced dehydration on competitive running performance. *Med. Sci. Sports Exerc.* **1985**, *17*, 456–461. [CrossRef]
38. Greenleaf, J.E.; Sargent, F. Voluntary dehydration in man. *J. Appl. Physiol.* **1965**, *20*, 719–724. [CrossRef]
39. Evans, G.H.; Shirreffs, S.M.; Maughan, R.J. Postexercise rehydration in man: The effects of carbohydrate content and osmolality of drinks ingested ad libitum. *Appl. Physiol. Nutr. Metab.* **2009**, *34*, 785–793. [CrossRef]
40. Maughan, R. Optimizing Hydration for Competitive Sport. In *Perspectives in Exercise Science and Sport Medicine*; Lamb, D., Gisolfi, C., Eds.; Cooper Publishing Group: Carmel, IN, USA, 1997.
41. Maughan, R.J.; Shirreffs, S.M. Dehydration, rehydration and exercise in the heat: Concluding remarks. *Int. J. Sports Med.* **1998**, *19*, S167–S168. [CrossRef]
42. Maughan, R.J.; Shirreffs, S.M. Dehydration and rehydration in competative sport. *Scand. J. Med. Sci. Sports* **2010**, *20*, 40–47. [CrossRef]
43. Shirreffs, S.M. Restoration of fluid and electrolyte balance after exercise. *Can. J. Appl. Physiol.* **2001**, *26*, S228–S235. [CrossRef] [PubMed]
44. Shirreffs, S.M.; Maughan, R.J. Volume repletion after exercise-induced volume depletion in humans: Replacement of water and sodium losses. *Am. J. Physiol. Physiol.* **1998**, *274*, F868–F875. [CrossRef] [PubMed]
45. Robertson, G. Abnormalities of thirst regulation. *Kidney Int.* **1984**, *25*, 460–469. [CrossRef] [PubMed]

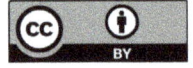

© 2019 by the authors. Licensee MDPI, Basel, Switzerland. This article is an open access article distributed under the terms and conditions of the Creative Commons Attribution (CC BY) license (http://creativecommons.org/licenses/by/4.0/).

MDPI
St. Alban-Anlage 66
4052 Basel
Switzerland
Tel. +41 61 683 77 34
Fax +41 61 302 89 18
www.mdpi.com

Nutrients Editorial Office
E-mail: nutrients@mdpi.com
www.mdpi.com/journal/nutrients

www.ingramcontent.com/pod-product-compliance
Lightning Source LLC
LaVergne TN
LVHW071950080526
838202LV00064B/6716